Biological Aspects
of Affective Disorders

NEUROSCIENCE PERSPECTIVES

Editor: Peter Jenner
Pharmacology Group
Biomedical Sciences Division
King's College London
Manresa Road
London SW3 6LX

Forthcoming titles in this series:

Roger Horton and Cornelius Katona (eds), Biological Aspects of Affective
Disorders
Judith Pratt (ed), The Biological Bases of Drug Tolerance and Dependence
Trevor Stone (ed), Adenosine in the Nervous System

Biological Aspects
of Affective Disorders

edited by

R.W.Horton
Department of Pharmacology & Clinical Pharmacology
St George's Hospital Medical School
London, UK

and

C.L.E. Katona
Department of Psychiatry
University College & Middlesex School of Medicine
London, UK

ACADEMIC PRESS
Harcourt Brace Jovanovich, Publishers
London   San Diego   New York
Boston   Sydney   Tokyo   Toronto

ACADEMIC PRESS LIMITED
24/28 Oval Road,
London NW1 7DX

United States Edition published by
ACADEMIC PRESS INC.
San Diego, CA 92101

A catalogue record for this book
is available from the British Library

ISBN 0–12–356510–3

Typeset by P & R Typesetters Ltd, Salisbury, UK
Printed and Bound in Great Britain by
the University Press, Cambridge

Contents

Contents

9   Genetic aspects of affective disorders
Larry Rifkin and Hugh Gurling

Contributors

Janis L. Anderson   Laboratory for Circadian & Sleep Disorders Medicine Brigham & Women's Hospital and Harvard Medical School, 221 Longwood Avenue, Boston, MA 02115, USA

Dennis S. Charney   Department of Veterans Affairs Medical Center & Department of Psychiatry, Yale University School of Medicine, West Haven, Connecticut 06515, USA

S.C. Cheetham   Boots Pharmaceuticals Research Department, R3, Pennyfoot Street, Nottingham NG2 3AA

Pedro L. Delgado   Department of Veterans Affairs Medical Center & Department of Psychiatry, Yale University School of Medicine, West Haven, Connecticut 06515, USA

J.M. Elliott   Department of Pharmacology & Toxicology, St Mary's Hospital Medical School, Norfolk Place, London W2 1PG

Hugh Gurling   Molecular Psychiatry Laboratory, Academic Department of Psychiatry, University College & Middlesex School of Medicine, Riding House Street, London W1P 7PN

R.W. Horton   Department of Pharmacology & Clinical Pharmacology, St George's Hospital Medical School, London SW17 0RE

C.L.E. Katona   Department of Psychiatry, University College & Middlesex School of Medicine, London W1N 8AA

Stephen Merson   St Charles' Hospital, London W10 6DZ

James C. Pryor   Department of Psychiatry, Vanderbilt University School of Medicine, Nashville, Tennessee 37232, USA

Larry Rifkin   Molecular Psychiatry Laboratory, Academic Department of Psychiatry, University College & Middlesex School of Medicine, Riding House Street, London W1P 7PN

Sir Martin Roth   Professor Emeritus of Psychiatry, Academic Department of Psychiatry, University of Cambridge, Addenbrooke's Hospital, Hills Road, Cambridge CB2 2QQ

Trevor Silverstone   Professor of Clinical Psychopharmacology, Medical College of St Bartholomew's Hospital, University of London, London EC1

Fridolin Sulser   Departments of Psychiatry & Pharmacology, Vanderbilt University School of Medicine, Nashville, Tennessee 37232, USA

Peter Tyrer   St Charles' Hospital, London W10 6DZ

Anna Wirz-Justice   Chronobiology Laboratory, Psychiatrische Universitätsklinik, Wilhelm Klein Strasse 27, CH-4025 Basel, Switzerland

Series Preface

The driving force for the production of this series lies in my own inability to keep up with the advances occurring in those areas of neuroscience in which I am especially interested. So many times I have been frustrated by being unable to find a current review of an important research area. Even when I resort to bothering colleagues who are experts in a particular field, I am told, more often than not, that such an overview does not exist. In my own area of expertise I frequently send away students empty-handed who have asked me to direct them to a definitive article on a well researched topic.

Although regretable, perhaps this situation is not surprising since the neurosciences are one of the most diverse and rapidly advancing areas in the biological sphere. By definition research in the neurosciences encompasses anatomy, pathology, biochemistry, physiology, pharmacology, molecular biology, genetics and therapeutics. Indeed, there are few individuals capable of maintaining a grasp of the literature in all these aspects of their own research interests let alone in other fields.

My answer was to establish *Neuroscience Perspectives* and to develop gradually a series of individual edited monographs dealing in depth with issues of current interest to those working in the neuroscience area. Each volume is being designed to bring a multidisciplinary approach to the subject matter by pursuing the topic from the laboratory to the clinic. As a consequence I have asked the editors of the individual volumes to produce a balanced critique of their topic which will be read, understood and enjoyed by as wide an audience as possible within the realm of neuroscience.

The choice of the topics for the series is a difficult matter. In the first instance these were largely dictated by my own interests or by my awareness of important and fundamental work being undertaken by colleagues. More recently, I have been recruiting subject matter and editors through attending a variety of diverse symposia in the neuroscience area. However, the choice of topics should reflect the needs of the audience reached by the series. So I invite you to let me know of areas which you feel are of importance and to give me suggestions for individuals who would be keen to edit a book for *Neuroscience Perspectives*.

Finally, it only remains to thank those individuals at Academic Press who have already worked for several years to develop *Neuroscience Perspectives*. In particular, Dr. Carey Chapman who has the unenviable task of recruiting the editors that I suggest and then harassing them for the completed work. My hope is that the series will fill the gap that I perceive and provide for my colleagues in the neurosciences a collection of interesting books which will become reference volumes in their field. I hope you will enjoy *Neuroscience Perspectives*.

Peter Jenner

Preface

Biological research in the affective disorders has been an international growth industry for several years. Researchers in the field come from a wide variety of scientific disciplines and there has been relatively little integrative work, particularly between preclinical and clinical approaches.

This volume attempts to bring together up-to-date reviews from a number of distinguished research groups, in order to provide a comprehensive introduction to our current understanding of the clinical features and management of patients with depression and mania, as well as of the biological abnormalities that may underlie their disease.

Roth provides a comprehensive review of the classification of affective disorders, incorporating not only his own distinguished contribution but also the theoretical framework of current European and American classificatory systems. Merson and Tyrer address the practicalities of physical treatment, and Silverstone provides an account of the clinical features and biological aspects of mania, a relatively neglected area of research.

Pryor and Sulser describe the evolution of this monoamine hypothesis which has dominated our thinking since the early 1960s and is likely to do so into the 21st century. Research on neurotransmitter abnormalities in depression has used three main strategies, which are covered in the next three chapters. Studies of peripheral blood components have been widely used as accessible models for neurones: Elliott describes the rationale for such work and summarises results to date. Delgado and Charney describe the neuroendocrine challenge tests that have been developed as 'windows' through which neurotransmitter function has been examined; and Cheetham et al. describe the current state of post-mortem brain research, the most direct and yet under-utilised approach to brain abnormalities in depression.

The final chapters review emerging research using more novel approaches likely to become increasingly fruitful in the coming years. Anderson and Wirz-Justice provide a lucid guide to the complex theoretical framework of research into abnormal biological rhythms in depression. Rifkin and Gurling review the most fundamental of recent advances: the shift of focus from neurotransmitter to genetic substrate.

We have chosen areas in which important research is certain to continue. We have not included areas which, though of undisputed clinical importance have yet, in our view, to 'come of age' as areas of biological research. In particular, it is likely that the next few years will see important advances in the application of novel neuroimaging techniques in affective disorder. Our primary aim is that this volume should serve as a sourcebook for young researchers from all disciplines contributing to our evolving understanding of the biology of depression.

We would like to thank Dr. Carey Chapman of Academic Press for her patience and encouragement.

R.W. Horton and C.L.E. Katona

CHAPTER 1

CLASSIFICATION OF AFFECTIVE AND RELATED PSYCHIATRIC DISORDERS

Sir Martin Roth

*Academic Department of Psychiatry, University of Cambridge,
Addenbrooke's Hospital, Hills Road, Cambridge CB2 2QQ, UK*

Table of Contents

BIOLOGICAL ASPECTS OF AFFECTIVE DISORDERS
ISBN 0-12-356510-3

1.1 Introduction

The introduction by Meduna of the first effective physical treatment for depressive illness in the 1930s and its later transformation into electro-convulsive therapy (ECT) by Cerletti and Bini provided a powerful stimulus to enquiries into the classification of depressive and related forms of psychiatric disorder. The new treatment proved highly successful in certain forms of depression, less successful in others, and in a proportion of patients with affective disorders symptoms were unrelieved or exacerbated. In these cases the therapy was contraindicated. It seemed essential to differentiate classes of patients in whom the treatment could be expected to promote recovery from those in whom little or no alleviation of symptoms would follow.

A reliable classification for purposes of prediction became an even more pressing need with the discovery of pharmacological treatments for depression. The antidepressant action of iproniazid was discovered by Crane (1957) and Kline (1958) and the first report of the efficacy of imipramine was published in 1958 by Kuhn. In the early clinical trials iproniazid was reported to be effective in endogenous depression (Kiloh *et al.*, 1960) and imipramine more successful in endogenous than in non-endogenous depression (Kiloh *et al.*, 1962), but a substantial proportion of those with neurotic depressions were improved. Numerous other trials followed.

Psychopharmacology soon provided one powerful means of testing the validity of models of classification within the domain of the affective disorders. However, findings from controlled trials of treatment alone could rarely provide decisive answers to questions posed and results had to be interpreted with caution.

Investigation of the effects produced by the new drugs also led to the formulation of pharmacological and biochemical hypotheses regarding the biological causes of disorders of affect. It became clear that their submission to stringent tests demanded the assembly of homogeneous cohorts of patients selected with the aid of reliable diagnostic criteria to ensure that significant findings would not be obscured by 'noise'.

It was in the halcyon years between 1949 and 1960 that most of the discoveries of contemporary clinical psychopharmacology were made. The imagination of many clinicians and basic scientists was stirred by the introduction into psychiatric practice of effective treatments for schizophrenia, depressive illness and anxiety disorders; in all these forms of illness the efficacy of the drugs previously available for the alleviation of suffering had been dubious or inadequate and their administration in some cases ascribed unacceptable hazards or side-effects.

It became increasingly apparent that more objective and replicable systems of diagnosis and classification were needed to promote scientific progress in psychiatry. Many ideas were advanced during this period. The most detailed and comprehensive taxonomy to evolve was the third version of the Diagnostic and Statistical Manual of the American Psychiatric Association (DSM-III; American Psychiatric Association, 1980). This classification, and the modified version that followed (DSM-III-R), was subjected to considerable criticism within the USA as well as in many other countries (Spitzer and Williams, 1983) but it succeeded in gaining worldwide acceptance by many psychiatrists in research and clinical practice.

Its beginnings can be traced to a set of diagnostic criteria, developed in the Department of Psychiatry at Washington University, St Louis, for a limited number of psychiatric disorders in relation to which there was sufficient evidence for criteria for inclusion and exclusion of cases to be formulated (Feighner et al., 1972). Definitions for depressive illness, anxiety states and some personality disorders were included. The central objective was to refine, objectify and improve replicability of diagnoses in clinical research. The Feighner criteria were followed by the Research Diagnostic Criteria (RDC) of Spitzer et al. (1978a, 1978b), again intended mainly for the use of investigators. After a period of field trials the publication of DSM-III followed in 1980. It provided operational criteria for diagnosis and a system of classification for all classes of psychiatric disorder. It had been endowed with a new identity as an instrument for everyday clinical practice as well as research.

Among the features claimed for the classification were its 'atheoretical' nature and its reliability as proved in the course of extensive field trials. The former represented a reaction against the psychoanalytic concepts of causation which had inspired DSM-II, the classification that had preceded DSM-III. The creators of DSM-III had come to regard these concepts as unfruitful, unscientific, conjectural and obsolete. They were therefore expunged from DSM-III.

As regards the second feature, the new diagnostic definitions were undoubtedly a forward step towards reliability and replicability of clinical observations. However, a high measure of agreement among a group of individuals with a common interest in creating a new diagnostic instrument does not establish scientific reliability in the more general context of clinical practice in a variety of settings. The influence of psychoanalysis may have been largely expunged, but it is open to question whether it is possible to create a theory-free taxonomy of psychiatric disorders. Certain theoretical concepts are clearly discernible, for example in the egalitarian categorical system into which the syndromes under Axis I are classified.

We shall encounter some of these undeclared theoretical assumptions as we consider the separate stages in the classification of affective disorders in the sections that follow.

4

1.2 Psychiatric classification and the hierarchical system

The hierarchical system of diagnosis has, in the past, formed part of the conceptual framework of European classifications and has been incorporated to some extent into DSM-III. It originated from the clinical descriptions of the various psychiatric disorders set down in Kraepelin's textbook and the classification that is implicit in his account of their interrelationships. Organic features manifest in the presenting mental state are at the top of the hierarchical system. When clouded consciousness, delirium, global cognitive impairment or other organic clinical features are observed in the course of examination of the mental state an organic syndrome is diagnosed; the features listed take precedence over those suggestive of normal 'functional' disorder, whether schizophrenic, depressive or neurotic. The category of organic mood disorders cannot be logically included at this level since they do not differ from non-organic mood disorders in respect of their phenomenology. Such cases should therefore be accorded one Axis I diagnosis of 'affective disorder' that accords with their psychiatric features and an entry that records the concomitant cerebral or somatic disease along Axis III (in the case of DSM-III-R).

Schizophrenia occupies the next rung of the hierarchy and features characteristic of it take precedence over paranoid symptoms associated with a delusional psychosis, such as paranoia, in which the typical hallucinations and other 'nuclear' features of schizophrenia are also found. These features in turn take precedence over features suggestive of psychotic or endogenous depression or manic-depressive psychosis. The clinical features of these conditions receive priority in diagnosis over neurotic depression (or dysthymia) and agoraphobic obsessional depressive or other neurotic symptoms and signs.

There are no hierarchical rules in operation between the different neuroses. However, neurotic disorders, as well as all the conditions above them in the hierarchical system, were given priority over personality disorders in the textbook of Mayer-Gross et al. (1954) and its later editions (1960, 1969 and 1977), which were influenced by the teaching of Kraepelin. There may be a close relationship between personality and neurosis, as believed by Kraepelin, Schneider, Jaspers and other founders of contemporary clinical psychiatry. This issue is taken up at a later stage. A diagnosis of personality disorder should not however be allowed to preempt a diagnosis of neurosis (or indeed a depressive paranoid or schizophrenic psychosis). A personality diagnosis and an illness diagnosis may both be relevant in certain cases and the neuroses in particular. This is explicitly recognized in DSM-III by the creation of a separate dimension, namely Axis II, for diagnosis of personality profile or special traits.

The diagnostic rules within the hierarchical system are not sacrosanct. The entities have to be regarded as hypotheses open to challenge and the system open to modification in the light of new findings. DSM-III makes no explicit reference to hierarchical theories or rules, although some of them have been clearly taken over from the Kraepelinian system. This is evident from the construction of some of the diagnostic decision trees included in DSM-III-R.

1.3 Levels of classification of affective and anxiety disorders (Figure 1)

In the sections that follow, classification of affective disorders is considered at a number of different levels, which correspond to the sequential steps in the process of logical inference followed in the course of arriving at a definite diagnosis. The system is a revised and updated version of an earlier scheme derived from a synthesis of old and new concepts (Roth, 1977, 1978a, 1978b; Roth and Barnes, 1981) and brought into relationship with DSM-III. The scheme incorporates findings published by the author and his colleagues in Newcastle and Cambridge since the 1960s in relation to endogenous depression (melancholia) and neurotic depression (dysthymia), the anxiety–depressive disorder relationship and the connection between these conditions and certain borderland psychoses (reviewed in Roth 1977, 1978a; Roth and Barnes, 1981; Roth 1990). European nomenclature has been used in the text and in Figure 1, which provides a diagrammatic outline of the classification. The terms employed in DSM-III-R and ICD-10 (draft) (World Health Organization, 1991), where there are corresponding syndromes, are given in the text and Figure 1.

1.4 Differentiation of depressive (or anxious) disorder from normal variation in mood (level I)

1.4.1 Normal affective states

The differentiation between normal affective response and clinical depression (or anxiety) is usually based on the severity and persistence of changes in mood in the case of clinical disorder and the presence in such disorder of a constellation of symptoms and signs which are not present in the moods experienced by most persons in response to stress and adversity.

6

1.4.2 Minor disorders and threshold conditions

1.4.2.1 Minor depression

The Research Diagnostic Criteria of Spitzer *et al.* (1978a) have provided operational diagnostic criteria for arriving at a diagnosis of 'minor depression'. The change in mood must be persistent and dominate the clinical picture or be of comparable severity with anxiety; clinical features which raise diagnostic possibilities other than primary depressions or some other disorder should be absent; the disorder must have lasted for 2 weeks for a 'definite' diagnosis; two other symptoms from a list of 16 depressive features have also to be present. For a variety of reasons (Katschnig, 1986) this does not promote a clear or satisfactory line of demarcation between normal depression of mood and depressive illness.

1.4.2.2 'Below threshold' and 'post-threshold' neurotic depression

The criteria developed by Wing and his colleagues have provided more objective and operational methods for defining the boundary lines of clinical depression. Those with scores of 1–4 on their Index of Definition (ID) (Wing and Sturt, 1978; Wing *et al.*, 1981) are judged as having mood change within the range of the norm ('sub-threshold'), while those who attain higher score are classed as having 'probable' (threshold, score 5) or 'definite' ('post-threshold', score 6–8) depressive illness. The scores on Wing's ID comprise the most unambiguous and best validated criteria of separation between normal change in mood and affective illness. They remain tentative and hypothetical, however, and should not be applied in an inflexible manner in clinical practice (Goodwin *et al.*, 1975).

There are drug responses that validate these differences. Amphetamine and cocaine serve as stimulants or mood elevators in a high proportion of normal subjects but are very feeble antidepressants.

1.5 Psychotic, endogenous and neurotic affective disorders (Level II)

1.5.1 Psychotic and endogenous depression

Decision-making at this level entails a differentiation between psychotic or endogenous affective disorder on the one hand and neurotic depressive or anxiety disorders on the other. The terms 'psychotic', 'endogenous' and

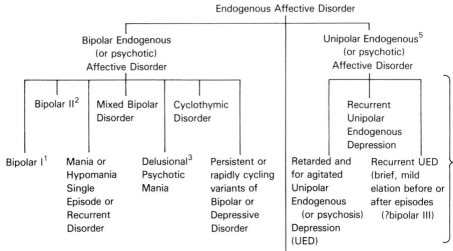

I
Normal Depression or Anxiety
(Levels 1 – 4 in the Index of Definition (ID)
of Wing et al. (1978)

Affective Disorder
(Levels 5 – 8 in Wing et al.'s ID)

Endogenous Affective Disorder

Bipolar Endogenous (or psychotic) Affective Disorder

Unipolar Endogenous[5] (or psychotic) Affective Disorder

Bipolar II[2] | Mixed Bipolar Disorder | Cyclothymic Disorder | Recurrent Unipolar Endogenous Depression

Bipolar I[1]

Mania or Hypomania Single Episode or Recurrent Disorder

Delusional[3] Psychotic Mania

Persistent or rapidly cycling variants of Bipolar or Depressive Disorder

Retarded and for agitated Unipolar Endogenous (or psychosis) Depression (UED)

Recurrent UED (brief, mild elation before or after episodes (?bipolar III)

Pseudoschizophrenic Mania[4]
Cycloid Psychosis (Leonhard, Perris)
Schizoaffective (Depressive) Psychosis
Acute Florid 'Mixed Psychosis'
Schizophreniform Psychosis
(Langfeldt) with paranoid depressive symptoms

Notes on Corresponding Syndromes in DSM-III-R and ICD-10 (Draft)

DSM-III-R

1. Bipolar Disorder. Subsumes, with some exceptions, all the variants shown here.
2. Mentioned as Bipolar II under heading of Atypical Bipolar Disorder.
3. Corresponds to Manic Episode with mood-congruent psychotic features as, specified under diagnostic criterion in DSM-III-R.
4. Corresponds to Manic Episode with mood incongruent psychotic features as described under criterion 4 in DSM-III-R.
5. A sub-group of major depression; those with 'melancholia' as specified in criterion 3 for 'depression with melancholia' and 'depression with psychotic features' respectively in DSM-III-R. Note that subdivision into endogenous (or 'psychotic') and 'neurotic' affective disorders shown at levels II and III does not exist in DSM-III-R.
6. Dysthymic Disorder. Except for criterion of duration (2 years).
7. Subsumed with varying degrees of severity. Under 'panic disorder' in DSM-III-R.
8. Hypochondriasis similar but makes no reference to the delusional or near delusional quality of the beliefs single or a very few diseases with the intensity of anxiety and/or depressive symptoms and grave suicidal risk.
9. Briefly mentioned in 'Atypical Somatoform Disorder' but near-delusional features and serious suicidal risk omitted.

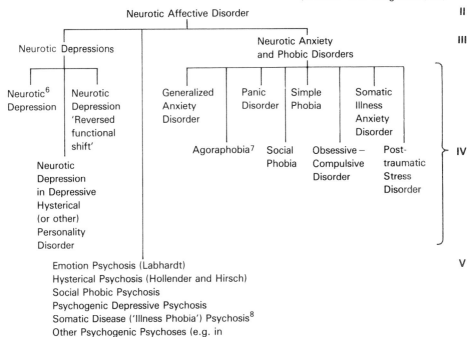

I
Normal Depression or Anxiety
(Levels 1 – 4 in the Index of Definition (ID)
of Wing *et al.* (1978)

Affective Disorder
(Levels 5 – 8 in Wing *et al.'s* ID)

Neurotic Affective Disorder   II

Neurotic Depressions   Neurotic Anxiety   III
                              and Phobic Disorders

Neurotic[6]   Neurotic   Generalized   Panic   Simple   Somatic
Depression   Depression   Anxiety   Disorder   Phobia   Illness
              'Reversed   Disorder   Anxiety
              functional   Disorder
              shift'   Agoraphobia[7] Social   Obsessive –   Post-   IV
Neurotic   Phobia   Compulsive   traumatic
Depression   Disorder   Stress
in Depressive   Disorder
Hysterical
(or other)
Personality
Disorder

Emotion Psychosis (Labhardt)   V
Hysterical Psychosis (Hollender and Hirsch)
Social Phobic Psychosis
Psychogenic Depressive Psychosis
Somatic Disease ('Illness Phobia') Psychosis[8]
Other Psychogenic Psychoses (e.g. in
  patients with dysmorphophobia)[9]

Notes on Corresponding Syndromes in DSM-III-R and ICD-10 (Draft)

ICD-10 (Draft)
1. Bipolar Affective Disorder.
2. Neither this or other bipolar subgroups specified.
3. Schizoaffective disorder, manic type.
4. Subsumed within schizoaffective disorder manic type.
5. Recurrent severe depressive disorder, endogenous and psychotic concept abandoned.
6. Dysthymia. Duration described merely as 'long standing'.
7. Subsumed as agoraphobia under 'phobic disorder' not as in DSM-III-R under panic disorder.
8. Hypochondriacal syndrome. Grouped under 'multiple somatisation disorder'. 'Fixed delusions' are an exclusive criterion.
9. Not mentioned as distinct category.

Figure 1 Classification of Affective and Anxiety Disorders.

'neurotic' have become controversial in recent years and are not employed or used in a restricted manner and without detailed definition in DSM-III-R. The concepts in question are indispensible for the orderly and logical classification of affective disorders. The terms that refer to them will therefore be briefly redefined here.

The term psychosis refers to a mental disorder in which thought, affect, behaviour and speech are so deranged that they incapacitate the individual from functioning in many aspects of his life. Psychotic patients are unable to discriminate between subjective experience and the testimony provided by the objective world. The boundaries of the self become blurred and, in consequence, stimuli that originate from the mind of the individual are believed to emanate from the outside world. For example, a schizophrenic patient experiences some thoughts as inserted into his or her mind by others who have usurped control over his or her thought processes, and is tormented by voices, believing them to emanate from distinct enemies and persecutors.

The patient with depressive psychosis has delusions of hopelessness, poverty, nihilism, deserved retribution and punishment, and the voices that utter these accusations and verdicts are those of relatives or strangers who may be alive or dead. These and other psychotic beliefs and experiences are largely resistant to all evidence from the real world that they are illusory.

The concept of psychosis is indispensable in legal and forensic psychiatry, as Scandinavian authors have repeatedly indicated. Without it, and the kindred clinical concept of 'endogenous' disorder, the classification of affective and many other disorders loses order and cohesion. 'Endogenous' as in endogenous depression does not refer so much to the absence of precipitating factors as to the emergence of a severely incapacitating disorder of mind in a stepwise manner or within a short period from a state of relatively normal mental functioning. The disorder is disproportionately severe and protracted in relation to any antecedent stress, which is trivial or absent, although it may be severe in some cases. Delusions and hallucinations are absent in Endogenous Depression ('Melancholia' in DSM-III-R) but there are usually kindred ideas of guilt, self-reproach and self-derogation, with limited or no insight into their morbid character. There are features which differentiate it qualitatively from the patient's premorbid patterns of thought and behaviour and from the patterns observable in the generality of normal persons. 'Neurosis' refers to all non-psychotic and non-endogenous emotional disorders. They are related to but distinct from personality disorders. At this level (II) neurotic affective disorder is a broad group which subdivides at level III into the Neurotic Depressions and Anxiety Disorders.

The greater part of the literature concerned with the dichotomy or continuity of 'endogenous' and 'neurotic' depressions has been concerned with both bipolar and unipolar depressions on the left side and neurotic depressions on the right side of the central partition at level III in Figure 1. But for reasons more fully discussed in the following section, the differentiation of psychotic from neurotic disorders has to be made at this level of decision-making.

1.6 Bipolar and unipolar depression and neurotic depression (dysthymia in DSM-III-R)

The history of the origins of the bipolar/unipolar dichotomy may clarify the issues involved in discrimination at this level. Leonhard (1957), who introduced the bipolar/unipolar concept, as did Angst (1966) and Perris (1966) who have been influential with Winokur and Clayton (1967) and Winokur *et al.* (1971) in re-establishing it, have confined this dichotomy to the endogenous psychoses. For example, in describing the unipolar disorders, Perris set an unequivocal demarcation line, insisting that depressive attacks must have been of endogenous or psychotic character to qualify for admission.

The main cause of confusion and disagreement in classification that is created by the elimination of psychotic features as a central criterion in the diagnosis of both bipolar and unipolar disorder can be described as follows. The bipolar cases constitute a small group amounting at most to about 20% of the total proportion of depressive disorders. Hence, when the restrictions implicitly imposed by Leonhard, Perris and Angst are ignored and differentiation between unipolar and bipolar groups is made prior to all other diagnostic judgements, the unipolar concept is liable to drift in clinical decision-making across the dividing line created at level III, drawn in Figure 1 between endogenous and neurotic disorders. The concept is then liable to be applied in diagnosis, not only to psychotic depressive but also to neurotic depressive, anxious and other neurotic disorders to the right of the central line of demarcation.

1.6.1 Criteria for the diagnosis of major depression (Table 1)

The explanation for this confusion is partly to be found in the diagnostic criteria for Major Depressive Episode in DSM-III-R (Table 1). Relatively non-specific physical symptoms, such as poor appetite, insomnia, loss of interest or pleasure *or* decrease in sexual drive and loss of energy and fatigue, are given the same weight as specific depressive features, such as psychomotor retardation, feelings of unworthiness, self-reproach or excessive or inappropriate guilt. The last three are compressed into a single feature and a high proportion of endogenous depressions meet the criteria. But so do many neurotic depressive

Table 1 Diagnostic criteria for Major Depressive Episode (DSM-III-R),

Note: A Major Depressive Syndrome is defined as criterion A below.

A. At least five of the following symptoms have been present during the same 2-week period and represent a change from previous functioning; at least one of the symptoms is either (1) depressed mood, or (2) loss of interest or pleasure. (Do not include symptoms that are clearly due to a physical condition, mood-incongruent delusions or hallucinations, incoherence, or marked loosening of associations.)

1. Depressed mood (or can be irritable mood in children and adolescents) most of the day, nearly every day, as indicated either by subjective account or observation by others.
2. Markedly diminished interest or pleasure in all, or almost all, activities most of the day, nearly every day (as indicated either by subjective account or observation by others or apathy most of the time).
3. Significant weight loss or weight gain when not dieting (e.g. more than 5% of body weight in a month), or decrease or increase in appetite nearly every day (in children, consider failure to make expected weight gains).
4. Insomnia or hypersomnia nearly every day.
5. Psychomotor agitation or retardation nearly every day (observable by others, not merely subjective feelings of restlessness or being slowed down).
6. Fatigue or loss of energy nearly every day.
7. Feelings of worthlessness or excessive or inappropriate guilt (which may be delusional) nearly every day (not merely self-reproach or guilt about being sick).
8. Diminished ability to think or concentrate, or indecisiveness, nearly every day (either by subjective account or as observed by others).
9. Recurrent thoughts of death (not just fear of dying), recurrent suicidal ideation without a specific plan, or a suicide attempt or a specific plan for committing suicide.

B. 1. It cannot be established that an organic factor initiated and maintained the disturbance.
   2. The disturbance is not a normal reaction to the death of a loved one (Uncomplicated Bereavement).

Note: Morbid preoccupation with worthlessness, suicidal ideation, marked functional impairment or psychomotor retardation, or prolonged duration suggest bereavement complicated by Major Depression.

C. At no time during the disturbance have there been delusions or hallucinations for as long as 2 weeks in the absence of prominent mood symptoms (i.e. before the mood symptoms developed or after they have remitted).

D. Not superimposed on Schizophrenia, Schizophreniform Disorder, Delusional Disorder, or Psychotic Disorder NOS (not otherwise specified).

patients who will fail to satisfy the restrictive and rather arbitrary criteria for dysthymia which has, in DSM-III-R, taken the place of Neurotic Depression on the other side of the dividing line at level III. It is noteworthy that, despite the exclusion of 'psychosis' as a general concept from DSM-III-R, it is possible to specify Major Depression as being 'with psychotic features', 'with melancholia' (broadly equivalent to endogenous depression) or 'without melancholia'.

Many patients with panic disorder, agoraphobia and other anxiety disorders which often exhibit a colouring of depressive symptoms also satisfy the criteria for diagnosis of Major Depression.

A part of the large literature regarding the co-morbidity of depressive disorder with panic disorder and agoraphobia and other anxiety disorders has probably been generated in this manner (Leckman *et al.*, 1983a, 1983b; Weissman *et al.*, 1984; Lesser, 1988). The problem of co-morbidity also extends to patients with eating disorders, such as bulimia nervosa, who often try to conceal their symptoms but in whom there is a considerable prevalence of depressive states, complicated in some cases by suicidal behaviour, particularly in the phases of overeating and increase in weight.

Failure to diagnose one of these specific neurotic syndromes as the primary disorder may be facilitated by the embarrassment and humiliation associated with such conditions as the house-bound agoraphobic state or regular self-induced vomiting. Selective assent may be unwittingly given to those questions posed by the psychiatrist that seek to explore the possibility of a major depressive episode, which carries considerably less stigma than phobic avoidance behaviour or eating disorder.

1.6.2 Differentiation of bipolar and unipolar endogenous depressions from neurotic depressions (Level III)

At this juncture the evidence bearing on the dysfunction between the endogenous forms of depression (or 'melancholia' or autonomous depression) on the one hand and neurotic forms of depression on the other requires consideration. In DSM-III-R, depressive and anxiety disorders are classified as distinct categorical entities. However, before renewed interest was directed towards the anxiety disorders some two decades ago, there is reason to believe that many were diagnosed as suffering from depressive states. This was reflected in the prominent agoraphobic and anxiety symptoms described in the so-called 'atypical depressions' of 30 years ago (West and Dally, 1959).

The discussion in this section will be limited to the validity of the distinction between the endogenous depressions (Kendell, 1976) to the left of the dividing line at level III and the non-endogenous depressions ('neurotic depression' or 'dysthymia') to the right of it. The relationships of anxiety and depressive disorder are discussed in a later section.

The history of this controversy has been reviewed by a number of authors (Kiloh and Garside, 1963; Kendell, 1968; Klerman, 1971) and only brief reference will be made to it here. Mendels and Cochrane (1968), reviewing seven factor analytic studies, concluded that there was a sufficient consensus to support the independence of the 'endogenous' and neurotic groups of disorders. Evidence has also been adduced that the endogenous states respond more favourably to pharmacological and electroconvulsive treatments for depression than the non-endogenous forms (Kiloh and Ball, 1961; Kiloh et al., 1962; Kiloh and Garside, 1963; Carney et al., 1965; Hickie et al., 1990). New observations in support of a clear partition at level III between these groups of disorders has come from recent investigations.

Parker et al., (1990) in Sydney have isolated a cluster of features subsumed under 'retardation', which has long been stressed as a central feature of melancholia and its two subgroups, psychotic and endogenous depression. Using multivariate analyses they have defined a 'Core' group of 15 signs differentiating 'psychotic/endogenous' and 'non-endogenous' depressives in two separate samples. The scores proved to be highly correlated with clinical DSM-III and RDC diagnoses of melancholia, suggesting that this syndrome could be defined by objective phenomenological features.

A separate investigation of ECT response in 35 depressed patients, (Hickie et al., 1990) demonstrated that psychomotor disturbances assessed by this Core rating system significantly predicted the response to electroconvulsive treatment in patients with a retarded form of melancholic illness. Although items assessing psychomotor agitation proved ineffective in prediction, the agitated depressives as a class showed the best response to ECT, suggesting that a larger number of measures of agitation might improve the predictive value of the Core ratings. These findings provide an important body of validation for the separation of endogenous (bipolar and unipolar) from the non-endogenous (or 'neurotic') forms of depression, and as retardation was predictive of outcome, whereas delusions and hallucinations were not, they also lend some support for the kinship of endogenous psychotic and melancholic forms of depression.

About a fifth of both endogenous and neurotic depressive disorders have been shown, in two recent studies from Australia (Kiloh et al., 1988) and the Maudsley Hospital in London (Lee and Murray, 1988), to pursue a chronic course after a mean interval of 15–18 years. In the Australian study only 20% of the 133 patients treated had remained well; 12% were chronically incapacitated and almost a third had died. The remaining 38% had suffered repeated attacks requiring readmission more often in the endogenous than in the neurotic depressions. The follow-up study of Lee and Murray yielded similar results: 89 Maudsley patients were found to have developed disorders with prominent schizophrenic features. None of the Australian cases revealed a diagnosis of schizophrenic or schizoaffective disorders. The prognosis of endogenous depression does not therefore appear as favourable as had been previously believed. But it does not follow that in prospective studies, in which methods of treatment had been predefined, patients regularly seen, compliance determined and provisions made for prophylactic treatment to be administered in refractory and relapsing cases, the outcome would prove as disappointing as in these two enquiries.

As far as the implications for classification are concerned, one recently reported finding has an important bearing on the distinction between the endogenous and neurotic depressions. A recent postscript from the Australian study has reported a significant difference between these two groups that validates the distinction between them. A further analysis of the follow-up findings in Sydney (Andrews *et al.*, 1990a) has shown that, whereas in neurotic depression 20% of the variance in outcome was accounted for by personality factors, in the endogenous depressions the figure was only 2%.

1.6.3 Similarities and differences between bipolar and unipolar endogenous depression (Level III)

The groups have been broadly differentiated from each other on the strength of a wide range of criteria drawn from age of onset, personality differences and a number of biochemical and physiological variables, as well as the course of the disorder and the heredity (Angst, 1966; Perris, 1966; Winokur and Clayton, 1967). Of these features, only the last two have been firmly established.

As far as heredity is concerned, as originally pointed out by Angst (1966), the first-degree relatives of unipolar probands nearly always prove to suffer from unipolar disorder if affected. In contrast, the first-degree relatives of bipolar probands who develop an affective illness might manifest either unipolar or bipolar disorder.

This difference between the bipolar and unipolar groups in respect of heredity has subsequently been confirmed in most enquiries (reviewed by McGuffin and Katz, 1986). Morbid risks in first-degree relatives of bipolar cases have been found to be in the region of 19%, as compared with a mean risk of 9.7% in unipolar cases. Twin and adoption studies have confirmed the importance of hereditary factors in bipolar disorders and their substantially smaller contribution in unipolar illness (McGuffin, 1988).

In a phenomenological sense there is little difference between the clinical profile of the depressive syndrome in bipolar and unipolar cases. It comprises a distinctive form of depression of mood qualitatively different from normal depression and from the forms of sadness and despondency experienced by the patient in healthy phases of life. There is diurnal variation, with depression usually at a peak in the morning, early morning waking but excessive sleep in some cases, psychomotor retardation or agitation or a combination of both, pessimistic, guilt-laden and self-derogatory ideas (present in delusional form in psychotic cases), loss of pleasure and interest in all or most activities, decline in motivation and drive and in sexual desire and interest, loss of self-esteem and confidence, loss of weight (increase in weight less often), thoughts of death or suicide, or suicidal attempts which had been planned and were potentially lethal. Attention has been mainly devoted at this level (III) to depressive illness because it is the most common manifestation of bipolar as well as unipolar disorder. It will be evident that all disorders in which some (or all) attacks are indubitably manic and associated with other disorders of affect, whether depressive or anxious, have to be classed with the endogenous or psychotic affective disorders.

The only alternative to the view that recognizes at least one categorically distinct group of affective disorders, usually depressive in manifestation, is one which recognizes no lines of demarcation and accordingly conceives of affective illnesses as extending without discontinuity from the cyclical depressive and manic disorders at one extreme at levels III and IV to the anxiety neuroses and beyond at the other.

It was a unitarian view such as this that was advanced by Lewis (1934,1936) regarding all affective disorders (Mapother and Lewis, 1941). He divided them into three types, each with a major and minor form: (1) Mania and Hypomania, (2) Melancholia and its more mild variant neurasthemic depression, and (3) Agitated depression, which was conceived as the severe version of the minor syndrome anxiety neurosis. The three groups of conditions were conceived as having no distinct boundaries between them but as merging insensibly with each other, forming a unitary class of disorders of affect, the variants of which differed only in quantitative respects. All the categories of psychiatric disorders reviewed in this chapter were therefore subsumed within a single entity. The line of demarcation between psychosis and neurosis disappears and the distinction between depressive and anxiety neuroses suffers a similar fate. Further, any attempts to define aetiopathological differences between the syndromes delineated are implicitly judged fruitless. All are conceived as reaction types in the sense of Adolf Meyer and, as such, devoid of any specific diagnostic or biological significance. According to Meyer's concept the manic-depressive reaction type ('thymergasia'), schizophrenic reaction type ('parergasia') and the psychoneurotic reaction type ('merergasia') could each occur under different external or internal circumstances in the same individual.

As Lewis's case histories, which were published as an Appendix to one of his papers (Lewis, 1936) were given in great detail, they enabled Kiloh and Garside (1977) to submit his unitary theory to independent critical tests with the aid of principal components and cluster analyses. Each of these methods showed that the patients could be separated by their scores on the relevant dimensions into at least two clearly distinct groups. This result is particularly germane for the separation proposed at this level of classification into those patients with endogenous affective illness of whatever complexion on the one hand and those with neurotic illness who are predominantly depressed or anxious on the other.

1.7 Bipolar endogenous depression (Level IV)

At this level the bipolar endogenous states are divided into a number of subgroups.

1.7.1 Bipolar I

This first group of bipolar affective disorders is manifest in attacks, both of severe elation and depression of endogenous or psychotic type, within the first few years of the first attack. The sequence of manic and depressive attacks may be alternating or irregular but there are intervals of remission between attacks, particularly during the earlier years of the disorder. This has come to be known as the type I syndrome. Endogenous depression with or without psychotic features (delusions and/or hallucinations) that vary in severity is the most common manifestation in the downward swings. Psychomotor behaviour is more often retarded than agitated. Attention has already been drawn to recent evidence for the diagnostic and predictive significance of psychomotor retardation. Eleven cluster and factor analytic investigations of depressive states have yielded a symptom constellation approximating to the 'retarded depressive syndrome' (Ashfield and Moray, 1990).

1.7.2 Bipolar II

This form of bipolar disorder is dominated by recurrent major depressive episodes. These are punctuated by mild bouts of non-psychotic elation and excitement which may follow bouts of depression or may occur spontaneously between them. A syndrome with these features has been accorded separate status by some workers (Angst, 1978; Fieve and Dunner, 1985) and has been widely described in recent years as Bipolar II (Endicott *et al.*, 1985; Cassano *et al.*, 1989). Phases of elation may not come to clinical attention because behaviour may superficially appear normal, but observation over a period often serves to define episodes characterized by excitement, irritability, disinhibition, and social indiscretions that are at variance with the subject's normal patterns of conduct.

A diagnosis of personality disorder may be erroneously made when the attacks commence in adolescence, when alcoholic excess, drug dependence, sexual promiscuity, prodigal expenditure and aggressive behaviour often predominate. A careful history reveals the onset to have been relatively abrupt and the conduct as out of character for the patient. There are some observations to support the theory that this disorder is associated with a particularly high risk of suicide (Akiskal *et al.*, 1989; Cassano *et al.*, 1989). Most cases meet the criteria for DSM-III-R cyclothymic disorder.

1.7.3 Bipolar III

This is a recently formulated and therefore tentative concept. Recurrent attacks of depression are associated with a history of bipolar disorder in first-degree relatives. Hypomanic episodes do not evolve spontaneously but may be precipitated during treatment with tricyclic or other antidepressants (Akiskal, 1983). This group has also been described as unipolar type II (Kupfer *et al.*, 1975), as distinct from unipolar I in which all affected first-degree relatives suffer from unipolar disorder. The status of the condition as a bipolar axis I disorder awaits further validation.

1.7.4 Recurrent mania

The next group comprises recurrent mania which is widely recognized as having a familial and genetic kinship with bipolar rather than unipolar illness. Exploration of the mode of onset, termination and course of episodes of elation often reveals short periods of mild or moderate depression and retardation and diminished drive prior to the onset of elation or following recovery in a proportion of patients.

1.7.5 'Mixed' bipolar disorder

In these psychoses manic and depressive features coexist in the same attack. Their interaction generates complex pictures: elation, grandiosity and boastfulness are manifest simultaneously or give way within minutes to depression, bouts of weeping, delusions of guilt or explosive anger. In addition to emotional turmoil, there is marked restlessness, aggressive and impulsive behaviour, overactivity and insomnia. Fits of laughter dissolve into floods of tears. Suicidal tendencies present a special risk since the constraint exerted by retardation and inhibition in pure depressive illness is removed in 'mixed' cases. Paranoid delusions and others of a mood-incongruent nature will be manifest; litigious behaviour is then a common feature. Schizophrenia is difficult to exclude in some cases but the previous record of psychiatric illness, the family history and treatment response are often helpful. Phenothiazines are often ineffective but lithium carbonate or a combination of lithium and butyrophenone brings symptoms under control in a high proportion of cases. When there is little or no response to drug treatment and the patient is threatened with exhaustion, a course of electroconvulsive therapy is strongly indicated and frequently succeeds where other measures have failed.

1.7.6 Paranoid manic psychosis

Although 'mixed' cases sometimes receive a diagnosis of schizophrenia, this is even more likely to happen in the 'paranoid' form because elation of mood may be inconspicuous or absent. The picture of mood disorder is dominated by irritable, aggressive, overbearing behaviour with paranoid delusions of a persecutory kind but also mood-incongruous delusions, such as being spied upon by special apparatus, thought insertion, passivity feelings and other first rank symptoms or auditory and/or visual hallucinations in a small proportion. Previous and succeeding attacks may be manifest as typical mania in some cases but the syndrome may present in a minority as the chronic phase of treatment resistant mania. Intermittent elation in the early stages, the character of previous attacks, the family history and the absence of negative schizophrenic features should raise the possibility of a manic illness. The record of premorbid adjustment is also helpful, since many patients have been energetic, outgoing, assertive and successful prior to the onset of affective disorder. However, *solitary* 'first rank' or 'nuclear' features do not warrant a diagnosis of schizophrenia. This group is represented as 'paranoid (psychotic) mania' with the bipolar disorders (level IV). The variant in which elation of mood and hyperactivity are absent or inconspicuous and the picture dominated by paranoid and a few or inconsistent schizophrenic features figures on level V as pseudoschizophrenic mania.

1.7.7 Cyclothymic disorder (DSM-III-R) (Table 2)

Both in DSM-III-R and in ICD-10 this is described as an instability of mood of at least 2 years duration in which there are numerous periods in which some symptoms characteristic of both depressive and manic disorder have been present but have not reached a severity and duration that meets the

Table 2 Diagnostic criteria for Cyclothymia (DSM-III-R).

A. For at least 2 years (1 year for children and adolescents), presence of numerous Hypomanic Episodes (all of the criteria for a Manic Episode, except criterion C that indicates marked impairment) and numerous periods with depressed mood or loss of interest or pleasure that did not neet criterion A of Major Depressive Episode.

B. During a 2-year period (1 year in children and adolescents) of the disturbance, never without hypomanic or depressive symptoms for more than 2 months at a time.

C. No clear evidence of a Major Depressive Episode or Manic Episode during the first 2 years of the disturbance (or one year in children and adolescents).

Note: After this minimum period of Cyclothymia, there may be super-imposed Manic or Major Depressive Episodes, in which case the additional diagnosis of Bipolar Disorder or Bipolar Disorder NOS (not otherwise specified) should be given.

D. Not superimposed on a chronic psychotic disorder, such as Schizophrenia or Delusional Disorder.

E. It cannot be established that an organic factor initiated and maintained the disturbance, e.g. repeated intoxication from drugs or alcohol.

criteria for major depression or manic episode. Remissions lasting for months at a time may be interposed between episodes of mood disturbance. As the upswings are often pleasurable and may promote social success or, in the gifted, creative achievement, they tend to arouse less concern in relatives and others than the depressive episodes. The range of symptoms manifest is too narrow in any one attack to meet criteria for a clinical diagnosis but the whole span of features is drawn upon in the course of successive episodes, with the exception of psychotic features such as delusions, hallucinations or disorder of thought and speech.

In the past, cyclothymia has been described with the personality disorders as a variant of the norm rather than an illness. Its appearance in DSM-III and DSM-III-R has probably been influenced by reports that in more than half the cases a favourable response is made to lithium (Peselow *et al.*, 1982). Further evidence regarding this claim is needed and the decision as to whether treatment with drugs should be instituted should therefore be weighed with particular caution.

1.8 Expanded bipolar spectrum

The syndromes under this heading are quoted from the observations of Cassano, Akiskal and their colleagues, in a consecutive series of 405 out-patients with major depression. A number of the conditions are variants of axis I disorders whose main features have already been described above. The others are mainly temperamental or personality disorders and therefore candidates for admission to the group of Axis II disorders. The clinical syndrome of the 'Expanded Bipolar Spectrum' has been classified into 'Episodic' and 'Persistent or Intermittent' groups (Akiskal *et al.*, 1989; Cassano *et al.*, 1989).

1.8.1 'Episodic' group

Under this heading Cassano and Akiskal include Bipolar II and Bipolar III disorder, which have already been described. In Bipolar III, major depression occurs in association with a family history of bipolar illness but hypomanic disorder is liable to be triggered by treatment with tricyclic compounds. This group formed only 1.3% of Cassano and Akiskal's 405 successive patients with depression. As some authorities (Angst, 1982) have been led by their enquiries to question whether these drugs can cause a true switch from depression to manic illness, the validity of the 'Bipolar III' concept remains uncertain at the present time.

The schizomanic form of schizoaffective disorder, and a proportion of the schizodepressive cases in which there is evidence from clinical features and genetics (Tsuang *et al.*, 1977; Tsuang and Simpson, 1984) for a kinship with affective disorder, particularly of bipolar type, are also included in the 'episodic' group of the expanded spectrum.

1.8.2 Persistent and intermittent group

1.8.2.1 Chronic mania

This refers to those forms of chronic mania in which, as the elated state subsides, persecutory, grandiose and bizarre delusions persist and predominate against a background of a burnt out affective state, which is liable to be mistaken for paranoid schizophrenia. This syndrome is therefore similar to the paranoid form of bipolar disorder already described above.

1.8.2.2 Cyclothymia

This figures in DSM-III as an axis I syndrome and has already been described above. The status of this condition is ambiguous at the present time. The mood swings are described both in DSM-III-R and ICD-10 (draft) as insufficiently severe to meet criteria for Bipolar affective disorder or recurrent depressive illness. This renders the disorder indistinguishable from 'cyclothymic' personality. However, Akiskal (1983) have claimed a favourable response to treatment with lithium in about 60% of patients.

There are large numbers of cyclothymic persons in whom mood swings are mild, elated phases, pleasurable and associated with increased productivity, while in depressive swings there is merely a limited lessening of achievement. Since it presents as a specific form of personality disorder, it is most appropriately recorded along Axis II of DSM-III-R rather than as an Axis I syndrome. The extent to which a representative sample of patients with cyclothymic disorder are at risk of developing clinical depression or mania and the features of those at risk need to be defined to resolve the present ambiguity in the nosological status of cyclothymia.

1.8.2.3 Protracted 'mixed' states

The complex states that evolve in these disorders prove, in a proportion of cases, refractory to treatment over long periods. Most cases of 'mixed' disorder pursue an episodic course; it is the chronic forms of the disorder that have been selected for inclusion here with the persistent cases. More evidence is required regarding the results achieved with the aid of lithium together with carbamazepine, for which successes have been claimed.

Three 'temperamental disorders' are included as persistent or intermittent members of the spectrum.

1.8.2.4 The irritable temperament

This is characterized by a moody, irritable, querulous state punctuated by short periods of normal or cheerful mood. 'Irritability' is a long established feature of manic-depressive disorder to which Mayer–Gross devoted an important paper in 1936. However, the reliability of a personality diagnosis on the basis of the features described and its predictive value for future attacks of bipolar disorder are undetermined.

1.8.2.5 Subaffective dysthymia

This temperamental disorder is considered by Cassano *et al.* (1989) and Akiskal (1983, 1990) as having associations with bipolar and unipolar disorder.

The essential features were described by Kraepelin (1921) under the heading of 'depressive temperament', manifest at an early age in the form of a gloomy, despondent, guilt-ridden and despairing mood associated with an earnest outlook and low self-esteem. It was regarded by him as a *forme fruste* of manic-depressive psychosis. A full description of the clinical profile has been provided under the title the 'depressive personality' by Slater and Roth (1969).

Subaffective dysthymia comprises both anxious and depressive symptoms (Akiskal, 1978). It is closely related to long-standing personality characteristics; persistent low-grade depression, pessimism with feelings of guilt, self-denial and joylessness predominate. A certain amount of validation for the affinities of the condition with bipolar disorder has been adduced from family history and treatment response (Rosenthal *et al.*, 1981) but more evidence from prospective long-term enquiries is needed to define its nosological status more clearly.

1.8.2.6 The hyperthymic temperament

This condition has been elaborated (Akiskal, 1983; Akiskal *et al.*, 1989; Cassano *et al.*, 1989) from the earlier descriptions of Kretschmer (1936) and Schneider (1958) as another constituent of the persistent form of the bipolar spectrum. It begins before the age of 21 years and is characterized by irritability associated with cheerfulness, overoptimism, extraversion, confidence, boastfulness, grandiose behaviour and large funds of energy. Those affected are inclined to be gregarious, novelty seeking, impulsive and promiscuous. Carping and captious criticism of others is a common associated feature.

1.8.2.7 Continuous and rapidly cycling variants of bipolar disorder

These variants of bipolar I and bipolar II disorder present difficult management problems, particularly as they carry considerable suicidal risk. Long-term treatment of typical bipolar cases with antidepressant drugs has been described (Akiskal *et al.*, 1989; Cassano *et al.*, 1980; Angst and Dobler-Nikola, 1984, 1985) as one of the causes of the phenomenon but this explanation is in dispute. A combination of lithium and carbamazepine has been recommended in treatment (Wehr *et al.*, 1988), and in those with a regular rapid alternation of major psychotic depression and mania or hypomania lithium combined with thyroxine has been described as effective (Cowdy *et al.*, 1983).

Women predominated among the recurrent depressives in the material of Cassano and Akiskal, and men among those with mania, hypomania and the hyperthymic temperament. The bipolar II syndrome made up 26.9% of the 405 cases of mood disorder and was therefore the most common bipolar syndrome among Cassano and Akiskal's large group of out-patients. It was judged as being closest to recurrent depression and as bridging the gap between unipolar and bipolar illness. This is also the view of Angst *et al.* (1980) and comes close to Kraepelin's unitary concept of affective disorder.

A large number of new and stimulating observations has therefore been contributed in relation to the subdivision of bipolar disorder. Further investigation can be expected to simplify the classification and refine the indications for treatment with prophylactic regimens and antidepressive drugs. Occam's Razor should perhaps be borne in mind in such enquiries: 'Entities should not be multiplied unnecessarily'.

Most of the conditions in the expanded 'bipolar' spectrum of Cassano *et al.* and Akiskal *et al.* refer to personality disorders and are not therefore included in Figure 1. The only Axis I syndrome not previously dealt with in the text is the 'rapidly cycling' variant of bipolar disorder, which is included.

1.9 Distinction between unipolar and bipolar disorders

One of the most important findings recorded in the course of Cassano and Akiskal's investigations relates to recurrent unipolar affective disorder. It resembles bipolar II in respect of age of onset (37.5 years), age of first hospitalization (38.6 years) and the number of admissions to hospital (1.7). This group has the lowest rate of complete remission between episodes (46.9%) and the percentage of patients who fulfilled DSM-III-R criteria for melancholia (80.5%) was slightly above that for the bipolar group. Moreover, this group, in which the great majority presented an 'endogenous' profile, constituted nearly half of the total sample (46.2%). The findings validate the original proposal of Leonhard, which confined the unipolar/bipolar concept to the psychotic/endogenous group of depressions alone. It also suggests that by confining the concept of 'melancholia' to a special subgroup of Major Depression, DSM-III-R converted unipolar disorder into a heterogeneous syndrome and blurred the boundary line between one of the most highly prevalent forms of depressive illness and both the anxious and depressive forms of neurotic illness.

Perris (1974) held that for a diagnosis of bipolar disorder both manic and depressive episodes were needed, whereas for unipolar disorders at least three depressive episodes must have occurred, with complete remission after each. Evidence has recently accrued that a further proportion of the unipolar depressions thus defined prove at a later stage to be bipolar.

Utilizing their new concept and criteria, Cassano and Akiskal were able to classify one in three patients in their consecutive series of depressed patients as belonging to the bipolar spectrum. This ratio is higher than other figures recorded for the proportion of depressives who meet criteria for bipolar disorder. The implications of the finding are important and independent enquiries in representative samples of patients are indicated.

1.10 Neurotic depression (dysthymia in DSM-III-R)—Level IV (Table 3)

Being a depressive neurosis, this form of affective disorder continues to be widely diagnosed in Europe but it has been deleted from DSM-III and DSM-III-R and the concept of 'dysthymia' substituted.

The conclusion reached by Akiskal (1978) and Klerman et al. (1979) that 'neurotic depression' should be declared obsolete, on account of its diagnostic ambiguity and uncertain prognostic value, fails to provide any satisfactory alternative general concept for the non-endogenous depressions. The recent report of Andrews et al. (1990b), to which reference has already been made, that 20% of the variance in the outcome of neurotic depressions was accounted for by personality factors, as against 2% in endogenous cases, provides some fresh evidence in validation of the concept. The alternative solution of a proliferation of diagnostic entities of an ambiguous and overlapping kind ('minor depression', 'anxiety depression', 'subaffective dysthymia', etc.), which has followed the elimination of 'neurotic depression' from DSM-III, does not seem to offer a satisfactory solution for the problem of classification in this important clinical territory.

In DSM-III-R (American Psychiatric Association, 1987), dysthymia (Table 3) ('neurotic depression') is defined as a persistently depressed mood that lasts most of the day, or is present over longer periods than it is absent, during a minimum of 2 years. For a DSM-III-R diagnosis at least two of the following six symptoms must be present: poor appetite or overeating, insomnia or hypersomnia, low energy or fatigue, low self-esteem, poor concentration or difficulty in making decisions, and pessimism. A dysthymic patient cannot be without these symptoms for more than 2 months at a time. Exclusion criteria in DSM-III-R include the presence of a major depressive episode during the first 2 years of the illness, a manic or hypomanic episode at

Table 3 Diagnostic criteria for Dysthymia.

A. Depressed mood (or can be irritable mood in children and adolescents) for most of the day, more days than not, as indicated either by subjective account or observation by others, for at least 2 years (1 year for children and adolescents).

B. Presence, while depressed, of at least two of the following:

1. Poor appetite or overeating
2. Insomnia or hypersomnia
3. Low energy or fatigue
4. Low self-esteem
5. Poor concentration or difficulty making decisions
6. Feelings of hopelessness.

C. During a 2-year period (1 year for children and adolescents) of the disturbance, never without the symptoms in A for more than 2 months at a time.

D. No evidence of an unequivocal Major Depressive Episode during the first 2 years (1 year for children and adolescents) of the disturbance.

Note: There may have been a previous Major Depressive Episode, provided there was a full remission (no significant signs or symptoms for 6 months) before development of the Dysthymia. In addition, after these 2 years (1 year in children and adolescents) of Dysthymia, there may be superimposed episodes of Major Depression, in which case both diagnoses are given.

E. Has never had a Manic Episode or an unequivocal Hypomanic Episode.

F. Not superimposed on a chronic psychotic disorder, such as Schizophrenia or Delusional Disorder.

G. It cannot be established that an organic factor initiated and maintained the disturbance, e.g. prolonged administration of an antihypertensive medication.

any time, psychotic symptoms or the aftermath of schizophrenia and the perpetuation of mood disturbance by a specific organic factor or substance.

There are early onset and late onset forms according to whether the disorder began before or after the age of 21 years. The symptoms differ from those of major depression only in terms of severity and duration.

Among associated features, previous personality disorder or long-standing difficulties in adjustment are consistently present and chronic psychosocial stressors are also common. Dysthymia may evolve as the chronic phase of unremitting affective disorder. There is a marked predominance of women.

Dysthymia has long been recognized in European psychiatry but regarded as a form of deviant personality. Kurt Schneider described it under the heading of 'depressive psychopathy' without any implication of anti-social conduct. He listed the following traits as characteristic: (1) quiet, passive, non-assertive; (2) gloomy, pessimistic, incapable of fun; (3) self-critical, self-reproachful and self-derogatory; (4) sceptical, hypercritical and complaining; (5) conscientious and given to self-discipline; (6) brooding and given to worry; and (7) preoccupied with inadequacy, failure and negative events to the point of morbid enjoyment of one's failures.

Schneider (1958, 1959) dissented from the view of Kraepelin that this personality was related to manic depressive illness in all its manifestations and was a 'fundamental' state from which acute manic depressive episodes could 'rise like mountain peaks from a structurally similar plain'. The truth probably lies between these two viewpoints. The profile delineated by Schneider is a personality disorder but there is much evidence to suggest that a proportion of those affected are liable to develop a superimposed affective disorder which often responds to treatment. When alleviation follows, as it often does, the adverse features of the premorbid personality may be more muted and a period of improved adjustment and greater pleasure and satisfaction from life follows but the basic personality profile is unchanged. The question that remains unanswered is the prevalence of such a complication in 'dysthymic' or 'depressive' personalities.

It will be clear that we have to some extent covered similar ground here to that in the section on 'subaffective dysthymia' conceived as a temperamental or personality disorder. The verdict that emerges from the evidence is that dysthymic disorders comprise closely related personality deviations and syndromes of affective illness. Both require sharper definition. The view that the 'depressive personality' (or subaffective dysthymia) is closely related to bipolar disorder has to be regarded as tentative and hypothetical.

1.10.1 Other concepts of premorbid personality in neurotic depression

The focus in DSM-III-R on the syndrome of 'dysthymia' should not be allowed to overshadow earlier contributions to definition of the premorbid personality profiles of patients with 'neurotic' or 'non-endogenous' forms of depression. A certain consensus about the most common personality predispositions in the non-psychotic forms of depression has emerged. The syndrome of 'hostile depression' has been independently identified by Overall et al. (1966), Kiloh et al. (1972) and Lorr et al. (1973). These profiles bear a certain resemblance to the 'hysteroid dysphoria' of Klein and Davis (1969), the angry depressives of Grinker *et al.* (1961), the self-pitying constellation of Rosenthal and Gudemann (1967) and the chronic characterologic syndrome of Schildkraut (1970). More than half a century ago Gillespie (1929) subdivided non-endogenous depressions into 'psychoneurotic depressions' and 'depressions in constitutional psychopaths'. This latter term is reminiscent of Schneider's concept of 'depressive psychopathy'.

Despite the increasing interest shown by investigators in several countries (Cassano *et al.*, 1989; Akiskal, 1990; Andrews *et al.*, 1990a, 1990b; Hirschfeld *et al.*, 1990) in the premorbid personality setting of the depressive and anxiety disorders, a paucity of factual observations leaves the clinical picture of the most common forms of depressive anxiety and other emotional disorders in an incomplete state. The lack of reliable and valid measures of personality constitutes an impediment to enquiry but it could be surmounted to some extent by a wider approach to investigation than that which is confined to standardized measures of personality. A more systematic and stringent approach to the delineation of the developmental history and adjustment record in interpersonal relationships, occupation and social, sexual and marital life of patients with these disorders would be likely to yield findings that enrich description and refine discrimination.

1.11 Anxiety disorders

The anxiety disorders are divisible into the groups shown at level IV in Figure 1.

1.11.1 Generalized anxiety disorder

The picture may be dominated by psychic or somatic symptoms or there may be a combination of the two. There are usually prominent symptoms of autonomic disturbance and general tension and the psychic symptoms of apprehension which are subjectively experienced as portending some awesome and distressing ordeal to be faced, but not yet. These are often described as free floating in character and as having no particular theme or object. It is doubtful whether any anxiety states are ever so empty of specific content. It is common for patients to have minor phobic symptoms, such as variable avoidance behaviour of agoraphobic kind which only rarely restricts the patient's movements; there may also be disinclination to attend social gatherings, which can also be overcome with an effort.

1.11.2 Somatic illness anxiety disorder

In formulating criteria for diagnoses of the specific anxiety disorders a special mention is merited by patients in whom fears of disease constitute a leading feature. These have been described as 'illness phobias' in some classifications but, whereas phobic patients experience a fear-laden aversion (which they recognize as irrational) for some specific situation or object into the morbid nature of their symptoms, usually with insight, these patients fluctuate between doubt and a quasidelusional conviction that they suffer from malignant, cardiac, venereal or other life-threatening disease. The symptoms are more common in men and fears of having contracted acquired immune deficiency syndrome (AIDS), which are devoid of foundation, are frequently encountered at the present time. Reassurance and evidence that the diseases feared are absent exert only fleeting effects or make no impression.

A similar syndrome is described under the heading of 'hypochondriasis' in DSM-III but it lays insufficient stress on the tense, unremitting anxiety in the clinical picture, the general feelings of malaise which are closely associated with the symptoms, the strong colouring of depression with despair that enters in many cases and the suicidal risk carried by the disorder. Although these are indubitably anxiety disorders, in some cases a diagnosis of 'anxiety psychosis' is appropriate.

1.11.3 Agoraphobia

In this condition there is intense fear of leaving the familiar and secure setting of home and avoidance of a situation from which escape might be difficult or help inaccessible in the event of panic or mounting feelings of anxiety or feelings of helplessness. Shops, crowds, gatherings, travelling by public transport, queues, restaurants, hairdressers, churches or theatres are some of the settings avoided. Other situations, such as fear or panic at traffic lights in experienced and competent drivers, are less easily explained. There is increasing limitation of normal activity until the patient is virtually housebound. However, most agoraphobics are able to venture into all the places they are compelled to avoid when alone, provided they are accompanied by a spouse, a parent or some other relative or friend. In a substantial proportion of patients symptoms follow or are markedly exacerbated by the first panic attack, but this is far from invariable.

Kindred perceptual disturbance is common in severe agoraphobia (Roth, 1959, 1984; Roth and Harper, 1962; Uhde et al., 1985; Cassano et al., 1990). It is experienced subjectively as a sense of blunted emotion, distortion or perception and the experience of moving like an automaton or clockwork toy. The experience of a divided self, comprising an observing and observed self in a world that seems remote and inaccessible, is another experience. Typical agoraphobic symptoms are prominent, attacks of panic are common in unfamiliar situations.

1.11.4 Panic disorder

Panic disorder, defined in terms of number of symptoms and attacks and their frequency, figures as a major syndrome in DSM-III-R and agoraphobias of variable severity are subgroups subsumed in it. In ICD-10 (draft), agoraphobia is given independent status. Panic disorder is characterized by discrete panic attacks which are described in DSM-III as erupting in a sudden and spontaneous manner, that is, without provocation. The attacks are associated with feelings of extreme fear and tension and such symptoms as palpitations, shortness of breath, chest pain, dizziness, feelings of unreality, perspiration, trembling and fears of imminent collapse, death or insanity. The attacks are usually of a few minutes duration. As they may mimic organic disorders, such conditions as thyrotoxicosis and phaeochromocytoma have to be borne in mind and excluded.

The account in DSM-III carries the implicit assumption that the panic attacks are primary and causal. There is, however, evidence that agoraphobia has a considerably higher prevalence in community samples than panic disorder (Weissman, 1988), and many agoraphobics do not suffer from and have not experienced panic attacks. There is evidence that panic attacks of this disorder commonly prove to have antecedent cognitive sources (Argyle and Roth, 1989a, 1989b) and fear provoking somatic symptoms as the starting point in others (Clark, 1986).

1.11.5 Social phobia

The fears are experienced in a wide variety of social settings where the individual feels himself to be the object of special attention or critical scrutiny. He experiences tremor, perspiration, inability to converse and fears of an embarrassingly urgent need to micturate or empty the bowels. These symptoms may compel patients to take flight from such situations and after a few such experiences avoidance of social events may become complete.

In 'specific social phobia' there is inability to write, speak or eat in the presence of others, or to micturate in a public lavatory. In musicians, artists and other performers, public appearance may be fraught with such overwhelming anticipatory anxiety that a successful career has to be abandoned.

1.11.6 Simple phobia

This is the most circumscribed and least incapacitating of the anxiety disorders. Fear is directed towards a single specific object or situation which has to be avoided or confronted with considerable anxiety. Only a minority seek medical attention since many sufferers find strategies for circumventing exposure to the object in question.

1.11.7 Obsessive–compulsive neurosis

There are recurrent and intrusive, senseless ideas, thoughts and impulses of an irrational nature. The central feature is the preoccupation with aggressive, blasphemous, sexual ideas or risks of infection or contamination. The morbid nature of the idea is recognized and persistent attempts are made to resist its intrusion. The compulsions are repetitive rituals of a cleansing, symbolic or expiatory nature or aimed at warding off some danger. Again, there is insight into and resistance against the morbid behaviours. Many authorities consider that obsessive–compulsive disorder is so specific and sharply delineated from other anxiety disorders that it should not be classed within this category.

1.11.8 Post-traumatic stress disorder

The anxiety follows some overwhelming trauma such as natural disaster, exposure to battle, earthquake, terrorist attack or rape under certain conditions and is characterized by repeated re-enactment in consciousness or in dreams of the original trauma, the experience of psychic numbing which renders the individual unable to feel love or affection or to derive pleasure from life, a sense of detachment from the environment, avoidance of all situations reminiscent of the traumatic event and symptoms of anxiety and depression.

1.12 Anxiety and depression

1.12.1 Relationship of anxiety to depressive disorders (Level IV)

This subject has been discussed in detail elsewhere (Roth, 1978a; Roth and Barnes, 1981). In a series of enquiries (Kerr et al., 1972; Roth et al., 1972; Schapira et al., 1972; Mountjoy and Roth, 1982a, 1982b; Roth and Mountjoy, 1982; Caetano et al., 1985) that drew upon clinical observations made with the aid of a structured standardized interview, follow-up studies and measures of personality, endogenous and neurotic depressive disorders were found to be relatively distinct from anxiety and phobic neuroses. There was some overlap between the groups but symptoms such as suicidal tendencies, diurnal variation of mood, early waking, retardation proved relatively specific for depression, while panic attacks, severe agoraphobic symptoms, depersonalization, derealization and perceptual distortion and dependent personality characterized the anxiety and phobic groups. The conclusion that the anxiety and depressive groups of patients were distinct from each other was based on the following groups of observations.

1. The results from the discriminating statistical analyses and the scale of 13 items derived from them (Gurney *et al.*, 1972) (Table 4) distinguished the two groups of patients and corresponded closely to the original clinical diagnosis. Similar conclusions have been reached by other investigators (Downing and Rickels, 1974; Prusoff and Klerman, 1974).
2. In the earlier studies endogenous depressions had been included in the depressive group. In later enquiries confined to patients with anxiety and phobic disorders and neurotic depressions alone, analyses of features recorded in the course of a structured clinical interview and the scores registered on a range of rating scales for anxiety and depressive states yielded essentially similar results to the enquiries described under (1) above (Mountjoy and Roth, 1982a, 1982b; Roth and Mountjoy 1982; Caetano *et al.*, 1985).
3. Independent follow-up studies showed outcome in depressed patients to be significantly superior to that in anxiety disorders. The assessments were blind so that the results provided independent validation for the separation of the groups.
4. There had been little cross-over between anxiety, phobic and depressive states in the follow-up period.
5. The indices that best predicted outcome in anxiety disorders proved to differ markedly from those that achieved the best forecast of outcome in depression. This result is incompatible with the unitary theory.

Recent investigations into personality setting of anxiety and depressive disorders have been undertaken on a fresh clinical population of 150 acute in-patients. The patients' self-ratings on the Maudsley personality inventory of the Cattell's 16PF were studied (Caetano, 1981; Caetano *et al.*, 1985). The distribution of these self-ratings showed that 84% of the patients could be assigned to the groups of anxiety state or depressive disorder on the basis of their current symptoms. They could also be classified into these same groups on the basis of independent personality measures.

A further enquiry of clinical ratings of personality, early life experience, developmental history and previous adjustment, elicited in the course of a

Table 4 Items in anxiety–depression index.

Item	Score	
Neurotic traits in childhood	3 or more	+10
	2 or less	+5
	None	0
Dependence	Present	+6
	Absent	0
Physical stress	Severe	+16
	Mild/moderate	+8
	None	0
Panic attacks	3 or more per week	+20
	2 or less per week	+10
	None	0
Situational phobias	Marked	+6
	Mild/moderate	+3
	None	0
Derealization	Marked and/or persistent	+2
	Mild	+1
	None	0
Anxiety symptoms	6 or more	+12
	3 to 5	+6
	Less than 3	0
Depressed mood	Severe	−18
	Mild/moderate	−9
	None	0
Early waking	Present	−4
	Absent	0
Suicidal tendencies	Attempt	−12
	Ideas	−6
	None	0
Retardation	Present	−6
	Absent	0
Obsessional symptoms	Marked	+4
	Mild	+2
	None	0
Neurotic (MPI)*	0–8	−15
	0–16	−12
	17–24	−9
	25–32	−6
	33–40	−3
	41–48	0

Ranges: anxiety +11 to +78; doubtful −3 to +10; depressive −55 to −2.
* (Maudsley Personality Inventory)

standardized interview, achieved a similar degree of discrimination between the two groups (M. Roth and C. Q. Mountjoy, unpublished data). Cross-validation by independent observers is required but it is clear from the available evidence that measures of premorbid personality and adjustment are indispensible complements to observations derived from examination of the present mental state in any enquiries arrived at refining the diagnosis and classification of depressive and anxiety disorders.

1.12.2 The co-morbidity of depressive disorders with panic and agoraphobic disorders

In DSM-III mood disorders and anxiety disorders are treated as entirely distinct conditions. The implication that anxiety disorders do not constitute mood or affective states is open to question, nor have the problems posed by the recent findings in relation to co-morbidity of the disorders been satisfactorily resolved.

It is inevitable that a condition as disabling as panic, or panic with agoraphobia, should be complicated after a period by depressive symptoms. These would add their own quota of certain anxiety symptoms which are inherent features of depressive states. The wide range of methodologies that have been employed to investigate the association makes it difficult to interpret the findings.

A group of investigators at Yale (Leckman et al., 1983a; Weissman et al., 1984) investigated the first-degree relatives of probands with major depression. They found that adult relatives of subjects with depression and panic disorder had raised rates of both major depression and anxiety states, as well as alcoholism. However, this pattern of morbidity risks was not found in probands with both depression and agoraphobia. This is not surprising. Panic attacks are a relatively common feature in patients with severe and moderate depression and both syndromes, as well as the secondary depressive effects of panic, might therefore occur in the first-degree relatives of patients with major depression. On the other hand, agoraphobia is a relatively distinct disorder which arises as a complication only in that small minority of depressed patients whose predisposition to an agoraphobic syndrome remains latent until depressive attacks supervene. In such patients agoraphobia is of relatively late onset in the fourth decade or at a later age.

An informative body of findings from Iowa (Noyes et al., 1986) showed that relatives of probands with panic disorder had a significantly higher prevalence of panic disorder (but not primary depression) than control subjects. There was a slight increase of secondary depression, most likely an expression of the demoralization that results from frequent anxiety disorders.

In a Cambridge study of 90 patients with panic disorder (Argyle and Roth, 1989a, 1989b), anxiety symptoms predominated in 74 cases. In these patients depression had appeared following the onset of panic symptoms and was most likely secondary depression of the 'demoralization' type. In 16 patients depression dominated the clinical picture. In this group, depression had preceded the panic attacks in nine cases; the panic attacks had evolved as a secondary development in most of these patients. This interpretation was supported by the later onset of panic disorder in this smaller second group; a mean of 31.7 years as compared with 27.7 years in those with 'demoralization' depression.

In the view of this author a certain part of the co-morbidity in panic-agoraphobic disorder and depression may be explained in terms of secondary complication by depressive symptoms. Some of the findings which are at variance with this conclusion have been recorded in investigations in which the secondary cases were not interviewed personally, information being obtained indirectly from an informant (Munjack and Moss, 1981). Reliable discrimination of anxiety and depressive disorders is difficult to achieve on the basis of descriptions of the emotional disorder in first-degree relatives obtained indirectly from other members of the family or from friends.

The conclusion, reached by some workers, that there is a common diathesis for depression and panic-agoraphobic disorder is not justified for the present. Panic is an inherent feature of a proportion of cases of severe depressive illness and there are features of panic disorder that can also satisfy DSM-III criteria for major depression. It is therefore to be expected that one or both should be found in first-degree relatives. Diagnoses of depressive illness made with the aid of the DSM-III-R criteria for major depression alone may identify no more than secondary effects of anxiety, panic and other forms of emotional illness (Argyle and Roth, 1989b). This may have been instrumental in the genesis of a substantial part of the co-morbidity of major depression with panic-agoraphobic disorders.

1.13 Atypical psychoses related to the affective and anxiety disorders

The lines drawn between levels III and V are intended to indicate that there is some evidence for a kinship between affective disorder and certain atypical psychoses which may have features suggestive of schizophrenic illness, a 'mixed' psychosis or some other form of psychotic disorder. These disorders in the borderlands of affective disorder are heterogeneous in respect of their clinical picture, presumptive aetiology and their relationships to typical affective disorders. This is reflected by a bewildering variety of names such as 'schizoaffective', 'cycloid', 'schizomanic', the 'mixed' psychoses in the sense of Kraepelin, 'hysterical psychosis', some of the 'psychogenic psychoses' commonly diagnosed in the Scandinavian countries, the 'emotion psychosis' of Labhardt and Rohr, and 'anxiety psychosis'. It is however possible to group them on the basis of the available evidence into two main classes.

The first group on the right comprises schizomanic disorders in which markedly incongruous paranoid and other delusional beliefs may be found in florid cases. Follow-up investigations (Brockington and Leff, 1979) have shown a kinship with manic rather than schizophrenic disorder, although patients spend rather more time in hospital than ordinary manic cases.

The cycloid psychosis of Leonhard (1957) refers to a condition with a blend of schizophrenic and affective symptoms. The attacks are usually recurrent but there are periods of remission between attacks. According to Perris (1974), the psychosis shows a familial homotypicality, with first-degree relatives exhibiting a closely similar form of disorder. Affinity with bipolar disorder is suggested by the cyclical course, the phenomenology, which includes prominent endogenous depressive features, and the claim by Perris (1974) that lithium is an effective treatment in some cases, although this has not yet received independent confirmation.

Under the heading the 'psychogenic psychoses', those with predominantly affective symptoms should also be included. Scandinavian authors (Strömgren, 1968) refer to delusional depressive symptoms, mania, stupor and ideas of guilt in the psychogenic depressive psychoses. However, the hereditary background of these conditions is not that of typical endogenous or psychotic affective disorder (Welner and Strömgren, 1958; Strömgren, 1974).

On the left-hand side there are disorders which have some affinity with the anxiety states or neurotic depressive disorders. Social phobic states may evolve in their severe form into a paranoid psychotic disorder in which ideas of self-reference are converted into fixed paranoid delusions which impute critical, derisory and offensive comments by those they encounter when they enter social groups. A psychotic syndrome of this nature seems to be recognized in Japan (Takahashi, 1989) but identical cases have been described in the UK (Roth, 1978a).

Another syndrome which deserves to be named 'anxiety psychosis' is that which develops from irrational fears that the symptoms experienced arise from serious or life-threatening disease. This evolves in a substantial minority from doubt-laden fears into near or delusional or fixed delusional conviction of malignant or venereal disease impervious to reassurance or objective evidence.

Insight is in abeyance. 'Hypochondriases' in DSM-III fails to convey the full phenomenological picture of this disorder.

Some 'psychogenic' psychoses emerge in the setting of long-standing neurotic illness or personality disorder following exposure to stress which impinges, however, on Achilles' heels in the personality. A monograph by Labhardt (1963) has been devoted to cases of this nature. The symptomatology comprises paranoid hallucinatory, and at times catatonic symptoms, transient clouding of consciousness, anxiety with severe autonomic disturbance, agitation and prominent hysterical symptoms. The stresses at onset are frequently onerous and life threatening, but the family history reveals no increase in morbid risk for schizophrenia. The psychosis runs a brief and favourable course and recovery is stated to occur in most cases within about 8 weeks of the onset of symptoms.

In a comparative study of patients with typical schizophrenia and patients with schizophreniform and related atypical disorders (McClelland et al., 1966), the latter group proved to differ not in terms of 'nuclear' features but precipitating factors, abrupt onset, hysterical symptoms, depersonalization and a strong depressive colouring, which were the features of greatest discriminating value. Anxiety and phobic features figured in the premorbid picture in a proportion of cases. The link with neurotic anxiety and depressive states or neurotic personality disorder is also substantiated by phenomenological and genetic enquiries (Welner and Strömgren, 1958), which showed that first degree relatives of schizophreniform patients had a low prevalence of schizophrenic illness; in contrast affective psychosis, anxiety neuroses and neurotic depressive disorders were relatively common in the first degree relations.

The atypical psychoses that have some kinship with the affective and anxiety disorders can be divided into two relatively distinct groups. The first comprises the psychoses that develop against the background of anxiety, phobia or obsessional disorder. These have received relatively little attention, although they appear to be of particular importance in the light of their benign prognosis. The most closely studied syndromes are the 'hysterical' psychoses (Hirsch and Hollender, 1981), the 'emotion' psychoses of Swiss authors (Labhardt, 1963; Rohr, 1961) and the psychoses that develop against a background of severe social phobia or kindred form of phobic disorder (Roth, 1979; Takahashi, 1989). These disorders run their course within a few years or, more rarely, months and are usually followed by a more or less complete remission from the delusions, although social phobias continue. Subsequent attacks follow the same pattern and are manifest either in a relapse into psychotic disorder of a closely similar nature or in a return to the pre-existing pattern of neurotic illness. The 'anxiety psychosis' dominated by near-delusional convictions of grave illness described above has received little attention. These syndromes may be subsumed under the heading of Anxiety and Hysterical Psychoses, although depression as well as anxiety features are prominent in the acute phase.

The second group comprises the 'schizomanic' disorder (Brockington *et al.*, 1980) and those schizodepressives that commence after the age of 40 and whose course and hereditary associations, as inferred from family studies (Tsuang *et al.*, 1977), show them to have affinities with the affective psychoses or endogenous disorders. The 'cycloid' disorders (Leonhard, 1961; Perris, 1974; Cutting *et al.*, 1978) may be variants of this group in the light of the presently available evidence; although Perris regards them as a distinct, third form of psychosis.

The relationships of these atypical psychotic disorders are indicated by the lines that lead from the parent group between levels III to V of neurotic affective disorders on the right side of Figure 1 in the case of anxiety and hysterical psychoses, and on the left side in the case of the conditions which are related to the endogenous bipolar and unipolar affective disorders.

1.14 Conclusions

1.14.1 Need for openness and experiment in relation to systems of classification

There are a number of systems of classification of the affective disorders in existence at the present time, not merely DSM-III-R and ICD-10 but also a variety of other schemes for different disorders, as in the case of the bipolar disorders which have been discussed at length in this chapter. The psychogenic or reactive psychoses are widely accepted in the Scandinavian countries and criticized in others, although they are represented in the draft version of ICD-10. The unipolar–bipolar dichotomy should, in the view of some investigators, be brought back into line with the unitary concept of manic–depressive disorder advanced by Kraepelin.

Far from being a symptom of incoherence of thought among psychiatrists, such voices of dissent from official systems of classification differences should be given the fullest encouragement when they are informed by ideas derived from empirical observation.

There is no system of classification of the affective disorders in existence which is based at every point upon an adequate body of factual observation. Each of the categories and the concepts from which they have been derived are in the nature of hypotheses which should be open to challenge and refutation. It is the extent to which they survive such challenge that should determine whether they are retained intact or need to be discarded or modified.

DSM-III-R and ICD-9 (ICD-10 remains in draft form) have much achievement to their credit. The danger is that they may be allowed to harden into doctrinal and closed systems of diagnosis and classification in scientific practice. The dangers created have to be considered separately under these two headings.

1.14.2 Conflict between taxonomic orthodoxy and the objectives of scientific enquiry

As far as scientific investigation is concerned, the creators of classification and scientific investigators are to some extent at cross purposes. The committees charged by official bodies to prepare a new or revised classification have to make unambiguous decisions, often about complex and controversial issues. At times, the available data regarding a problem in classification are insufficient for a firm judgement but the committees *are compelled* to arrive at a conclusion.

The objectives of the scientist and his attitude to problems are in diametrical opposition to such practices. His task is to ferret out and lay bare the contradictions and ambiguities he discovers within classification schemes. Stringent investigation into phenomenology, treatment response, heredity and other biological variables may yield results that require lines of demarcation between disorders to be redrawn. Some boundary lines may have to be erased and others substituted.

A good example is provided by the concept of 'Unitary Psychosis', revived by a number of eminent investigators (Kendell and Gourlay, 1970; Crow, 1986, 1988). This challenges the way in which the psychoses are subdivided in every known system of classification. Many investigators are critical of this concept but its exponents have advanced some thought-provoking and possibly fruitful ideas. Those interested in the classification of affective disorders must follow the progress of this controversy and evaluate any fresh data that emerge with an open mind.

In short, while those who have been entrusted with the task of creating new national and international classifications will be disposed to defend their main concepts, those engaged in scientific investigations into affective disorders will, if their work proves creative, tend to subvert them. If fundamental advances were to be made about the causes of manic–depressive disorder or one of the highly prevalent forms of anxiety disorder, it is probable that existing classifications of affective disorders would have to undergo radical revision. Hence the need for openness and flexibility in official systems of classification of affective (and other) disorders.

1.14.3 Conflict between official classification and clinical practice

The application of classification systems in clinical practice poses problems of a different kind. Of course, official national and international systems of classification, and even novel ones such as DSM-III which have gained wide acceptance, have to be largely devoted at present to the classification of the syndromes whose symptoms and signs can be elicited and observed during the course of examination of the patient's present mental state. This is the only part of the clinical examination of psychiatric patients which has been standardized, and it is only these syndromes (recorded on Axis I of DSM-III) that have achieved acceptable levels of interobserver reliability in diagnosis. To a certain extent they have also been validated by observations on course and outcome of treatment response, hereditary basis and, in small part, by other biological variables. This is the explanation for the fact that the large body of publications that have drawn upon DSM-III or ICD-9 for diagnostic criteria in clinical or neurobiological investigations is dominated by cross-sectional concepts and syndromes such as bipolar disorder, major depression and Panic Disorder. Personality diagnoses and concomitant disorders are rarely mentioned in research publications unless they are used as exclusion criteria in attempts to recruit a homogeneous group of patients. Yet a categorical diagnosis expressed in terms of an Axis I syndrome represents a truncated version of the concept of affective disorder that continues to inform the clinical practice of most psychiatrists throughout the world. Categorical diagnosis in the clinic is set in the context of patients' previous history, premorbid personality, social status, physical disability and social achievement, and relationships between these different aspects are explored and expressed. This is what is meant by a clinical formulation, a synthesis of all relevant features that is an essential foundation for decisions regarding the management of patients with affective disorder and attempts to predict their outcome.

1.14.4 Rift between the new and old concepts of disorders of affect

The assumption that the symptoms and signs elicited in the course of examination of the present mental state represent the patient's illness in its entirety (a view which is implicit or stated explicitly in much contemporary clinical literature of the affective disorders) represents a radical departure from the conceptualization of these disorders in classical descriptive psychiatry. This refers to the concepts of Kraepelin, Jaspers, Schneider, Mayer-Gross, Sjöbring and Slater. The conceptual disparity is most marked in relation to what were called the 'neurotic depressions' and the kindred disorders. Neurotic disorder was conceived as being inextricably entwined with one or other form of personality disorder. In Slater's concept of the 'Neurotic Constitution', neuroses were conceived as exaggerations or parodies or maladaptive versions of inherent personality traits. The neurotic personality was regarded as a major causal factor in the genesis of neurotic illness. As already indicated, Kraepelin regarded even manic–depressive illness as being frequently rooted in the life-long 'depressive temperament'. An increasing body of recent observations has testified to the importance of premorbid personality for the diagnosis, management, prediction of outcome and the 'understanding' of neurotic anxiety and depressive disorders (Andrews *et al.*, 1990b; Roth, 1990).

Hirschfeld (1990) has recently adduced evidence that individuals who suffer from 'Dysthymia' are extremely disturbed personalities, characterized by increased neuroticism and introversion, which persist after they have recovered from the disorders of their affective life. Other studies have shown that neuroticism and extroversion scores and other personality variables differentiate depressive disorders from anxiety neuroses (Kerr *et al.*, 1970; Caetano *et al.*, 1985). Tyrer reported that depressive and dependent personality disorders were more common in anxious than in depressive patients (Tyrer *et al.*, 1983).

These and other observations have provided a starting point for taking a new look at a number of issues in relation to the classification of affective disorders which remain controversial, despite decades of clinical and biological investigation. The differentiation between psychotic and neurotic affective disorders needs to be examined afresh with the aid of the best available measures of personality profile and adjustment patterns as well as cross-sectional features of presenting mental states. Further investigations should be undertaken into the bipolar–unipolar dichotomy to determine whether the greater genetic loading of the former than the latter is reflected in differences in personality structure as well as the clinical picture in depressive states.

There is some evidence to suggest that the disorders at level V represented on the neurotic side (right) of the diagram, namely the psychogenic, anxious, hysterical and 'emotion' psychoses, and the 'social phobic' psychoses differ in respect of personality profile from the paranoid–manic, pseudo-schizophrenic, cycloid and schizophreniform disorders on the left extreme end of Figure 1.

The group represented on the left-hand side appears to have a kinship with endogenous affective psychoses and bipolar or manic depressive psychosis in particular. That on the right-hand side seems to be more closely related to anxiety, hysterical and non-endogenous depressive forms of illness; that is, 'neurotic' conditions and their concomitant personality disorders.

Attention has already been drawn to the finding that personality factors accounted for a far higher proportion of the variance in outcome in neurotic than in the endogenous depression (Andrews *et al.*, 1990b). There was a tenfold difference between the two groups in respect of the part played by personality factors in shaping outcome. It would therefore appear worthwhile investigating whether the contribution of personality to outcome also differentiates the atypical psychoses which develop in the context of neurotic disorder and associated personality factors from those atypical psychoses whose kinship appears to be with endogenous and psychotic depressive states. Such enquiries may shed light not only on the classification of atypical psychoses which have become increasingly prominent in clinical practice in the past fifteen to twenty years; they could be expected to shed some light on the aetiological origins of these disorders and thus provide further guidelines regarding the forms of pharmacological treatment most likely to alleviate their symptoms. Conventional forms of antipsychotic treatment with neuroleptic drugs alone prove ineffective in a substantial proportion of these atypical forms of psychotic disorder.

References

Akiskal, H.S., Bitar, A.H., Puzantian, V.R. *et al.* (1978) *Arch. Gen. Psychiatry* **35**, 756–766.

Akiskal, H.S. (1983) In *Psychiatry Update: The American Psychiatric Association Annual Review*, vol. 2 (ed. Grinspoon, L.), pp 271–292. Washington, DC, American Psychiatric Press.

Akiskal, H.S. (1987) *Psychiatr. Ann.* **17**, 32–37.

Akiskal, H.S., Walker, P.W., Puzantian, V.R., King, D., Rosenthal, T.L. & Dranon, M. (1983) *J. Affective Disorders* **5**, 115–128.

Akiskal, H.S., Cassano, G.B., Musetti, L., Perugi, G., Tundo, A. & Mignani, V. (1989) *Psychopathology* **22**, 268–277.

Akiskal, H.S. (1990) In *Dysthymic Disorder* (eds Burton, S.W. & Akiskal, H.S.), pp 1–12. London, Royal College of Psychiatrists.

American Psychiatric Association (1980) *Diagnostic and Statistical Manual of Mental Disorders*, 3rd edn (DSM-III). Washington DC, American Psychiatric Association.

American Psychiatric Association (1987) *Diagnostic and Statistical Manual of Mental Disorders*, 3rd edn (revised) (DSM-III-R). Washington DC, American Psychiatric Association.

Andrews, G., Stewart, G., Morris-Yates, A., Holt, P. & Henderson, S. (1990a) *Br. J. Psychiatry* **157**, 6–12.

Andrews, G., Neilson, M., Hunt, C., Stewart, G. & Kiloh, L.G. (1990b) *Br. J. Psychiatry* **157**, 13–18.

Angst, J. (1966) *Zur Atiologie und Nosologie Endogenen Depressiver Psychosen*. Berlin, Springer-Verlag.

Angst, J. (1978) *Arch. Psychiatr. Nervkrank.* **266**, 65–73.

Angst, J. (1982) *Psychopathology* **18**, 140–154.

Angst, J. & Dobler-Nikola, A. (1984) *Eur. Arch. Psychiatry Neurol. Sci.* **234**, 21–29.

Angst, J. & Dobler-Nikola, A. (1985) *Eur. Arch. Psychiatry Neurol. Sci.* **234**, 408–416.

Angst, J., Frey, R., Lohmeyer, B. & Zerbin-Rudin, E. (1980) *Hum. Genet.* **55**, 237–254.

Argyle, N. & Roth, M. (1989a) *Psychiatr. Dev.* **3**, 175–186.

Argyle, N. & Roth, M. (1989b) *Psychiatr. Dev.* **3**, 187–209.

Brockington, K.R., Wainwright, S. & Kendell, R.E. (1980) *Psychol. Med.* **10**, 73–83.

Brockington, I.F. & Leff, J.P. (1979) *Psychol. Med.* **9**, 91–99.

Caetano, D. (1981) PhD thesis, University of Cambridge.

Caetano, D., Roth, M. & Mountjoy, C. (1985) In *Psychiatry*, vol. 1. In (eds Pichot, P., Berner, P., Wolf, R. & Thau, K.), pp 513–524. New York, Plenum Press.

Carney, M.W.P., Roth, M. & Garside, R.F. (1965) *Br. J. Psychiatry* **111**, 659–674.

Cassano, G.B., Akiskal, H.S., Musetti, L., Perugi, G., Soriani, A. & Mignani, V. (1989) *Psychopathology* **22**, 278–288.

Cassano, G.B., Perugi, G. & Musetti, L. (1990) *Psychiatr. Ann.* **20**, 517–521.

Clark, D.M., Salkovskis, P.M., Gelder, M.G. *et al.* (1986) In *Panic and Phobias* (eds Hand, I. & Wittchen, H.F.), pp 149–158. Berlin, Springer–Verlag.

Clark, D.M. (1986) *Behav. Res. Ther.* **23**, 585–600.

Clark, D.M. (1986) *Behav. Res. Ther.* **4**, 461–470.

Cowdy, R.W., Wehr, T.A., Zis, A.P. & Goodwin, F.K. (1983) *Arch. Gen. Psychiatry* **40**, 414–420.

Crane, G.E. (1957) *Psychiatr. Res. Rep.* **8**, 142–182.

Crow, T.J. (1986) *Br. J. Psychiatry* **149**, 675–683.

Crow, T.J. (1988) *Br. J. Psychiatry* **153**, 675–683.

Cutting, J.C., Clare, A. & Mann, A.H. (1978) *Psychol. Med.* **8**, 637–648.

Downing, R.W. & Rickets, R. (1974) *Arch. Gen. Psychiatry* **30**, 312–317.

Dunner, D.L. (1987) *Psychiatr. Ann.* **17**, 18.

Endicott, J., Nee, J., Andreasen, N., Clayton, P., Keller, M. & Coryell, W. (1985) *J. Affective Disord.* **8**, 17–28.

Feighner, J.P., Robins, E., Guze, S.B., Woodruff, R.A., Winokur, G. & Munoz, R. (1972) *Arch. Gen. Psychiatry* **26**, 57–63.

Fieve, R.R. & Dunner, D.L. (1985) In *The Nature and Treatment of Depression* (eds Flach & Draghi), pp 145–166. New York, Wiley.

Gillespie, A.H. (1929) *Guys Hosp. Rep.* **79**, 306–344.

Goodwin, F.K., Post, R.M. & Sack, R. (1975) In *Neurobiological Mechanisms of Adaptation and Behaviour* (ed. Mendell, A.J.), pp 96–97. New York, Raven Press.

Grinker, R.R., Miller, J., Sabshin, M. *et al.* (1961) *The Phenomena of Depression.* New York, Harper & Row.

Gurney, C., Roth, M., Garside, R.F., Kerr, T.A. & Schapira, K. (1972) *Br. J. Psychiatry* **121**, 162–166.

Hickie, I., Parsonage, B. & Parker, G. (1990) *Br. J. Psychiatry* **157**, 65–71.

Hirsch, S.R. & Hollender, M. (1981) *Am. J. Psychiatry* **120**, 1066–1074. *Am. J. Psychiatry* **120**, 1066–1074.

Hirschfeld, R.M.A. (1990) In *Dysthymic Disorder* (eds Burton, S.Q. & Akiskal, H.S.), pp 69–77. London, Royal College of Psychiatrists.

Katschnig, H. (1986) In *Life Events and Psychiatric Disorders: Controversial Issues* (ed. Katschnig, H.), pp 74–106. Cambridge, Cambridge University Press.

Kendell, R.E. (1968) *The Classification of Depressive Illness*, Maudsley Monograph No. 18. London, Institute of Psychiatry.

Kendell, R.E. (1976) *Br. J. Psychiatry* **129**, 15–28.
Kendell, R.E. & Gourlay, J. (1970) *Br. J. Psychiatry* **117**, 261–266.
Kerr, T.A., Schapira, K., Roth, M. & Garside, R.F. (1970) *Br. J. Psychiatry* **116**, 11–19.
Kerr, T.A., Roth, M., Schapira, K. & Gurney, C. (1972) *Br. J. Psychiatry* **121**, 167–174.
Kiloh, L.G. & Ball, J.R.B. (1961) *Br. Med. J.* **5220**, 168–171.
Kiloh, L.G. & Garside, R.F. (1963) *Br. J. Psychiatry* **109**, 451–463.
Kiloh, L.G. & Garside, R.F. (1977) *Aust. N.Z. J. Psychiatry* **11**, 149–156.
Kiloh, L.G., Child, J.P. & Latner, G. (1960) *J. Ment. Sci.* **106**, 1425–1428.
Kiloh, L.G., Ball, J.R.B. & Garside, R.F. (1962) *Br. Med. J.* **1**, 1225–1227.
Kiloh, L.G., Andrews, G., Neilson, M. *et al.* (1972) *Br. J. Psychiatry* **121**, 183–196.
Kiloh, L.G., Andrews, G. & Neilson, R.M. (1988) *Br. J. Psychiatry* **153**, 752–757.
Klein, D. & Davis, J. (1969) *Diagnosis and Drug Treatment of Psychiatric Disorders*, pp 180–185. Baltimore, Williams & Wilkins.
Klerman, G.L. (1971) *Arch. Gen. Psychiatry* **24**, 305–319.
Klerman, G.L., Endicott, J., Spitzer, R. *et al.* (1979) *Am. J. Psychiatry* **136**, 57–70.
Kline, N.S. (1958) *J. Clin. Exp. Psychopathology* **19** (Suppl. 1), 72–78.
Kraepelin, E. (1921) *Manic-Depressive Insanity and Paranoia* (trans. Barclay, R.M.) Edinburgh, E. & S. Livingstone.
Kretschmer, E. (1936) *Physique and Character* (trans. Miller, E.). London, Kegan Paul, Trench, Trubner and Co.
Kuhn, R. (1958) *Am. J. Psychiatry* **115**, 459–464.
Kupfer, D.J., Pickard, D., Himmelhoch, J.M. & Detre, T.P. (1975) *Arch. Gen. Psychiatry* **32** 866–871.
Labhardt, F. (1963) *Die Schizophrenieahnlichen Emotionspsychosen: Ein Beitrag zur Abgrenzung Schizophrenieartiger Zustandsbilder.* Berlin, Springer–Verlag.
Leckman, J.F., Merikangas, K.F., Pauls, D.L., Prusoff, B.A. & Weissmann, M.M. (1983a) *Am. J. Psychiatry* **140**, 880–882.
Leckman, J.F., Weissmann, M.M., Merihangas, M.M. *et al.* (1983b) *Arch. Gen. Psychiatry* **40**, 1055–1060.
Lee, A.S. & Murray, R.M. (1988) *Br. J. Psychiatry* **153**, 741–751.
Leonhard, K. (1957) *Aufteilung der Endogenen Psychosen.* Berlin, Akademie Verlag.
Lesser, I.M. (1988) *J. Anx. Disord.* **2**, 3–15.
Lewis, A.J. (1934) *J. Ment. Sci.* **80**, 277–378.
Lewis, A.J. (1936) *J. Ment. Sci.* **82**, 488–558.
Lorr, M., Pokorny, A.D. & Klett, C.J. (1973) *J. Clin. Psychol.* **29**, 290–294.
McClelland, H.S., Roth, M., Neubauer, H. & Garside, R.F. (1966) In *Proceedings of the IVth World Congress of Psychiatry*, 5–11 September, Madrid (ed. Lopez Ibor, J.J.). Excerpta Medica Foundation.
McGuffin, P. (1988) *Br. J. Psychiatry* **153**, 591–596.
McGuffin, P. & Katz, R. (1986) In *The Biology of Depression* (ed. Deakin, J.F.W.), Gaskell Psychiatry Series, pp 26–52.
Mapother, E. & Lewis, A.J. (1941) In *A Textbook of the Practice of Medicine*, 6th edn. (ed. Price, F.W.), pp 1851–1863. Humphrey Milford, Oxford University Press, London.
Mayer–Gross, W., Slater, E. & Roth, M. (1954) *Clinical Psychiatry* (revised editions 1960, 1969, 1977). London, Baillière, Tindall & Cassell.
Mendels, J. & Cochrane, C. (1968) *Am. J. Psychiatry* **124** (Suppl.), 1–11.
Mountjoy, C.Q. & Roth, M. (1982a) *J. Affective Disord.* **4**, 127–147.
Mountjoy, C.Q. & Roth, M. (1982b) *J. Affective Disord.* **3**, 149–161.
Munjack, D.J. & Moss, H.R. (1981) *Arch. Gen. Psychiatry* **38**, 869–871.

Noyes, R. Jr., Crowe, R.R., Harris, E.L., Hamra, B.J., McChesney, C.M. & Chaudry, D.R. (1986) *Arch. Gen. Psychiatry* **43**, 227–232.

Overall, J.E., Hollister, L.E., Johnson, M. *et al.* (1966) *J.A.M.A.* **195**, 946–950.

Parker, G., Hadzi-Pavlovic, D., Boyce, P. *et al.* (1990) *Br. J. Psychiatry* **157**, 55–65.

Perris, C. (1966) *Acta Psychiatr. Scand.* **42** (Suppl. 194), 118–152.

Perris, C. (1968) *Acta Psychiatr. Scand.* **194**, 15–44.

Perris, C. (1974) *Acta Psychiatr. Scand.* (Suppl. 253)

Peselow, E.D., Dunner, D.L., Fieve, R.R. & Lautin, A. (1982) *Am. J. Psychiatry* **39**, 747–752.

Prussof, B. & Klerman, G.L. (1974) *Arch. Gen. Psychiatry* **30**, 302–309.

Rohr, K. (1961) *Arch. Psychiatr. Nervenkr.* **201**, 626–647.

Rosenthal, S.H. & Gudemann, J.E. (1967) *Arch. Gen. Psychiatry* **16**, 241–249.

Rosenthal, T.L., Akiskal, H.S., Scott-Strauss, A. *et al.* (1981) *J. Affective Disord.* **3**, 183–192.

Roth, M. (1959) *Proc. R. Soc. Med.* **52**, 587–596.

Roth, M. (1977) In *Neuro-transmission and Disturbed Behaviour* (eds Van Praag, H.M. & Bruinvels, J.), pp 109–157. Utrecht, Scheltema Holkema.

Roth, M. (1978a) *Pharmakopsychiatr. Neuropsychopharmakol.* **11**, 27–42.

Roth, M. (1978b) In *Psychiatric Diagnosis: Exploration of Biological Predictors* (eds Akiskal, H.S. & Webb, W.L.), pp 9–47. Spectrum Publications Inc.

Roth, M. (1979) In *Neuropsychopharmacology* (eds Saletu, B., Berner, P. & Hollister, L.), pp 17–36. Oxford, Oxford University Press.

Roth, M. (1984) *Psychiatr. Dev.* **1**, 31–52.

Roth, M. (1990) *J. R. Soc. Med.* **83**, 609–614.

Roth, M. & Barnes, T.R.E. (1981) *Compr. Psychiatry* **22**, 54–77.

Roth, M. & Harper, M. (1962) *Compr. Psychiatry* **3**, 215–226.

Roth, M. & Mountjoy, C.Q. (1982) In *Handbook of Affective Disorders* (ed. Paykell, E.S.), pp 70–92. Edinburgh, Churchill Livingstone.

Roth, M., Gurney, C., Garside, R.F., Kerr, T.A. & Schapira, K. (1972) *Br. J. Psychiatry* **121**, 146–171.

Schildkraut, J.J. (1970) *Neuropsychopharmacology and the Affective Disorders*. Boston, Fable Brown.

Schneider, K. (1958) *Psychopathic Personalities*. Springfield IL, C.C. Thomas.

Schneider, K. (1959) *Clinical Psychopathology* (trans. Hamilton, M.W.), New York, Grune & Stratton.

Shapira, K., Roth, M., Kerr, T.A. & Gurney, C. (1972) *Br. J. Psychiatry* **121**, 165–181.

Slater, E. & Roth, M. (1969) *Clinical Psychiatry*. London, Baillière, Tindall & Cassell.

Spitzer, R.L. & Williams, B.W. (1983) In *International Perspectives on DSM-III* (eds Spitzer, R.L., Williams, M.B.W. & Skodol, A.E.), pp 339–354. New York, American Psychiatric Press.

Spitzer, R., Endicott, J. & Robins, E. (1978a) *Research Diagnostic Criteria for a Selected Group of Functional Disorders*, 3rd edn. New York, New York State Psychiatric Institute.

Spitzer, R., Endicott, J. & Robins, E. (1978b) *Arch. Gen. Psychiatry* **35**, 773–782.

Strömgren, E. (1968) Reactive psychoses. *Acta Jutlandica* **40**, 4.

Strömgren, E. (1965) *Acta Psychiat. Scand.* **41**, 483–485.

Takahashi, T.(1989) *Comp. Psychiatry* **30**, 45–52.

Tsuang, M.T. & Simpson, J.C. (1984) *Schizophr. Bull.* **10**, 14–25.

Tsuang, M.T., Dempsey, G.M., Dvoredsky, A. & Struss, A. (1977) *Biol. Psychiatry* **12**, 331–338.

Tyrer, P., Casey, P. & Gall, J. (1983) *Br. J. Psychiatry* **142**, 404–408.

Uhde, T.W., Boulenger, J.P., Roy-Bryne, P.P., Geraci, M.F., Vittone, B.J. & Post, R.M. (1985) *Prog. Neuropsychopharmacol. Biol. Psychiatry* **9**, 39–51.

Weissman, M.M. (1988) In *Handbook of Anxiety*, vol. 1 (eds Roth, M., Noyes, R. & Burrows, G.D.), pp 83–100. Amsterdam, Elsevier.

Weissman, M.M., Prusoff, B.A., Gammon, G.B., Merikangas, K.R., Leckmann, J.F. & Kidd, K.K. (1984) *J. Am. Acad. Child Psychiatry* **23**, 78.

Wehr, T.A., Sack, D.A., Rosenthal, N.E. & Cowdry, R.W. (1988) *Am. J. Psychiatry* **145**, 179–184.

Welner, J. & Strömgren, E. (1958) *Acta Psychiatr. Neurol. Scand.* **33**, 377–399.

West, S.D. & Dally, P.J. (1959) *Br. Med. J.* **1**, 1491–1494.

Wing, J. & Sturt, E. (1978) *The PSE-ID-CATEGO System: A Supplementary Manual.* London, Institute of Psychiatry.

Wing, J.D., Cooper, J. E. & Sartorius, N. (1979) *The Measurement and Classification of Psychiatric Symptoms.* London, Cambridge University Press.

Wing, J.K., Bebbington, P., Hurry, J. & Tennant, C. (1981) In *What is a Case? The Problem of Definition in Psychiatric Community Surveys* (eds Wing, J.K., Bebbington, P. & Robins, L.N.), pp 45–61. London, Grant McIntyre, Medical Scientific.

Winokur, G. & Clayton, P. (1967) In *Recent Advances in Biological Psychiatry* (ed. Wortis, J.), pp 35–50. Plenum, New York.

Winokur, G., Cadoret, R.J., Dorzal, J. & Baker, M. (1971) *Arch. Gen. Psychiatry* **24**, 135–144

Winokur, G., Behar, D., van Valkenburg, C. *et al.* (1978) *J. Nerv. Ment. Dis.* **166**, 764–768.

Winokur, G., Tsuang, M.T. & Crowe, R.R. (1982) *Am. J. Psychiatry* **139**, 209–212.

World Health Organization (1990) *ICD-10 (draft).* World Health Organisation, Geneva.

CHAPTER 2

PHYSICAL TREATMENTS FOR DEPRESSION

Stephen Merson and Peter Tyrer

Stephen Merson, MRCPsych., Clinical Research Fellow & Honorary Registrar.
Peter Tyrer, MD., MRCP., FRCPsych., Senior Lecturer in Community Psychiatry,
St Charles' Hospital, London W10 6DZ, UK

Table of Contents

Much of the interest in depression shown by basic scientists and clinicians in the last 40 years has flowed from evidence that physical treatments for depressive illness are not only effective but in many cases the preferred therapy for the disorder. Thus, changes in the classification of depression (see Chapter 1), the burgeoning interest in the biochemistry of depression, and the epidemiology of depressive disorders and their causal influences (exemplified by studies of life events), all owe at least some of their inspiration to the development of successful physical treatments. This may tempt contradiction, but it is worth reminding ourselves that for the first 30 years of this century depressive disorders were virtually forgotten diagnoses. Aubrey Lewis (1934) rescued them from obscurity by clinical description and Cerletti and Bini (1938) began the era of physical treatments by their introduction of electroconvulsive therapy (even though depression was not the original indication for the treatment).

2.1 Indications for physical treatment

'Physical treatment' is a rather unfortunate description which implies marked personal activity when it is in fact a very passive process. It covers the range of treatments that are given in order to correct some presumed physical, or organic, abnormality in the patient. In the case of depression the distinction is often made between understandable sadness and unhappiness in response to an event, usually a loss, which is considered unsuitable for physical treatment and, at the other extreme, a condition manifest by severe depressive symptoms and psychomotor changes in the absence of obvious precipitants (at least immediate ones) and which is presumed to be caused by a biochemical abnormality requiring reversal by pharmacological treatment or electroconvulsive therapy (ECT). This explains the attraction of a dichotomous classification of depression for psychiatrists; it has face validity and can be a useful guide to practice. Unfortunately the decision to give treatment is often made before adequate assessment so that diagnosis becomes a tautologous exercise that justifies rather than indicates the treatment.

The indications for physical treatment can be summarized under a series of headings, all beginning with the letter 's': specific symptoms, severity, suicide, stupor and speed. They are worth discussing separately but together they make a major contribution towards the continuum of symptomatology in depression. This continuum also reflects the relative indications for psychological and physical treatments which follow opposite exponential curves with varying degrees of overlap, particularly marked in the middle range (Figure 1).

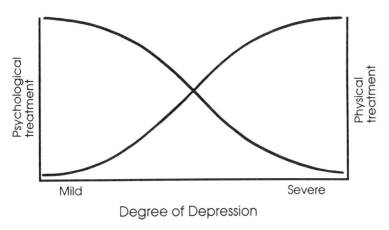

Figure 1 Scope of physical and psychological treatment of depressive illness.

2.1.1 Specific symptoms

There is a popular belief that certain symptoms of depression, particularly certain 'somatic' symptoms, are specific indicators for physical treatment in depression (Table 1). These symptoms include marked anorexia, weight loss, loss of libido, a characteristic pattern of sleep disturbance with waking in the early morning, and a diurnal mood swing. These symptoms, which are perhaps better described as 'endogenomorphic' (Klein, 1974) rather than 'somatic', because they cover more than bodily symptoms, are often found in more severe depressive illness and it is difficult to know whether they should be

Table 1 Depressive symptoms indicating response to physical treatment.

Distinct quality of altered mood
Diurnal variation of mood
Weight loss
Reduced appetite
Middle and late insomnia
Motor retardation
Motor agitation
Hopelessness
Guilt

regarded as specific indicators for physical treatment independent of severity. Studies of antidepressant drugs have shown that all symptoms of depression respond to antidepressants (Morris and Beck, 1974; Bielski and Friedel, 1976) and the relative specificity of somatic symptoms may be spurious, as these, being marked in severe depression, may be the first to improve when clinical response begins.

There have also been several studies of psychological treatments, particularly cognitive therapy, suggesting that they are effective in the treatment of relatively severe depression (Rush *et al.*, 1977; Blackburn *et al.*, 1981; Teasdale *et al.*, 1984). The recently completed large-scale study of depression carried out by the National Institute of Mental Health in the USA also showed that cognitive therapy and interpersonal psychotherapy were both as effective as imipramine in treating moderate depressive illness (Weissmann *et al.*, 1987; Klerman, 1988). However, it would be wrong to infer from this that cognitive therapy and other psychological treatments are effective against the whole range of depressive symptoms because these treatments have not been tested in the most severe forms of depression.

Similar suggestions have been made with the regard to the outcome of ECT (e.g. Hobson, 1953) but, again, in the absence of comparable control groups with similar symptoms it is impossible to be certain whether these symptoms do indeed respond specifically to ECT or whether they have the best outcome irrespective of the nature of treatment.

2.1.2 Severity and stupor

As indicated in Figure 1, the more severe the depressive illness the greater the indication for physical treatment. This is shown at its most extreme in the now relatively rare condition of depressive stupor, in which psychomotor retardation is so pronounced that the sufferer is fixed in immobility despite being fully conscious. States in which there are depressive delusions (e.g. of hopelessness, unworthiness and guilt) and hallucinations (usually auditory and of a derogatory nature) are also such strong indications for physical treatment that this treatment could be regarded as mandatory, if only because in these cases there is little or no insight and all forms of psychological treatment are largely ineffective.

2.1.3 Suicide

Suicidal thinking is the depressive symptom that therapists most fear; it is the only one that makes all other features immutable if it is executed successfully. Although it is roughly correlated with the severity of depression it is by no means always so, and the classical situation, whereby successful suicide only takes place after partial treatment of a severe depressive illness has enabled the sufferer to execute the suicidal act, is well known.

The presence of suicidal symptoms may also be a major influence in choosing physical treatment (see below) as many antidepressants have significant dangers in overdose. In some instances it may be a reason for avoiding drug treatments altogether. This is particularly relevant in patients with impulsive suicidal thoughts, such as those commonly associated with emotionally unstable personality disorders, commonly known as borderline personality disorders in the USA (American Psychiatric Association, 1980).

However, when suicide is considered to be a significant risk and is clearly part of a depressive illness, treatment in hospital under supervision is desirable and in such cases the physical treatment, whether it is antidepressants or ECT, can be carefully monitored.

2.1.4 Speed

Although antidepressants have an unfortunate latent period before the onset of clinical response (see below), this period is usually longer for psychological treatments. ECT has the advantage of showing its beneficial effects within 2 weeks (Medical Research Council, 1965; Freeman et al., 1978; Gregory et al., 1985) and will be the treatment of choice when the clinician considers a rapid response to be essential. Of course, severe depression is associated with terrible suffering and this should always be shortened as soon as is humanly possible. However, in some cases this becomes even more important, for example when patients refuse to eat or drink or are so suicidal that they have to be supervised for every minute of the day. The same will apply in depressive stupor.

2.2 Assessing the need for physical treatment

For patients with severe depression there is no difficulty in deciding that physical treatment is currently the most appropriate form of management (Figure 1). There is much greater difficulty in selecting the physical therapy mode when the severity of the depression is moderate because, under these circumstances, psychological treatments can be regarded as equally appropriate.

The first necessity is to carry out a good history and mental state examination, which will detect all the important items discussed above. This will be followed by classification of the type of depressive illness (see Chapter 1). Other associated diagnoses must also be taken into account at this time. For example, an additional diagnosis of borderline personality disorder (or emotionally unstable personality disorder in ICD-10) may make the clinician wary of prescribing any form of physical therapy to an out-patient because of the dangers of overdose and the likelihood of spontaneous recovery. There may also be some clear cause for the depressive illness that obviates the need for physical treatment. These could include one of the many drugs known to precipitate depressive illness, including α-adrenergic blocking hypotensive drugs, steroids and some antibiotics (Edwards, 1989), or a major life event such as bereavement.

The issue of compliance is also important. Poor compliance may be predicted if the patient argues strongly against a physical treatment being given. Because of recent concern about dependence on benzodiazepines, many people regard all psychotropic drugs as 'tranquillizers' and this belief can persist despite much explanation. In instances where the degree of depression is moderate and the attitude towards physical treatments is poor it is preferable to choose a psychological treatment. The same situation can occur in reverse where the patient thought suitable for psychological treatment is insistent that only medication can help the problem. This issue is not taken sufficient account of in clinical trials because all patients selected for such studies have to meet the criterion that they are prepared to accept any of the possible treatments available. There is a significant minority of patients that will not show such agnosticism and it is usually better to work with the patient in their preferred mode of treatment wherever possible, rather than to be constantly at odds.

Compliance tends to be poor in depressive illness because of the delay in response and only about 50% of patients regarded as sufficiently depressed to require antidepressants complete what can be described as a full course of therapy (Johnson, 1981). If a patient is to be treated as an out-patient, great care must be taken to ensure that the patient appreciates both the timing and nature of unwanted and desired effects of the drug, otherwise compliance is more likely to be poor.

It is also a useful exercise before the first prescription is given to try and determine for how long a treatment is likely to be continued. Unfortunately there is still a great deal of guesswork in this exercise. There is good evidence that, once improvements from a depressive illness have been achieved with antidepressant drugs (or ECT), relapse is likely to occur within a few months if the treatment is withdrawn, and that such relapse can be prevented by maintenance therapy of the antidepressant in somewhat lower dosage. Thus, the finding that over 40% of patients relapse within 4 months after discontinuation of active drug treatment (and its replacement by placebo) has led to the notion that maintenance treatment needs to be continued until the episode, which, having been symptomatically improved by treatment, remits spontaneously (Mindham et al., 1973; Prien and Kupfer, 1986). The exact duration of the depressive episode is assumed to vary in a normal distribution, with a mean duration of 4–6 months, and this time span is therefore suggested as the optimal duration of such maintenance treatment.

This leaves the question of the duration of prophylactic treatment, aimed at the prevention of future episodes of illness. There is abundant record of the natural history of depressive illness from before the days of effective drug treatment to make clear that such illness tends to be recurrent (Angst *et al.*, 1973; Zis and Goodwin, 1979; Lee and Murray, 1988). Equally, there is sufficient evidence from controlled study to show that prophylactic treatment is effective. This evidence is particularly strong in the case of the role of lithium salts in the prevention of manic, and to a lesser extent depressive, episodes in bipolar affective illnesses (Prien *et al.*, 1973). However, there is accumulating evidence in the prophylaxis of unipolar illness that both tricyclic drugs and lithium salts are effective, and recent work with 5-hydroxytryptamine (5-HT) reuptake inhibitors argues for their prophylactic use (Schou, 1979; Prien *et al.*, 1984; Montgomery *et al.*, 1988). Therefore, in the depressed patient with a history of previous severe depression but not of mania, prophylaxis with one of these drugs is almost mandatory. There is insufficient scientific data to suggest for what period this is required, since most controlled studies of prophylaxis have not extended beyond 2 years; the most reliable guide to the clinician, as so often in psychiatric prognosis, remains the previous history, particularly with regard to the frequency of previous illnesses and the degree of morbidity associated with them. Doses used have, at least in the case of tricyclic drugs, tended to be lower than those used in treatment of the acute illness, but there is no clear scientific backing for this practice and effective prophylactic dosage remains an area deserving of some further study.

2.3 Drug treatments

2.3.1 Tricyclic antidepressants

These drugs have been the mainstay of antidepressant treatment for the past 30 years, although their pre-eminence is now under threat. The original tricyclic antidepressant, imipramine, was closely followed by amitriptyline and a host of similar drugs that only differed marginally in the degree of their sedative effects (Table 2).

Comparison of the many clinical trials that have been carried out with antidepressant therapy in the past 30 years has demonstrated that tricyclic antidepressants are undoubtedly effective in the treatment of moderate and severe depressive disorder but are not so efficacious as ECT (Medical Research

Table 2 Tricyclic antidepressant drugs (in descending order of sedative effect).

	Year of introduction	Standard daily dose for treatment of depression (mg)
Trimipramine	1966	150
Amitriptyline	1961	150
Dothiepin	1969	150
Clomipramine	1970	150
Desipramine	1963	150
Nortriptyline	1963	100
Protriptyline	1966	60
Imipramine	1959	150
Doxepin	1969	300
Lofepramine	1983	210

Council, 1965). There are three main problems with the older antidepressants: they have a delay in the onset of their clinical action of up to 4 weeks, they have a high incidence of generally unpleasant anticholinergic unwanted effects, and they are dangerous in overdosage. Comparison of fatal poisoning rates (see below) shows that the antidepressants with the highest incidence are all old tricyclic antidepressants. This does not mean, however, that all antidepressants with the tricyclic nucleus are similarly affected. Lofepramine, a new antidepressant that is also a tricyclic compound, has a low incidence of anticholinergic effects and is extremely safe in overdose (Pugh et al., 1982).

Another tricyclic antidepressant, clomipramine, also has a low incidence of fatalities from overdosage but is none the less a toxic compound. The reasons for this are far from clear. Fatality rates of drugs depend on indications for which they are given, and over the last 20 years there has been a perception amongst prescribers that the old compounds are the only antidepressants of proven efficacy and therefore should be given to the most severely depressed patients. If this were true, it would support the fatality rate but lead to an erroneous conclusion that the old antidepressants were more dangerous. If, however, antidepressants were prescribed almost at random for different indications, then the fatality rates would be a much greater index of toxicity. One other interesting explanation, put forward by Montgomery & Montgomery 1982, is that some antidepressants, particularly those that selectively inhibit 5-HT reuptake, also inhibit suicidal thoughts and acts. This could explain why clomipramine has such a low fatality rate even though it is known to be a toxic antidepressant (Montgomery, 1989).

The delay in antidepressant action with the tricyclic compounds is not adequately explained. Although, from animal studies, it is generally believed that antidepressants act by raising central levels of catecholamines and 5-HT, mainly by inhibiting the reuptake of both these amines from the synaptic cleft, this effect is virtually immediate, and certainly complete in 24 h. It has also been shown, however, that down-regulation of β-adrenoreceptors follows after some delay as a consequence of having higher central catecholamine levels (see Chapter 3). It is therefore reasonable to argue that in depressive illness central β-receptors are supersensitive, and in order for depression to be relieved this supersensitivity has to be reduced by raising central noradrenaline and 5-HT levels (Tyrer and Marsden, 1985). However, even this hypothesis does not explain why it takes up to 4 weeks before the clinical effects of tricyclic antidepressants are shown.

2.3.2 Monoamine oxidase inhibitors

Although the early studies of monoamine oxidase inhibitors (MAOIs) in depressive illness suggested definite efficacy, this was not so marked as with tricyclic antidepressants (Medical Research Council, 1965; Greenblatt et al., 1964). However, much of the poor performance of MAOIs can be explained by the poor design of the trials, which did not give the drugs for an adequate length of time and in sufficient dosage (Paykel, 1979). For example, phenelzine, the most commonly prescribed MAOI, needed to be given for at least 4 weeks in a dosage of 60 mg daily in order to show satisfactory superiority over placebo; in a dose of 30 mg daily over this period it is no better than placebo (Ravaris et al., 1976).

Because of the well-known adverse effects of MAOIs (see below), these drugs are now used rarely in the treatment of depression. This is understandable because they are of somewhat lesser efficacy than tricyclic antidepressants when given in conventional dosage, and now that there are many more antidepressants available MAOIs are seldom likely to be drugs of first choice. Even so, they remain as effective antidepressants of the same clinical value as other compounds when given in adequate dosage (Paykel et al., 1982).

However, when anxiety is a major symptom associated with depression, and other associated symptoms such as phobias are present, it may be reasonable to consider treatment with an MAOI (Robinson et al., 1973). Although the main result of their pharmacological action is similar to that of tricyclic antidepressants (i.e. they raise central catecholamine levels by inhibiting the breakdown of the amines through their effects on monoamine oxidase), their clinical effects do not always accord with this. In particular, there are studies which suggest that patients who do not respond to tricyclic antidepressants may do so to MAOIs, and vice versa (Pare, 1965; Pare and

Mack, 1971), suggesting that there is a place for both kinds of drug. This may be particularly relevant when a clinician is faced with a problem of resistant depression (see below).

2.3.3 New antidepressants

There are many antidepressants in this group and they have no common features, apart from the fact they are not tricyclic antidepressants. Many of them are no longer new; for example, maprotiline and viloxazine have been available for over 16 years. The different drugs and their main pharmacological properties are summarized in Table 3.

Selective noradrenaline reuptake inhibitors

Much has been made about the classification of antidepressants into selective noradrenaline and 5-HT reuptake inhibitors. Although this is of some interest to pharmacologists, there is nothing intrinsic in the selectivity of reuptake inhibition that should lead to any predictions about the efficacy of different antidepressants. Most antidepressants inhibit the reuptake of both noradrenaline and 5-HT to varying degrees, and even those that are particularly selective still inhibit the reuptake of the other catecholamines to some extent. However, there are some differences, mainly concerning unwanted effects, that differentiate the drugs in this group.

Maprotiline is the most selective noradrenaline reuptake inhibitor available on prescription. It has no special advantages but is an effective antidepressant that is probably of similar efficacy to the tricyclic compounds (Montgomery et al., 1980). Viloxazine is similarly effective but has never been particularly popular in the UK, although it is widely used in continental Europe.

Table 3 Pharmacological properties of new antidepressant drugs.

	5-HT reuptake inhibition	Noradrenaline uptake inhibition	Other action
Viloxazine	−	+ +	
Maprotiline	−	+ +	
Nomifensine	−	+ +	Dopamine agonist
Trazodone	+	−	
Fluoxetine	+ +	−	
Zimelidine	+ +	−	
Mianserin	(+)	−	α_2 and histamine antagonist

Mianserin is an unusual compound that is neither a noradrenaline nor 5-HT reuptake inhibitor. It is an antagonist at presynaptic noradrenergic receptors. It has attracted particular popularity in the treatment of the elderly depressed patient because of the low incidence of anticholinergic effects.

Selective 5-HT reuptake inhibitors

Zimelidine was the first antidepressant introduced as a specific 5-HT reuptake inhibitor. Although it appeared to be an effective antidepressant (Aberg-Wistedt, 1982), it was withdrawn in 1984 because of its idiosyncratic side-effects, notably the Guillain–Barré syndrome. Several other compounds with very similar effects have been introduced recently, of which fluvoxamine, fluoxetine and paroxetine are the best known. Again, these drugs are probably similar in efficacy to tricyclic antidepressants but have few anticholinergic effects. However, they all seem to have gastrointestinal side-effects, including anorexia, and this may be sufficiently pronounced to lead to weight loss rather than weight gain, one of the most common problems with tricyclic antidepressant therapy. However, it should not be assumed that this effect is a consequence of specific inhibition of 5-HT reuptake, as the same symptoms are also prominent with viloxazine.

These antidepressants have many points in their favour. They are undoubtedly effective as antidepressant drugs, they are generally better tolerated, and much safer in overdosage. Fluoxetine has a possible advantage of a very long half-life (over 100 h), so that a drug can be given less frequently than once a day if necessary. This could aid the community treatment of patients who might be unreliable about taking medication.

Despite these advantages there are still some important question marks hanging over these new compounds. They do have a higher incidence of what Rawlins (1981) has described as type B (bizarre) unwanted effects, rather than the type A (augmented) effects of tricyclic antidepressants, which are predictable, dose related and not usually serious. The more bizarre side-effects include blood dyscrasias (mianserin), neurological symptoms (zimeldine) and haemolytic anaemia (nomifensine), and have been sufficiently serious to lead to the removal of zimelidine and nomifensine from the market. It is highly unlikely that new antidepressants as a group should have a particular predilection to serious and unpredictable and unwanted effects and it is a matter of considerable concern.

The second area of concern is the efficacy of these compounds. Clinical trials of new antidepressants are now well executed and involve much larger numbers of patients than were treated in the original studies with tricyclic compounds. However, the patient population is somewhat different. In the early studies with amitriptyline and imipramine, there were no effective antidepressant treatments (apart from ECT) and so it was ethical to compare the new compounds with placebo in severely depressed patients. Once these studies had established that the new compounds were indeed effective antidepressants, it became unethical to select severely depressed patients for clinical trials. The consequence of this is that the population used to test the new antidepressants is undoubtedly depressed but much less severely ill than those tested in the original trials. This of course does not mean that the compounds would not be effective in severe depression but the necessary gap in testing may have led to the assumption that they are not as powerful.

2.3.4 Lithium salts

Although the major use of lithium is in the prophylaxis of bipolar affective disorders and, to a lesser extent, in the treatment of mania (Tyrer, 1985), there is some evidence that lithium also has antidepressant properties (Worrall et al., 1979). This finding is not as surprising as it may have first appeared to many clinicians. There are no substances used as prophylactics in medicine that are not themselves therapeutic for the conditions they prevent and so it would be unusual if lithium was completely devoid of antidepressant effect. However, because of the large number of other effective compounds that are available, the use of lithium is normally only considered for resistant depression (see below).

2.3.5 Other drugs with antidepressant properties

Many other drugs have been claimed to be effective in the treatment of depressive illness without being regarded in anyway as primarily antidepressants. They include the anticonvulsant carbamazepine, often regarded as a 'limbic stabilizer' with effects in both depression and mania (Post et al., 1986), benzodiazepines (Tiller et al., 1989), L-tryptophan (Thomson et al., 1982) and the energizing antipsychotic drug, flupenthixol, when given in low dosage (Young et al., 1976). Benzodiazepines are effective antianxiety drugs in the short term and because anxiety is highly correlated with at least the minor degrees of depression it is not surprising that depression often improves concurrently with anxiety. This is clear from many rating scales for depressive illness, which, in order to reflect the reality of depression in clinical practice, had to include some anxiety items (e.g. Hamilton, 1967; Montgomery and Asberg, 1979).

Carbamazepine is usually considered for the treatment of resistant bipolar depressive illness; L-tryptophan is more popular as an adjunct to other antidepressant treatment (including MAOIs) rather than as sole treatment.

Interest in newer antidepressant drugs shows no sign of abating and there is now a 'third generation' of drugs under development that may shortly be released for clinical practice (Pinder, 1990). These include specific α_2-antagonists such as idazoxan, reversible MAOIs such as moclobemide, selective phosphodiesterase inhibitors such as rolipram, and drugs which act on peptide metabolism such as captopril. Despite this ingenuity there is no evidence that any of these compounds act more quickly or are to any significant degree more effective than existing antidepressants.

2.4 Electroconvulsive therapy (ECT)

One of the consequences of improved antidepressant drug therapy and the wider range of compounds available is a lessened use of ECT. This trend has also been accelerated by earlier detection of depressive illness and by public campaigns against ECT, primarily motivated by aesthetic revulsion. Despite this, ECT remains superior to all other antidepressant treatments in its speed of action (significant improvement occurring after only two treatments) and its efficacy (Freeman et al., 1978; Johnstone et al., 1980; Gregory et al., 1985). Although unilateral ECT is undoubtedly superior to bilateral treatment in producing fewer unwanted effects, particularly memory disturbance (see below), there are doubts about its efficacy when compared with bilateral ECT. Although many trials have shown no difference in efficacy (D'Elia and Raotma, 1975), those that have shown a difference have all demonstrated superiority for bilateral treatment (Abrams, 1986), with one study suggesting that the speed of response is faster in the bilaterally treated patients (Gregory et al., 1985).

ECT should be reserved for the severely depressed patient, particularly when the condition is thought to be life threatening, and for other patients with moderate or severe depression who have failed to respond to antidepressant drugs. If the degree of depression is life threatening, compulsory treatment may sometimes be indicated. Although in the past prolonged courses of treatment were often given, there is little evidence that more than 12 treatments or a frequency of treatments above three times a week is of any greater efficacy.

There are no satisfactory studies demonstrating the value of prophylactic ECT (e.g. given once monthly). It would seem reasonable to predict that prophylactic ECT would be as effective as other antidepressant treatments, but whether the frequency of treatment required could be as little as once a month is far from clear. When ECT is compared with other forms o' antidepressant treatment its effects appear to be relatively short liv'

(Johnstone *et al.*, 1980), and effective prophylaxis may therefore require a frequency of administration which would preclude compliance.

2.5 Psychosurgery

Psychosurgery now has a very small part to play in psychiatric treatment. It has never been subjected to a satisfactory controlled trial, partly because of ethical problems and also because its use had already diminished substantially by the time that adequate trial methodologies were developed. It is therefore impossible to be certain whether psychosurgery is effective. Certainly it can be of value in patients with obsessional neurosis, particularly those with recurrent rituals, and those with persistent anxiety and recurrent depressive illness, but it is impossible to say whether this treatment is superior to other forms of antidepressant therapy. Techniques have improved in recent years and are designed specifically to sever pathways to the inferior frontal lobe (Kelly, 1976; Bridges and Bartlett, 1977). However, despite this, the use of the treatment is declining so rapidly that depressive illness can be considered one of the indications for psychosurgery only in exceptional circumstances.

2.6 Practicalities of treatment

As can readily be seen, the features of depressive illness influence the clinician in his choice of a physical method of treatment for a particular patient. Some clinical factors will also influence the selection of a particular agent. Before examining the practicalities of administering physical treatments it is therefore worthwhile considering such other factors which affect the exact choice of antidepressant agent. Foremost amongst these are the presence of a high risk of suicidal behaviour and the coexistence of cardiovascular disease.

icidal thoughts are common in those suffering from depressive illness, ir root in ideas of hopelessness, self-blame and worthlessness, or in ape the unpleasant subjective experience of depressed mood. rmacotherapy undoubtedly prevents suicidal acts over the rtunate paradox of the use of antidepressant drugs erdose may give to the patient a means to completed , at least for the tricyclic drugs, is principally a function of their cardiotoxicity, due both to membrane-stabilizing and anticholinergic effects. One of the major thrusts of new antidepressant drug development has been an attempt to reduce this cardiotoxicity (and toxicity in general), and in this respect, unlike the attempts to increase efficacy, there has been notable success. The new antidepressant drugs, with the probable exception of maprotiline, have less inherent cardiotoxicity. In particular, the recently introduced tricyclic drug lofepramine is relatively safe in overdose, and thus cardiotoxicity is not a universal accompaniment of the tricyclic structure. There are data, from the nationwide collection of information about the extent of drug prescription and fatalities associated with their use, which consistently support what would be expected from knowledge of the drugs' pharmacological properties. Thus, the older tricyclics (amitriptyline, imipramine, dothiepin), as well as maprotiline, are approximately twice as likely to be implicated in fatal self-poisoning than an MAOI, and four times as likely as mianserin and viloxazine (Leonard, 1986; Cassidy and Henry, 1987). However, the fact that clomipramine, a tricyclic drug known to be highly cardiotoxic, is implicated in relatively few fatalities suggests that these findings are influenced by other factors, such as diagnostic practice and prescribing habits.

The cardiovascular effects of antidepressant drugs at therapeutic doses as opposed to toxic doses are well documented (Orme, 1984). As might be expected, the tricyclic drugs have the most marked effects of all the antidepressant drugs on cardiovascular function and this is mediated through three discernible pharmacological pathways. Anticholinergic effects lead to tachycardia and accompanying accelerated atrioventricular conduction, which is partially compensated by a quinidine-like action delaying atrioventricular conduction, and a direct effect reduces myocardial contractility. In addition, a peripheral α-adrenergic blockade produces a postural hypotensive effect, which is also seen with the use of MAOIs. The use of lithium salts is associated with a characteristic T-wave flattening seen on electrocardiogram, which, however, is of no clinical significance.

These pharmacological activities have led to some anxieties on the part of prescribing clinicians in using these drugs in patients with cardiovascular pathology, particularly following reports of an increase above the expected numbers of sudden deaths, presumed to be due to cardiac arrhythmias, associated with their use, although this finding has yet to be replicated (Moir et al., 1972). However, a prospective and blind study of the use of dothiepin, imipramine and placebo in depressed patients with ischaemic heart disease failed convincingly to show significant adverse changes in left ventricular function or conduction, although the tachycardic and postural hypotensive effects were clear (Veith et al., 1982). It seems likely that concern about adverse cardiotoxic effects of the tricyclic drugs given in therapeutic do̅ has been overstated and their use need only be restricted in patiͤ

61

serious conduction defects (bundle branch block and heart block), cardiac failure and recent myocardial infarction.

Thirty years clinical use of tricyclic drugs has led to the accumulation of a large body of empirically derived information regarding their efficacy as antidepressant agents, and this has increasingly become substantiated by the results of controlled investigation. Similarly, knowledge has grown concerning the practicalities of the use of these drugs. We are not yet in a position to make comparably robust assertions regarding the use of the newer antidepressant drugs, although it is reasonable, from the detailed knowledge of their pharmacology and pharmacokinetics, to assume some similarities. It is certainly true that their use in clinical practice tends to follow the precedent set by the tricyclic drugs.

2.6.1 Drug dosage

Despite the well-established variation between individuals in their rates of metabolism of tricyclic drugs (principally by hydroxylation in the liver), it is still common practice for clinicians to prescribe fixed, and therefore to an extent arbitrary, doses of drugs. The capacity of individuals to hydroxylate is at least partially under genetic control (Alexanderson *et al.*, 1969) and leads to a large difference (up to tenfold) in the plasma level achieved at steady state after ingestion of given doses (Mahgoub *et al.*, 1977). Experimental work on the relationship between plasma drug level and therapeutic effects suggests that a linear relationship is not the case, for example with amitriptyline or nortriptyline, where the relationship follows an inverted U-shaped curve (Kraph-Sorensen *et al.*, 1976; Montgomery *et al.*, 1979). Thus, failure to respond may occur with high as well as low plasma levels. This has led some researchers to suggest the routine estimation of plasma clearance of an initial test dose of a tricyclic drug in order to detect those slow hydroxylators who may be expected to develop a high range of plasma levels, and consequent non-response (Montgomery *et al.*, 1979). Others recommend the measurement of plasma drug levels in patients who fail to respond as expected, those who develop excessive adverse effects with modest doses, and the elderly, where differences in pharmacokinetics may be significant (Braithwaite *et al.*, 1979a; Asberg, 1983).

Pharmacokinetic differences are important in the elderly because of reduced hepatic and renal clearance of drugs and their metabolites, and because of changes in the spaces of distribution available to both water and lipid soluble drugs (Braithwaite *et al.*, 1979b). For most drugs this means an increase in the drug half-life and a delay in achieving steady state plasma levels, as well as higher peak plasma levels. The latter results in a higher incidence of dose-related adverse effects, for example anticholinergic effects with tricyclic drugs, in the elderly, and may necessitate a lower starting dose, particularly in the cases of the tricyclic drugs and lithium salts.

2.6.2 Delay in therapeutic effect of drugs

One of the earlier clinical observations concerning the use of the tricyclic antidepressants was of consistent delay of 2 or more weeks in the onset of antidepressant effect following the establishment of steady-state plasma levels (at 3 or 4 days) (Blashki et al., 1971). Placebo-controlled studies suggest that the initial clinical improvement attributable to the operation of non-specific therapeutic (or placebo) factors may actually be less in those receiving active drug (perhaps due to adverse drug effects), until an antidepressant effect distinct from sedative effects becomes evident from the third week of treatment (Asberg et al., 1970; Oswald et al., 1972). There is some evidence from animal studies suggesting that this delay may be related to the time taken for intracellular proteins synthesized in the cell body to progress centrifugally (Schildkraut et al., 1970). Because response time to these drugs is so unpredictable it has become conventional to persist with drug treatment for 6 weeks at therapeutic dosage before accepting non-response. Drug trials consistently show that between 30 and 40% of patients with moderate depressive illness fail to respond symptomatically to an adequate course of antidepressant drug, and further treatment strategies are therefore required (Medical Research Council, 1965).

2.6.3 Drug withdrawal

Early realization that discontinuation of the tricyclic drugs led to the appearance, usually within 7–10 days, of symptoms such as insomnia, gastrointestinal disturbance, anxiety and perceptual disorders led to some debate as to whether these symptoms represent a distinct withdrawal syndrome or the early signs of a relapse of the affective illness for which treatment was initially prescribed. Recent prospective and placebo-controlled work has shown that abrupt cessation of tricyclic antidepressants is accompanied by a recognizable withdrawal syndrome, appearing as early as 48 h after discontinuation in a large minority of patients (Bialos et al., 1982). It is particularly likely to occur after prolonged treatment and after sudden withdrawal (Kramer et al., 1961). The symptoms may be partly due to a rebound cholinergic overactivity, but the occurrence of a relatively specific perceptual disorder argues for the involvement of other mechanisms (Charney et al., 1982). Uncontrolled work suggests that gradual withdrawal over several weeks may reduce both the frequency and the severity of the syndrome. Discontinuation of MAOIs, particularly when sudden, has been shown to be attended by a syndrome of sympathetic overactivity quite distinct from illness relapse in approximately one-third of patients (Tyrer, 1984).

2.6.4 Adverse effects

In the time that has elapsed between the introduction of the first generation of antidepressant drugs and the present day, the increase in sensitivity of the statutory licensing authorities has led to the paradoxical situation where the older drugs, which are tried and tested (at least in the minds of clinicians), have a range of adverse effects that might preclude the granting of a licence today. In contrast, the fate of newer drugs, whose efficacy is generally no greater or less than the standard drugs against which they are compared (usually imipramine or amitriptyline), depends to an increasing extent on their ability to demonstrate a safer profile at therapeutic and toxic dosage.

The early tricyclic drugs, being relatively dirty pharmacologically, have a wide range of unwanted effects that are evident early on in treatment and are important not only for the discomfort caused to the patient, but also because of the increased risk of non-compliance. The dose-dependent anticholinergic syndrome, including tremor, visual accommodation difficulty, dry mouth, urinary retention and constipation, which is an unwelcome addition to an already unpleasant state for a young patient, may represent a more serious hazard to an elderly patient with a concurrent medical condition and therefore demands caution and the use of lower doses. Sedative effects, particularly marked in those drugs with antihistaminergic activity, such as amitriptyline, trimipramine and mianserin, can be used for the benefit of the severely insomniac or agitated patient. The newer antidepressant drugs possess immediate adverse effects which differ from those of the tricyclic drugs, as one may expect from a knowledge of their range of pharmacological activities. Thus, the sedative effects of mianserin and the nausea, vomiting and syndrome of serotonergic overactivity seen with the 5-HT reuptake blocking drugs are predictable and, to an extent, dose dependent. All antidepressant drugs, with the probable exception of the now withdrawn drug, nomifensine, have been implicated in the provocation of epileptiform seizures in normal individuals and are therefore used with caution in known epileptics. Many of the newer antidepressant drugs are associated with the occurrence at low frequency of unpredictable and generally serious adverse effects, which may necessitate stopping treatment. The occurrence of serious blood dyscrasias, including aplastic anaemia, in association with mianserin provoked great caution in its use and the recommendation of routine serial blood counts (Committee on Safety of Medicines, 1986b). Use of lofepramine has recently been associated with reversible liver damage, including hepatitis and hepatic failure, and development of irreversible priapism with trazodone limits its use to women

(Committee on Safety of Medicines 1984, 1988). The risk of associated Guillain–Barré syndrome with zimelidine and of haemolytic anaemias with nomifensine have led to the withdrawal of two antidepressant drugs of proven efficacy (Committee on Safety of Medicines, 1983, 1986a). MAOIs share the anticholinergic actions of the tricyclic drugs, but their main restriction is due to food and drug interactions (Pare, 1985).

2.6.5 Drug interactions

Although, in principle, polypharmacy is best avoided, there are occasions when prescribing psychotropic drugs when it is difficult to avoid, whether due to deficiencies in diagnostic or treatment strategies. The drug treatment of concurrent medical conditions also generates several important drug interactions. Antidepressant drugs are frequently used in conjunction with hypnotics: benzodiazepines cause no significant interaction. The use of neuroleptic drugs with tricyclic drugs causes competition for hydroxylating liver enzymes and an increase in the plasma levels of both drugs (Johnstone, 1985). As with sympathomimetic drugs and tyramine-containing foods with MAOIs, after discontinuing use of MAOIs it is wise to leave a drug-free interval of at least 2 weeks, and often up to 4 weeks, before beginning treatment with a tricyclic or other antidepressant drug (Pare et al., 1982). The occurrence of hypertensive crises due to high levels of circulating pressor amines was initially noted when patients taking MAOIs ate certain foodstuffs (Blackwell et al., 1967). The main hazard is now known to occur when MAOIs are combined with indirectly acting sympathomimetic drugs, such as the freely available decongestants ephedrine and phenylethylamine (Pare, 1985).

2.6.6 Lithium salts

Lithium salts are most frequently used in the continuation and prophylactic phases of the treatment of bipolar affective disorders, and it is in this role that the guidelines for their use are most clearly established. They may also have a place in the treatment of unipolar depressive illness. Although the relationship between dose and plasma levels is roughly linear, there is a wide variation between individuals, depending mainly upon differences in renal clearance. For this reason, as well as the low therapeutic index (i.e. the ratio between toxic and therapeutic dosage), it is important to assess renal function prior to starting treatment, and thereafter to monitor closely the serum lithium level until steady-state conditions are reached. Serum trough levels, measured 10–12 h after a dose, of between 0.5 and 0.8 mmol/litre are required to ensure efficacy, although in the face of persistent adverse effects it is possible to achieve therapeutic effect in most patients with serum levels of between 0.4 and 0.5 mmol/litre (Baastrup *et al.*, 1970; Coppen *et al.*, 1971).

Lithium is generally well tolerated at non-toxic doses but toxicity appears at serum levels above 1.5 mmol/litre and may be precipitated by changes in dosage or preparation, or by interactions with other drugs. Important in this latter respect are the thiazide diuretics and the non-steroidal anti-inflammatory drugs, both of which reduce renal clearance of lithium and may thereby bring about states of lithium intoxication (MacNeil *et al.*, 1975). Toxicity is characterized by gastrointestinal disturbance, ataxia and visual disturbance, progressing to seizures, coma and death, and demands careful and urgent correction of fluid and electrolyte balance (Schou, 1980).

Long-term use of lithium has been associated with the development of hypothyroidism and goitre, for which an autoimmune aetiology has been postulated. There have been recent reports implicating lithium in the occurrence of extrapyramidal syndromes, both in the presence and absence of neuroleptic drugs, and it is wise in this instance to withdraw lithium (Hay and Simpson, 1982). Lithium salts are contraindicated in the first trimester of pregnancy due to a reported association with a high incidence of serious fetal cardiovascular abnormalities, particularly Ebstein's anomaly, and, in pregnant patients requiring continuation or prophylactic treatment, neuroleptic or antidepressant drugs may be used (Weinstein, 1980).

2.6.7 Electroconvulsive therapy

The history of electroconvulsive treatment is that of a fortuitously derived treatment, used in the absence of any viable alternative in the treatment of the most severe and life-threatening psychiatric disorders. As such, it has not, at least until relatively recently, received the scientific study which, for example, the antidepressant drugs have, and hence the practicalities of its use have been developed gradually and empirically. The replacement of sine waveforms by pulsed stimuli of shorter duration and the use of constant current in order to deliver a stimulus of known energy are examples of this process. Debate has occurred concerning the relative merits and risks of unilateral and bilateral electrode placement, and it now seems clear (at least at the currently used levels of stimulus energy) that unilateral placement is associated with a lower incidence of adverse effects (principally short-term memory disturbance), at the expense of either a loss or a delay in efficacy (Halliday *et al.*, 1968; Abrams, 1986; Weiner *et al.*, 1986). This could be explained by the hypothesis that effects are related not directly to the occurrence of a seizure but to the total energy of the electrical stimulus, i.e. that the seizure may be an epiphenomenon, and that seizures with unilateral placement occur at a lower energy threshold. The delay in efficacy with unilateral electrode placement can therefore be seen as the use of a lower energy stimulus over a longer period of time in order to achieve the equivalent therapeutic effect.

Whatever the underlying physiology, the relative places of unilateral and bilateral treatments in the treatment of depressive illness have become increasingly clear, in large part due to several well-designed trials carried out in the UK in the last 15 years. Both forms of ECT are of proven superiority to placebo, and the majority of studies show bilateral administration to be more efficacious then unilateral administration over a given study period (Lambourne and Gill, 1978; Brandon *et al.*, 1984; Gregory *et al.*, 1985). It is notable that many studies with a longer duration or follow-up period indicate that similar proportions of patients respond if the course of unilateral treatment is extended (e.g. Freeman *et al.*, 1978). With regard to adverse effects, there is good evidence that non-dominant hemisphere unilateral treatment is less associated with cognitive disturbance than bilateral treatment (Weiner *et al.*, 1986).

The question of the duration of treatment of ECT has not been adequately addressed. Practice has shown that 60–70% of severely depressed patients have shown some response by the sixth treatment, and this figure has become the conventional duration of a standard course of treatment. However, it is known that some patients will show no sign of response until much later and in such cases treatment is continued more on the grounds that not to treat would be unethical rather than on any firm scientific ground, until remission, possibly spontaneous, occurs (Medical Research Council, 1965; Freeman *et al.*, 1978).

Whilst the occurrence of a convulsion is not a guarantee of efficacy, failure to convulse is associated with failure to respond, and hence convulsion is taken as a clinical marker of an adequate physiological response to an electrical stimulus. The most frequent reasons for failure to convulse are faulty electrode placement or poor electrical contact, and concurrent use of anticonvulsant drugs, usually in the guise of a benzodiazepine administered as a hypnotic. Whilst there is no evidence that ECT is synergistic with other antidepressant treatments, there is no contraindication to the concurrent use of antidepressant drugs (other than anaesthetic cautions) and, indeed, it is logical to institute the continuation phase of treatment whilst the acute phase is being treated with ECT.

2.6.8 Psychosurgery

The relatively unstandardized early neurosurgical procedures for the treatment of psychiatric disorder, such as Freeman and Watts' standard leucotomy of the 1940s, have now been superseded by procedures ensuring a well-defined, localized and accurately placed stereotactic lesion in the ventromedial or subcaudate regions. Current techniques may employ radioactive seed implantation, cryogenic lesions, electrocoagulation or ultrasonics to produce such lesions (Bridges and Bartlett, 1977). The perioperative morbidity and mortality is no greater than that of other neurosurgical procedures and the high rates of adverse effects reported in early series are not reported with the use of the stereotactic method (Goktepe *et al.*, 1975). Epileptic seizures may occur in a sizeable minority of patients postoperatively but are only persistent enough to require anticonvulsant medication in about 2% of cases; persistent personality change, usually towards disinhibition or apathy but sometimes towards assertiveness, is reported in between 5 and 10% of cases (Birley, 1964; Sykes and Tredgold, 1964; Goktepe *et al.*, 1975).

2.7 Treatment of resistant depression

Most clinicians are aware of the concept of resistant depression, although it is difficult to define. The persistence of a significant degree of depressive symptomatology, sufficient to satisfy the Research Diagnostic Criteria for major depressive illness or the diagnosis of major depressive episode in DSM-III-R (American Psychiatric Association, 1987), despite a full course of antidepressant therapy (including psychological treatment such as cognitive therapy) for at least 8 weeks, would certainly satisfy the criteria, although the period of treatment can be reduced to as little as 4 weeks. Because of the success of antidepressants in treating acute depressive illness a relatively small number of patients have resistant depression. As a result, there are relatively few patients for research studies in any one centre and there is therefore really no satisfactory information about the best strategy for treating resistant depression. Whatever approach is chosen, it will depend at least to some extent on the personal preferences of the clinician, and in the present state of knowledge this is understandable and appropriate.

In this account we shall confine ourselves to the treatment of relatively severe depression. There has been increasing interest in chronic mild depression, stimulated by the work of Akiskal and his colleagues (1980), and this has led to the introduction of dysthymic disorder and the diagnosis in both DSM-III-R, and the provisional draft of ICD-10. Dysthymia is a low-grade depressive disorder, not following from a major depressive episode (i.e. not just a partially treated form of more severe depression), which is often associated with some degree of personality disturbance and which can persist for many years without ever causing major handicap. Thus the sufferer is able to continue working and rarely progresses beyond out-patient status in the psychiatric services. The treatments for dysthymic disorder include the antidepressants already mentioned in this review but also include the range of psychotherapies. In many cases a combination of drug and psychological treatments is often appropriate for this disorder. In the more severe depressions the place of psychological treatment is relatively small but can be given in addition to physical treatment. The main strategies involve (1) the use of different antidepressants alone, (2) ECT, either alone or in combination with other treatments, (3) combined antidepressant therapy, and (4) other approaches, such as sleep deprivation.

2.7.1 Change to another antidepressant

Most patients reaching the criteria for resistant depression would have been treated with a tricyclic antidepressant, probably in gradually increasing dosage. Before changing this it is probably worthwhile reducing the dosage because of evidence that there is a 'therapeutic window' of plasma antidepressant levels, above and below which response does not take place (Asberg, 1983). Assuming that the patient remains depressed despite altering the dosage of the antidepressant, it is first worthwhile considering changing to another compound. There is anecdotal evidence, to some extent fortified by research studies that do not formally address comparative efficacy, that antidepressants which selectively inhibit the reuptake of 5-HT are more effective than other compounds in resistant depression. This has been mainly stimulated by some evidence with clomipramine (which is a selective 5-HT reuptake inhibitor despite also being a tricyclic antidepressant) and by some evidence that a 'serotonin depression' exists within the affective disorders (Asberg et al., 1976). Clearly, if serotonin depression did exist and only accounted for a small proportion of significant depressive illness, it would still explain why a minority of patients who did not respond to conventional antidepressants might do so when treated with 5-HT reuptake inhibitors. There have been several studies showing that these drugs are effective in resistant depression (e.g. Reimherr et al., 1984; Tyrer et al., 1987; Delgado et al., 1988), so the approach is certainly worth considering.

2.7.2 ECT and other treatments

Although ECT is generally more effective than all other types of antidepressant treatment (Kendell, 1981), it is surprising that its use is often not considered for patients with resistant depressive disorders. This may be because ECT is frequently excluded by clinicians except when a depressive disorder is very severe and usually accompanied by delusions and other psychotic features. Nevertheless, in other forms of depression, particularly when confusional symptoms are prominent (Bulbena and Berrios, 1986) or when schizoaffective features are present (Ries *et al.*, 1981) ECT may be the preferred option. ECT may also be combined successfully with other antidepressant treatments, particularly antidepressant drugs. The most powerful combination (at least in terms of numbers of treatments) is that recommended many years ago by William Sargant and his colleagues (1966), in which ECT is given two or three times weekly in conjunction with combined antidepressant therapy (tricyclic antidepressants and monoamine oxidase inhibitors) and sedative–hypnotic drugs to maintain the patient in a sleeping state for at least 18 hours a day. This treatment has never been evaluated adequately but appears to be more effective in resistant affective disorder than most other psychiatric conditions (Sargant *et al.*, 1966).

2.7.3 Combined antidepressant treatment

Because different groups of antidepressants vary in their pharmacological actions it is understable that they may sometimes be used in combination in resistant depression. However, care has to be taken to avoid dangerous interactions. The best-known combined antidepressant therapy is that of a tricyclic antidepressant and a MAOI. Although this attracted serious criticism in the 1960s because of apparent fatal interactions, examination of the data suggests that the dangers were grossly overemphasized (Schuckit *et al.*, 1971) and that the combination was safer than originally thought. However, a great deal depends on which drugs are being combined and the order of their combination. In general, if the MAOI is added to the drug regimen of a patient already taking a tricyclic antidepressant there are no important problems, but if the tricyclic antidepressant is added to the treatment of a patient already on a MAOI there can be a significant potentiation of unwanted effects (Tyrer, 1982). The combination of amitriptyline and phenelzine appears to be particularly safe, as the pressor effects of tyramine (responsible for the 'cheese reaction') are less in patients receiving this combination than in those receiving the MAOI alone (Pare *et al.*, 1982).

Although studies of patients with moderate depression have failed to demonstrate any superiority for combined therapy when compared with the same antidepressants in single dosage (Young *et al.*, 1979; White *et al.*, 1982), there have been no satisfactory studies of combination therapy in resistant depression. The only study which has examined the efficacy of combined antidepressants (amitriptyline and phenelzine) in depression that had failed to respond to adequate doses of single antidepressants showed that the combination was only just inferior in efficacy to ECT (Davidson *et al.*, 1978).

Lithium carbonate (and other salts) may also be combined with tricyclic antidepressants and MAOIs in the treatment of refractory depression.

Although there are no satisfactory controlled trials demonstrating the efficacy of this combination, there have been many open studies testifying to its value (e.g. Nelson and Byck, 1982; Roy and Pickar, 1985; Schrader and Levien, 1985). The augmentation of the effect of antidepressants by lithium has also been demonstrated in a placebo-controlled study in patients treated with amitriptyline, mianserin and desipramine, with improvement usually occurring in the second week after the introduction of lithium (Heninger *et al.*, 1983).

Other forms of combination treatment that have been promoted for refractory depression include the addition of thyroid hormone, particularly in the form of tri-iodothyronine (T_3). In one study the improvement was shown within 3 days of starting hormone treatment (Goodwin *et al.*, 1982). As depressions are associated with a relative deficiency of cerebral catecholamines, including 5-HT, it is predictable that L-tryptophan and 5-hydroxytryptophan (5-HTP) might be expected to have antidepressant effects. There is good evidence that L-tryptophan is an effective antidepressant when given alone or in combination with other antidepressants (Thomson *et al.*, 1982), and also potentiates the effects of other antidepressants, including MAOIs (Pare, 1963). At the same time, however, it is possible that the potentiating effects of L-tryptophan may be similarly achieved by increasing the dose of the original antidepressant; this has not been formally tested. 5-HTP has also been shown to be an effective antidepressant (Mendlewicz and Youdim, 1980) but is not available for general clinical use.

Combinations of three or more antidepressant drugs have also been recommended for intractable depression. These 'cocktails', as they have come to be called, include lithium, tryptophan and MAOIs such as phenelzine, and the same combination together with the addition of tricyclic or newer antidepressant drugs. These have not been tested to any degree of accuracy and their efficacy is almost entirely anecdotal (Hale *et al.*, 1987). The most that can be said about them is that they are safe and relatively free of unwanted effects when doses are increased gradually.

It is important to realize that many of these agents, including lithium salts, carbamazepine and L-tryptophan, are also effective in mania; these drugs can therefore be used in the treatment and prophylaxis of depression in the context of bipolar affective disorder (Tyrer, 1989). The combination of antidepressants together with sleep deprivation treatment is also said to be beneficial. Sleep deprivation treatment was first used in the treatment of depressed patients following the observation that sleep deprivation led to a transient elevation of mood in normal subjects. The treatment has subsequently been used with depressed in-patient populations and involves the disruption of all sleep throughout a complete diurnal cycle by the use of activities and occupational diversions. This is repeated twice weekly until response or non-compliance occurs. Several uncontrolled studies have shown dramatic improvements in depressed patients hitherto refractory to standard courses of antidepressant drugs, often after as few as one or two treatments (Bhanji and Roy, 1975; Larsen *et al.*, 1976; Svendsen, 1976). The main practical difficulties are lack of adequate compliance, particularly in less severely depressed out-patients, and the relatively rare occurrence of episodes of hypomania. Although this has now gone out of fashion to some extent, its mechanism of efficacy, although still not known, is likely to be quite different from those of other antidepressant treatments. As sleep deprivation has been reported, like antidepressants, to down-regulate β-adrenergic receptors, it is reasonable to combine sleep deprivation with other forms of antidepressant treatment. In refractory depression the combination of sleep deprivation together with combined tricyclic antidepressants and MAOIs has been shown to be effective (Dessauer *et al.*, 1985), and it is also alleged that sleep deprivation may make patients more susceptible to the therapeutic effects of ECT (Kvist and Kirekegaard, 1980). However, these studies were not adequately controlled and it would be unwise to draw any firm conclusions from them.

A scheme for treating resistant depression is outlined in Figure 2. It is assumed that the depression is a chronic one and that a period of at least 4 weeks can be allowed to elapse before any type of treatment is rejected as unsatisfactory. In instances where the severity of the depression is such that more rapid treatment is necessary, it may be appropriate to move to

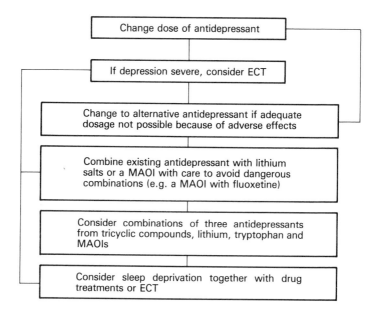

Figure 2 Strategy for treating resistant depression.

combination treatment before attempting the earlier ones. It may also be appropriate to consider psychosurgery when all other treatments have failed and the patient is left with severe and unremitting symptoms.

Finally, it is worth adding a cautious note that when patients with apparent depressive illness fail to respond to treatment the diagnosis may not be that of a primary depressive illness. The range of possible disorders masquerading as depression is a large one that includes physical disorders such as myxoedema and hidden neoplasms, dietary deficiencies such as pellagra, organic disorders of the brain, including early dementia, and other psychiatric disorders such as schizophrenia and various types of personality disorder. The clinician should therefore always question the diagnosis if patients fail to respond initially and to keep his or her diagnostic tentacles sensitive before continuing along the line of ever more powerful antidepressant treatment combinations.

References

Aberg-Wistedt, A. (1982) *Acta Psychiatr. Scand.* **66**, 50–65.

Abrams, R. (1986) *Convuls. Ther.* **2**, 253–257.

Akiskal, H.S., Rosenthal, T.L. & Haykal, R. F. (1980) *Arch. Gen. Psychiatry* **37**, 778–783.

Alexanderson, B., Evans, D.A.P. & Sjoqvist, F. (1969) *Br. Med. J.* **4**, 764–768.

American Psychiatric Association (1980) *Diagnostic and Statistical Manual of Mental Disorders*, 3rd edn. Washington DC, American Psychiatric Association.

American Psychiatric Association (1987) *Diagnostic and Statistical Manual of Mental Disorders*, 3rd edn. (revised). Washington DC, American Psychiatric Association.

Angst, J., Baastrup, P., Grof, P. *et al.* (1973) *Psychiatr. Neurol. Neurochirurgia (Amsterdam)* **76**, 489–500.

Asberg, M. (1983) In *Treatment of Depression: Old Controversies and New Approaches* (eds Clayton, P.J. & Barrett, J.E.), pp 95–96. New York, Raven Press.

Asberg, M., Cronholm, B., Sjoqvist, F. & Tuck, D. (1970) *Br. Med. J.* **4**, 18–21.

Asberg, M., Thoren, P., Traskman, L. *et al.* (1976) *Science* **191**, 478–480.

Baastrup, P.C., Poulsen, J.C., Schou, M. *et al.* (1970) *Lancet* **ii**, 326–328.

Bhanji, S. & Roy, G.A. (1975) *Br. J. Psychiatry* **127**, 222–226.

Bialos, D., Gilles, E., Jatlow, P. *et al.* (1982) *Am. J. Psychiatry* **139**, 325–329.

Bielski, R.J. & Friedel, R.O. (1976) *Arch. Gen. Psychiatry* **33**, 1479–1489.

Birley, J.F.T. (1964) *Br. J. Psychiatry* **110**, 211–221.

Blackburn, I.M., Bishop, S., Glen, A.I.M., Whalley, J.J. & Christie, J.E. (1981) *Br. J. Psychiatry* **139**, 181–189.

Blackwell, B., Marley, E., Price, J. & Taylor, B. (1967) *Br. J. Psychiatry* **113**, 349–365.

Blashki, T.G., Mowbray, R. & Davies, B. (1971) *Br. Med. J.* **1**, 133.

Braithwaite, R.A., Montgomery, S.A. & Dawling, S. (1979a) In *Drugs and the Elderly* (eds Cooks, J. & Stevenson, I.H.), pp 134–144. London, MacMillan.

Braithwaite, R.A., Montgomery, S.A. & Dawling, S. (1979b) *Clin. Pharmacokinet.* **4**, 129–136.

Brandon, S., Cowley, P., McDonald, C. *et al.* (1984) *Br. Med. J.* **288**, 22–25.

Bridges, P.K. & Bartlett, J.R. (1977) *Br. J. Psychiatry* **131**, 249–260.

Bulbena, A. & Berrios, G.E. (1986) *Br. J. Psychiatry* **148**, 87–94.

Cassidy, S. & Henry, J. (1987) *Br. Med. J.* **295**, 1021–1024.

Cerletti, U. & Bini, L. (1938) *Arch. Gen. Neurol. Psychiatr. Psychoanal.* **19**, 266–268.

Charney, D.S., Heninger, G.R., Sternberg, D.E. & Landis, H. (1982) *Br. J. Psychiatry* **141**, 377–386.

Committee on Safety of Medicines (1983) *Curr. Probl.* No. 11.

Committee on Safety of Medicines (1984) *Curr. Probl.* No. 13.

Committee on Safety of Medicines (1988) *Curr. Probl.* No. 23.

Committee on Safety of Medicines Update (1986a) *Br. Med. J.* **293**, 41.

Committee on Safety of Medicines Update (1986b) *Br. Med. J.* **293**, 688.

Coppen, A.J., Noguera, R., Bailey, J. *et al.* (1971) *Lancet* **ii**, 275–279.

Davidson, J., McLeod, M., Law-Yone, B. & Linnoila, M. (1978) *Arch. Gen. Psychiatry* **35**, 639–42.

Delgado, P.L., Price, L.H., Charney, D.S. & Heninger, G.R. (1988) *J. Affective Disord.* **15**, 55–60.

D'Elia, G. & Raotma, H. (1975) *Br. J. Psychiatry* **126**, 82–89.

Dessauer, M., Goetze, U. & Tolle, R. (1985) *Neuropsychobiology*, **13**, 111–116.

Edwards, J.G. (1989) In *Depression: An Integrative Approach* (eds Herbst, K. & Paykel, E.), pp 81–108. London, Heinemann.

Freeman, C.P., Basson, J.V. & Crighton, A. (1978) *Lancet*, **i**, 738–740.

Goktepe, E.O., Young, L.B. & Bridges, P.K. (1975) *Br. J. Psychiatry* **126**, 270–280.

Goodwin, F.K., Prange, A.J., Post, R.N., Muscettola, G. & Lipton, M.A. (1982) *Am. J. Psychiatry* **139**, 34–38.

Greenblatt, M., Grosser, G.H. & Wechsler, H. (1964) *Am. J. Psychiatry* **120**, 935–943.

Gregory, S., Shawcross, C.R. & Gill, D. (1985) *Br. J. Psychiatry* **146**, 520–524.

Hale, A.S., Proctor, A.W. & Bridges, P.K. (1987) *Br. J. Psychiatry* **151**, 213–217.

Halliday, A.M., Davison, K., Browne, M.W. & Kreeger, L.C. (1968) *Br. J. Psychiatry* **114**, 997–1012.

Hamilton, M. (1967) *Br. J. Soc. Clin. Psychol.* **6**, 278–289.

Hay, G. & Simpson, N. (1982) *Lancet* **ii**, 160–161.

Heninger, G.R., Charney, D.S. & Sternberg, D.E. (1983) *Arch. Gen. Psychiatry* **40**, 1335–1342.

Hobson, R.F. (1953) *J. Neurol. Neurosurg. Psychiatry* **16**, 275–81.

Johnson, D.A. (1981) *Acta Psychiatr. Scand.* **63** (Suppl. 290), 447–453.

Johnstone, E.C. (1985) *Br. J. Hosp. Med.* **34**, 198–201.

Johnstone, E.C., Deakin, J.F.W., Lawler, P., Frith, C.D., Stevens, M., McPherson, K. & Crow, T.J. (1980) *Lancet* **ii**, 1317–1320.

Kelly, D. (1976) *Br. J. Hosp. Med.* **16**, 165–174.

Kendell, R.E. (1981) *Br. J. Psychiatry* **139**, 265–269.

Klein, D.F. (1974) *Arch. Gen. Psychiatry* **31**, 447–454.

Klerman, G.L. (1988) In *Depression and Mania.* (eds Georgotas, A. & Cancro, R.), pp. 490–501. Amsterdam, Elsevier.

Kragh-Sorensen, P., Eggert-Hansen, C., Baastrup, P.C. & Hvidberg, E.F. (1976) *Psychopharmacologica*, **45**, 305–316.

Kramer, J.C., Klein, D.F. & Fink, M. (1961) *Am. J. Psychiatry*, **118**, 549–550.

Kvist, J. & Kirkegaard, C. (1980) *Acta Psychiatr. Scand.* **62**, 494–502.

Lambourne, J. & Gill, D. (1978) *Br. J. Psychiatry* **133**, 514–519.

Larsen, J.K., Lindberg, M.L. & Skovgaard, B. (1976) *Acta Psychiatr. Scand.* **54**, 167–173.

Lee, A.S. & Murray, R.M. (1988) *Br. J. Psychiatry* **153**, 741–751.

Leonard, B.E. (1986) *Lancet* **ii**, 1105.

Lewis, A.J. (1934) *J. Ment. Sci.* **80**, 1–42.

MacNeil, S., Hanson-Nortey, E., Paschalis, C. *et al.* (1975) *Lancet* **i**, 1295.

Mahgoub, A., Idle, J.R., Dring, G., Lancaster, R. & Smith, R.L. (1977) *Lancet* **ii**, 584–586.

Medical Research Council (1965) *Br. Med. J.* **1**, 881–86.

Mendlewicz, J. & Youdim, M.B. (1980) *J. Affective Disord.* **2**, 137–146.

Mindham, R.H.S., Howland, C. & Shepherd, M. (1973) *Psychol. Med.* **3**, 5–17.

Moir, O.C., Cornwell, W.B., Dingwall-Fordyce, I. *et al.* (1972) *Lancet* **ii**, 561–564.

Montgomery, S.A. (1989) In *Depression: An Integrative Approach* (eds Herbst, K. & Paykel, E.), pp 178–196. London, Heinemann.

Montgomery, S.A. & Asberg, M. (1979) *Br. J. Psychiatry* **134**, 382–389.

Montgomery, S.A. & Montgomery, D.B. (1982) *J. Affective Disord.* **4**, 291–298.

Montgomery, S.A., McAuley, R., Rani, S.J. *et al.* (1979) *Br. Med. J.* **1**, 230–231.

Montgomery, S.A., McAuley, R., Montgomery, D.B., Dawling, S. & Braithwaite, R.A. (1980) *Clini. Ther.* **3**, 292–298.

Montgomery, S.A., Dufour, J., Brion, S. *et al.* (1988) *Br. J. Psychiatry* **153** (Suppl. 3), 69–76.

Morris, J.B. & Beck, A.T. (1974) *Arch. Gen. Psychiatry* **30**, 667–674.

Nelson, J.C. & Byck, R. (1982) *Br. J. Psychiatry* **141**, 85–86.

Orme, M.L.E. (1984) *Br. Med. J.* **289**, 1–2.

Oswald, I., Brezinova, V. & Dunleavy, D.L.F. (1972) *Br. J. Psychiatry* **120**, 673–677.

Pare, C.M.B. (1963) *Lancet* **ii**, 527–528.

Pare, C.M.B. (1965) In *The Scientific Basis of Drug Therapy in Psychiatry* (eds Marks, J. and Pare, C.M.B.), pp 110–113. Oxford, Pergamon Press.

Pare, C.M.B. (1985) *Br. J. Psychiatry* **146**, 576–584.

Pare, C.M.B. & Mack, J.W. (1971) *J. Med. Genet.* **8**, 306–311.

Pare, C.M.B., Kline, N., Hallstrom, C. & Cooper, T.B. (1982) *Lancet* **ii**, 183–186.

Paykel, E.S. (1979) In *Psychopharmacology of Affective Disorders* (eds Paykel, E.S. & Coppen, A.), pp 193–220. Oxford, Oxford University Press.

Paykel, E.S., Rowan, P.R., Parker, R.R. & Bhat, A.V. (1982) *Arch. Gen. Psychiatry* **39**, 1041–1049.

Pinder, R.M. (1990) In *Antidepressants: Thirty Years On* (eds Leonard, B. & Spencer, P.), pp 334–348. London, CNS Publishers (in press).

Post, R.M., Uhde, T.W., Roy-Byrne, P.P. & Joffe, R.T. (1986) *Am. J. Psychiatry* **143**, 29–34.

Prien, R.F. & Kupfer, D.J. (1986) *Am. J. Psychiatry*, **143**, 18–23.

Prien, R.F., Klett, C.J. & Caffey, E.M. (1973) *Arch. Gen. Psychiatry* **29**, 420–425.

Prien, R.F., Kupfer, D.J., Mawsky, P.A. *et al.* (1984) *Arch. Gen. Psychiatry* **41**, 1096–1104.

Pugh, R., Bell, J., Cooper, A.J. *et al.* (1982) *J. Affective Disord.* **4**, 355–363.

Ravaris, C.L., Nies, A., Robinson, D.S., Ives, J.O. & Bartlett, D. (1976) *Arch. Gen. Psychiatry* **33**, 347–350.

Rawlins, M.D. (1981) *Br. Med. J.* **282**, 974–976.

Reimherr, F.W., Wood, D.R., Byerley, B., Brainard, J. & Grosser, B.I. (1984) *Psychopharmacol. Bull.* **20**, 70–72.

Ries, R.K., Wilson, L., Bokan, J.A. & Chiles, J.A. (1981) *Compr. Psychiatry* **22**, 167–173.

Robinson, D.S., Nies, A., Ravaris, C.L. *et al.* (1973) *Arch. Gen. Psychiatry* **29**, 407–413.

Roy, A. & Pickar, D. (1985) *Br. J. Psychiatry* **147**, 582–583.

Rush, A.J., Beck, A.T., Kovacs, M. & Hollon, S.D. (1977) *Cogn. Res. Ther.* **1**, 17–37.
Sargant, W., Walter, C.J.S. & Wright, N. (1966) *Br. Med. J.* **1**, 322–324.
Schildkraut, J.J., Winokur, A. & Applegate, C.W. (1970) *Science* **168**, 867–869.
Schou, M. (1979) *Arch. Gen. Psychiatry* **36**, 849–853.
Schou, M. (1980) In *Handbook of Lithium Therapy* (ed. Johnson, F.N.). Lancaster, MTP Press.
Schrader, G.D. & Levien, H.E.M. (1985) *Br. J. Psychiatry* **147**, 573–575.
Schuckit, M., Robins, E. & Feighner, J. (1971) *Arch. Gen. Psychiatry* **24**, 509–514.
Svendsen, K. (1976) *Acta Psychiatr. Scand.* **54**, 184–192.
Sykes, N.K. & Tredgold, R.F. (1964) *Br. J. Psychiatry* **110**, 609–640.
Teasdale, J.D., Fennell, M.J.V., Hibbert, G.A. & Amies, P.L. (1984) *Br. J. Psychiatry* **144**, 400–406.
Thomson, J., Rankin, H., Ashcroft, G.W. *et al.* (1982) *Psychol. Med.* **12**, 741–751.
Tiller, J., Schweitzer, I., Maguire, K. & Davies, B. (1989) *Br. J. Psychiatry* **155**, 483–489.
Tyrer, P. (1984) *J. Affective Disord.* **6**, 1–7.
Tyrer, P. & Marsden, C. (1985) *Trends Neurosci.* **8**, 427–431.
Tyrer, P., Marsden, C.A., Casey, P. & Seivewright, N. (1987) *J. Psychopharmacol.* **1**, 251–57.
Tyrer, P.J. (1982) In *Drugs in Psychiatric Practice*, (ed. Tyrer, P.J.), pp 249–279. London, Butterworths.
Tyrer, S.P. (1985) *J. Affective Disord.* **8**, 251–257.
Tyrer, S.P. (1989). *Br, J. Hosp. Med.* **42**, 184–194.
Veith, R.C., Raskins, M.A., Caldwell, J.H. *et al.* (1982) *N. Engl. J. Med.* **306**, 954–959.
Weiner, R.D., Rogers, H.J., Davidson, J.R.T. & Squire, L.R. (1986) *Ann. N Y. Acad. Sci.* **462**, 315–325.
Weinstein, M.R. (1980) In *Handbook of Lithium Therapy* (ed. Johnson, F.N.), pp 421–429. Lancaster, MTP Press.
Weissman, M.M., Jarrett, R.B. & Rush, J.A. (1987) In *Psychopharmacology: The Third Generation of Progress* (ed. Meltzer, H.Y.), pp 1059–1070. New York, Raven Press.
White, K., Razari, J., Simpson, G. *et al.* (1982) *Psychopharmacol. Bull.* **18**, 180–181.
Worrall, E.P., Moody, J.P., Peet, M. *et al.* (1979) *Br. J. Psychiatry* **135**, 255–262.
Young, J.P.R., Hughes, W.C. & Lader, M.H. (1976) *Br. Med. J.* **1**, 1116–1118.
Young, J.P.R., Lader, M.H. & Hughes, W.C. (1979) *Br. Med. J.* **2**, 1315–1317.
Zis, A.P. & Goodwin, F.K. (1979) *Arch. Gen. Psychiatry* **36**, 835–839.

CHAPTER 3

EVOLUTION OF THE MONOAMINE HYPOTHESES OF DEPRESSION

James C. Pryor[1] and Fridolin Sulser[1,2]

*Departments of[1] Psychiatry and[2] Pharmacology,
Vanderbilt University School of Medicine, Nashville, Tennessee 37232, USA*

Table of Contents

During the last 20 years, the biogenic amine hypotheses of affective disorders (catecholamine hypothesis and indoleamine hypothesis) have dominated research strategies in biological psychiatry. The original catecholamine hypothesis proposed that affective disorders result from abnormalities in central noradrenergic systems (noradrenaline (NA) deficiency in depression, functional excess of NA in mania), while the indoleamine hypothesis of depression postulated that abnormalities in central serotonergic function

BIOLOGICAL ASPECTS OF AFFECTIVE DISORDERS
ISBN 0-12-356510-3

(serotonin (5-HT) deficiency) may occur in selective subgroups of patients suffering from affective disorders. Results derived from acute pharmacological experiments have by and large provided data supporting both hypotheses. These amine hypotheses of affective disorders have stimulated considerable biological research on the psychobiology of depression and thus had heuristic value.

It is the aim of this chapter to review briefly the evolution of the monoamine hypotheses of affective disorders and to put them into perspective within the context of recent advances in our understanding of the molecular events in the cascade of amine receptor-mediated signal transduction and its modification by antidepressant treatments.

3.1 Origins of the monoamine hypotheses of depression

Edward Freis (1954) reported on five patients who were treated with 'high doses' of reserpine for hypertension and who went on to develop 'mental depression' of various severity. The depressions in these patients were described as a 'withdrawal from the environment, lethargy, and unhappiness, but not anxiety'. Suicidal ideation was also noted in two of the five patients. This first report was followed by a number of others, including that of Muller *et al.* (1955) who reported on seven cases of depression out of 97 patients treated with reserpine and other raulwolfia alkaloids for hypertension. In these cases, anxiety was a prominent component of the depressions, and two patients became actively suicidal. Five of the patients required electroconvulsive therapy (ECT) to remit the depressions. A period of 3–6 months treatment with reserpine preceded the onset of psychiatric symptoms, and five of the patients had psychiatric histories before being treated with reserpine. In 1957, the drug iproniazid was introduced as a treatment for mental disorders (Ayd, 1957). This drug was discovered during the search for more effective antitubercular drugs. While on iproniazid, patients with tuberculosis experienced some euphoria, which prompted its trial as an antidepressant (Delay *et al.*, 1952; Loomer *et al.*, 1957). In 1958, imipramine was introduced as a treatment for endogenous depression and found to be very effective (Kuhn, 1958). Because of the structural similarities between imipramine and chlorpromazine, imipramine was first tested as a potential antipsychotic agent. Its therapeutic value for the treatment of depression was an unexpected discovery.

No known mechanism of action was available at the time to explain the clinical observations made in patients taking reserpine, iproniazid, or imipramine. However, with the discoveries in the late 1950s and early 1960s of the importance of the chemistry and function of monoamines in the brain, a window into the function of the brain was opened.

Comprehensive reviews exist for the reader who is interested in the history of the early discoveries on the mode of action of reserpine, iproniazid, and imipramine on central noradrenergic systems (Zeller, 1982; Carlsson, 1983; Lehmann and Kline, 1983; Sulser and Mishra, 1983). The pharmacological discoveries (depletion of catecholamines and serotonin by reserpine-like drugs, increased availability of noradrenaline and/or serotonin by antidepressants, either through the blocking of monoamine oxidase (MAO) or the neuronal uptake of the amines by tricyclics) provided the scientific basis for the clinically relevant catecholamine and serotonin hypotheses of affective disorders.

3.2 Catecholamine hypotheses of affective disorders

Considering the pharmacological effects of psychotropic drugs, a fairly consistent relationship between drug effects on catecholamines and affective or behavioural states became evident. Thus, drugs which cause depletion or inactivation of NA centrally (reserpine-like drugs) produce sedation or depression, while drugs which increase or potentiate brain NA (monoamine oxidase inhibitors (MAOIs) and tricyclic antidepressants) were associated with behavioural stimulation or excitement, and generally exerted an anti-depressant effect in man (Bunney and Davis, 1965; Schildkraut, 1965; Schildkraut and Kety, 1967). Schildkraut credits Jacobsen (Jacobsen, 1964) for giving one of the earliest formulations of the catecholamine hypothesis of depression. Citing a number of studies on the effects of antidepressants in the reserpine-induced animal model of depression, Schildkraut concluded that both MAOIs and tricyclic antidepressants 'could reverse the effects of reserpine by increasing NA at brain adrenergic receptor sites' (Schildkraut, 1965). This statement forms the crux of the original catecholamine hypothesis. These early findings prompted clinical investigators to search for alterations in NA metabolism in affective disorders. In support of the original catecholamine hypothesis of affective disorders (NA deficiency hypothesis) was the finding of reduced excretion of the NA metabolite, 3-methoxy-4-hydroxyphenyl glycol (MHPG) in patients with bipolar depression and schizoaffective disorders; MHPG excretion was found to be increased during manic episodes in other patients (Schildkraut, 1978). This metabolite was felt to be mainly derived from the metabolism of NA in brain, although the true contribution of brain MHPG to its total excretion is anywhere from 20 to 70% (Maas et al., 1979). A retrospective review of treatment outcomes appeared to indicate that symptomatic patients who excreted less MHPG in the urine responded more favourably to the antidepressant imipramine (Maas *et al.*, 1972: Maas, 1975). Because imipramine blocks NA reuptake, it was theorized that this group of depressed patients could be characterized as NA deficient. Further, those patients who had normal or high levels of urinary MHPG appeared to respond more favourably to amitriptyline, which was originally shown to block 5-HT reuptake. Therefore, this group was hypothesized to be 5-HT deficient. However, these findings have proved inconsistent. In further studies there have been reports that urinary MHPG in depressed patients is increased, decreased, or the same as in normal controls (for review, see Maas, 1986). While diagnostic heterogeneity has been used to explain some of the discrepancies with regard to the studies on urinary MHPG, the influence of non-specific stress, diet, and other factors has to be considered. In any event, studies on urinary NA metabolites have to be interpreted cautiously and their relevance to central noradrenergic mechanisms remains questionable.

Cerebrospinal fluid (CSF) MHPG has also been studied because, at first glance, it would appear that measurements of CSF metabolites of NA might provide a better index of central noradrenergic activity (Koslow *et al.*, 1983: Maas *et al.*, 1984). Again, however, inconsistencies have been found. Much urine, blood, and CSF was collected and analysed in the following 20 years in an effort to establish that either the lack of or increase of a monoamine was associated with affective disorders. Also, if depression were solely the consequence of NA deficiency, loading with L-dihydroxyphenylalanine (L-dopa), the amino acid precursor of NA, would be expected to exert therapeutic efficacy. However, the use of L-dopa, both with and without peripheral decarboxylase inhibitors, has been unsuccessful in the treatment of depression (Goodwin *et al.*, 1970), although bipolar patients have developed hypomania during treatment.

Studies on enzymes involved in the synthesis or degradation of catecholamines have also failed to lend unequivocal support to the catecholamine hypothesis of affective disorders. Because of these inconsistent results, clinical studies of the function of central noradrenergic systems have shifted from studies of concentrations of NA metabolites in biological fluids to more dynamic assessment strategies, e.g. the use of pharmacological challenges and the evaluation of responsiveness of adrenergic receptors (for a comprehensive review, see Siever, 1987).

3.3 Serotonin hypotheses of affective disorders

In parallel to the emergence of the catecholamine hypothesis of affective disorders, serotonin (5-HT) neurotransmitter systems have been implicated in the pathophysiology of affective disorders (for reviews of the early data see Coppen and Wood, 1982; van Praag, 1982). Urinary and CSF 5-HT and/or its metabolites have often, but not uniformly, been found to be lowered in patients with affective illness, and drugs which increase serotonergic activity by and large exert antidepressant effects in patients.

Initial findings of a decrease in 5-HT in the brains of suicide victims, along with the suggestion that 5-HT systems were involved in behavioural syndromes in animals, fuelled speculation and further studies on the role of 5-HT in depression. Murphy *et al.* (1978) reviewed the current literature on the findings in suicide victims. In six studies, decreases in the concentrations of 5-HT in various brain regions were noted in suicide victims compared with controls; no differences were observed in three studies. Studies of the major metabolite of 5-HT, 5-hydroxyindole acetic acid (5-HIAA), in urine, CSF and brain suggest a role for 5-HT in affective disorders. Murphy *et al.* (1978) reviewed the literature on decreases in brain concentrations of 5-HIAA in suicide victims versus those of controls. In four studies there appeared to be a suggestion of a decrease in 5-HIAA in the suicide group (see also Chapter 6).

Precursor loading with either tryptophan or 5-hydroxytryptophan (5-HTP) has been employed for the treatment of depression. The addition of 5-HT precursors to standard antidepressant treatments (i.e. MAOIs), or substitution by 5-HT precursors, was beneficial in the overall treatment of depression. Early studies showed an apparent antidepressant effect of tryptophan in 'endogenous' depressed patients with a preferential effect in the treatment of bipolar depression. These findings could not be replicated later, however. Results of studies on the therapeutic value of 5-HTP were also equivocal. Most studies showed either no effect of 5-HTP alone or a modest improvement in antidepressant effects if continued with standard therapy (for review, see Meltzer and Lowy, 1987). Of note is a study of an apparent prophylactic effect of 5-HTP on depression. Patients who had been treated for depression were assigned to either placebo or 5-HTP in a 1-year cross-over design study. Those patients who received 5-HTP showed a much lower incidence of relapse than those in the placebo group. This response was most closely related to CSF 5-HIAA levels (van Praag and de Haan, 1981).

The early findings of decreased 5-HIAA concentrations in the CSF of depressed patients was exciting, and more importantly, fairly reproducible. Åsberg and colleagues (1976a) examined CSF from 68 patients with depression. Twenty-nine percent of these patients comprised a group with 'low' CSF 5-HIAA levels. There was no difference between these groups in terms of severity of depression. However, it was later noted that the group with low CSF 5-HIAA was more prone to attempt suicide by violent means than the group with normal 5-HIAA levels (Åsberg *et al.*, 1976b).

Other studies of psychiatric and non-psychiatric patients have suggested that low CSF 5-HIAA is not a marker for depression *per se*, but a marker for impulsivity (Brown *et al.*, 1979; Linnoila *et al.*, 1983; Roy and Linnoila, 1988). A correlation between decreased CSF 5-HIAA and impulsivity has been found across diagnostic categories, including depression, substance abuse and personality disorders. Low CSF 5-HIAA in depressed patients has been noted in Sweden to be a strong predictor of violent suicide to the point that all depressed in-patients at the Karolinska Institute undergo routine lumbar punctures and those with low CSF 5-HIAA concentrations must be followed up more closely than others (M. Linnoila, personal communication).

Although 5-HT seems to be important in the pathophysiology of mood disorders, the lack of specificity and robustness of some of the findings require further considerations. It is clear, however, that a simple 5-HT deficiency hypothesis does not explain the importance of 5-HT in the aetiology of affective disorders. Multiple interactions between 5-HT and other neuronal systems exist (see later) and, as pointed out by Meltzer and Lowy (1987) in a comprehensive review on the 5-HT hypothesis of depression: 'an impairment in the regulation of serotonergic neurotransmission in relation to other neurotransmitter systems may emerge as the most important factor in the aetiology of depression'.

3.4 Transmitters and regulators other than monoamines

Although not part of a review on the evolution of the monoamine hypotheses of affective disorders, the role of other neurotransmitter systems (e.g. dopamine (DA), acetylcholine) and neuropeptides (e.g. corticotrophin releasing factor, thyrotrophin releasing hormone, and somatostatin) in affective disorders must be considered. The interested reader is referred to relevant chapters in *Psychopharmacology, the Third Generation of Progress*, edited for the American College of Neuropsychopharmacology by Herbert Y. Meltzer (1987). Since glucocorticoids have been shown to modulate central aminergic receptor function, and glucocorticoid receptors have been identified in the cell bodies of NA and 5-HT-containing neurones, this class of regulators is discussed in more detail later.

3.5 Switch from acute presynaptic to delayed postsynaptic receptor-mediated events: monoamine receptor adaptation hypotheses of affective disorders

The inconsistencies of biochemical and pharmacological data derived from either plasma, urine, or CSF in relation to the original catecholamine and serotonin hypotheses of affective disorders are striking. This has raised serious questions as to the validity of these hypotheses. However, variability of study conditions, differences in diagnostic criteria, variable sensitivity of biological assays and large intraindividual variations in biochemical parameters may explain some of the inconsistent results.

Perhaps the strongest argument against the original form of the catecholamine hypothesis of depression is the fact that the pharmacological and biochemical changes produced by the antidepressant drugs occur within minutes. Clinical practice, however, indicates that antidepressants do not produce their mood altering effects for at least 10–14 days following initiation of treatment. This finding is true for ECT as well, in that it takes 3–5 treatments to produce mood elevating effects. Much of the improvement seen early on in the treatment of depression is probably associated with improvements in sleep caused by the antihistaminic properties associated with most traditional antidepressants (see Chapter 2).

Two discoveries made in the second half of the 1970s have contributed to a revision of the original amine hypotheses of affective disorders, and have shifted the research emphasis on the mode of action of antidepressant treatments from *acute* presynaptic to *delayed* postsynaptic receptor-mediated events. First, Vetulani and Sulser (1975) reported that chronic antidepressant treatments (pharmacotherapy and ECT) caused subsensitivity of the NA receptor-coupled adenylate cyclase system in brain. The second important discovery was the demonstration that this desensitization of NA receptor systems was linked to a decrease in the density of β-adrenoceptors (Banerjee et al., 1977). The delayed desensitization of the NA–β-adrenoceptor-coupled adenylate cyclase system in brain seems to be a biochemical action that is shared by most, if not all, clinically effective antidepressant treatments, including ECT and some of the newer 'second generation' antidepressants. This desensitization is linked in most, but not all, cases to a decrease in the density of β-adrenoceptors of the β_1 subtype (see recent reviews by Baker and Greenshaw, 1989; Sulser and Sanders-Bush, 1989). Chronic administration of antidepressant drugs reduces the β-adrenoceptor–cyclic AMP-mediated formation of melatonin in the rat pineal gland. These studies provide evidence of a *net* deamplification of the NA signal (Heydorn et al., 1982; Friedman et al., 1984). Thus, the down-regulation of the NA–β-adrenoceptor-coupled adenylate cyclase system does not merely reflect a compensatory mechanism to offset the increased synaptic availability of NA, while the overall rate of signal transduction is unchanged. While the data obtained in the rat on the *net* deamplification of the NA signal following chronic treatment with antidepressants are unequivocal, data on plasma melatonin obtained in man could at first glance lead to opposite conclusions (Checkley, 1988; Checkley et al., 1990). Although results obtained in the pineal gland cannot necessarily be extrapolated to the function of aminergic systems in brain, the discrepancies in the pineal data between the two species may cast some doubt on the general validity of the β-adrenergic receptor adaptation hypothesis. However, whereas melatonin stimulation in the rat is mediated via β-adrenoceptors, and desensitization following chronic treatment with antidepressant drugs in turn leads to a decreased formation of this indole compound, the type of receptors involved in melatonin formation is less clear in other species. For example, in hamsters and monkeys, the increase in melatonin is predominantly α_1-receptor mediated. If the regulation of melatonin in the human pineal occurs via both β- and α_1-adrenoceptors, the reported increased responsiveness following chronic treatment with desipramine and ($+$)-oxaprotiline (Checkley *et al.*, 1990) could actually reflect a down-regulation of β-adrenoceptors. A decrease in β-adrenoceptor function is known to be associated with an increase in α_1-adrenoceptor activity (Sulser, 1984). As the endogenous neurohormone is NA, it would, unlike isoproterenol, interact with both β- and α_1-adrenoceptors, with the net result being an *increase* in melatonin formation in this species.

The decrease in the density of β-adrenoceptors following chronic treatment with antidepressants appears to be quite specific for this class of psychotropic drugs (Sellinger *et al.*, 1980), and interestingly, includes drugs which more specifically affect the reuptake of 5-HT e.g. zimelidine, fluvoxamine and sertraline (Sulser, 1990). The finding that the antipsychotic drug chlorpromazine causes a down-regulation of β-adrenoceptors (Schultz, 1976) does not detract from the down-regulation hypothesis, as chlorpromazine increases, like tricyclics, the synaptic availability of NA due to inhibition of neuronal reuptake of NA. Chlorpromazine may well have antidepressant activity clinically, although this particular therapeutic action may be masked by other pharmacological effects of the drug (e.g. blockade of dopamine D-2 receptors).

Electrophysiological correlates of antidepressant-induced desensitization of postsynaptic β-adrenoceptor systems are of interest. Thus, a significant reduction in the sensitivity of cortical pyramidal cells and cerebellar Purkinje cells to NA occurs following chronic administration of both tricyclic antidepressants and MAOIs (Siggins and Schultz, 1979; Olpe and Schellenberg, 1980). The time-course of recovery from subsensitivity, as evidenced electrophysiologically, parallels the time-course of recovery of β-adrenoceptor subsensitivity, as evidenced biochemically.

Though many interactions between different receptor systems and within subtypes of receptors have been described, the interactions between serotonergic, β-noradrenergic and glucocorticoid receptor systems are of particular interest with regard to the monoamine hypotheses of depression. Ever since Dahlstrom and Fuxe (1964) mapped NA- and 5-HT-containing cell bodies and terminals in brain, a functional linkage between noradrenergic and serotonergic neuronal systems has been implied. Studies using psychopharmacological and electrophysiological approaches have generated robust support for this aminergic link. Thus, chronic administration of clinically effective antidepressants leads to an increase in the inhibitory response of forebrain neurones to microiontophoretically-applied 5-HT (de Montigny and Aghajanian, 1978). The supersensitivity to 5-HT (and/or DA), evidenced electrophysiologically or behaviourally, following the chronic administration of antidepressants or ECT is, however, prevented by lesioning of noradrenergic neurones (Green and Deakin, 1980; Gravel and de Montigny, 1987), thus clearly demonstrating the intimate interconnections of aminergic neuronal systems. Assuming that the noradrenergic β-adrenoceptor-mediated input from the locus coeruleus is inhibitory at dopaminergic and/or serotonergic effector sites, a down-regulation of β-adrenoceptor systems by antidepressants or ECT would cause a disinhibition or facilitation of dopamine- and 5-HT-mediated behaviours that would be prevented by lesions of the locus coeruleus. The following results could therefore be interpreted through this mechanism: (1) The increased behavioural responses to the 5-HT agonist 5-methoxy-N-dimethyltryptamine after chronic treatment with imipramine or amitriptyline (Friedman and Dallob, 1979); (2) the potentiation of apomorphine-induced aggressive behaviour following chronic treatment with antidepressants (Maj *et al.*, 1979); and (3) the above-mentioned enhanced sensitivity to iontophoretically-applied 5-HT following chronic treatment with antidepressants.

A number of studies have shown that an impairment of serotonergic neuronal activity caused by either neurotoxic lesions of serotonergic neurones or by inhibition of tryptophan hydroxylase by p-chlorophenylalanine (PCPA) renders central β-adrenoceptors resistant to down-regulation by antidepressants and ECT (Brunello *et al.*, 1982, 1985; Janowsky *et al.*, 1982; Drumbrille-Ross and Tang, 1983; Manier *et al.*, 1984; Nimgaonkar *et al.*, 1985). At first, these data have suggested a functional link between serotonergic and noradrenergic neuronal systems occurring at the level of β-adrenoceptors; they were of considerable clinical interest as it has been shown almost a decade ago that PCPA can nullify the therapeutic efficacy of antidepressants (Shopsin *et al.*, 1975; 1976). The demonstrated *co*-requirement of 5-HT for a down-regulation of β-adrenoceptors by tricyclic antidepressants suggested a rationale for the clinical observations that 5-HT precursors potentiate the antidepressant response to tricyclic antidepressants and MAOIs (Mendlewicz and Youdim, 1980; Coppen and Wood, 1982; van Praag, 1982). Recent results obtained by the use of non-linear regression analysis of agonist competition binding curves have, however, mandated a reinterpretation of these earlier data. An impairment of serotonergic neurones has been shown to *increase* β-adrenoceptors with low micromolar affinity for isoproterenol that masked the down-regulation of β-adrenoceptors with high nanomolar agonist affinity (Manier *et al.*, 1984, 1987; Offord *et al.*, 1988; Stockmeier and Kellar, 1988; Riva and Creese, 1989a). These up-regulated binding sites have now been identified as 5-HT_{1B} sites which increase following a reduction in the synaptic availability of 5-HT and are labelled by the β-adrenoceptor antagonist dihydroalprenolol (Gillespie *et al.*, 1989; Riva and Creese, 1989b; Stockmeier and Kellar, 1989). These developments have necessitated moving the '5-HT–NA link' from the β-adrenoceptor level to sites beyond the receptors (see section on future prospects).

3.6 Biochemical effector systems of the 5-HT–NA-linked signal transduction system

During the last few years, our understanding of aminergic receptor systems has increased spectacularly. Most of the adrenergic and serotonergic receptors have been cloned and their structure and orientation in the bilayer of the plasma membrane are known. These receptors are integral membrane proteins and characterized by seven hydrophobic transmembrane domains. They belong to the super-family of G-protein coupled receptors (Lefkowitz and Caron, 1988; Hartig, 1989). When β-adrenoceptors or 5-HT receptors bind NA or 5-HT respectively, they promote the binding of GTP to G-proteins. This in turn leads to regulation of activities of specific effector systems which include enzymes that synthesize cytoplasmic second messengers or ion channels that regulate the flux of specific ions. The function and structure of G-proteins has been comprehensively reviewed (Gilman, 1987; Ross, 1989). β-Adreno-ceptors are linked by G-proteins to adenylate cyclase with cyclic AMP as the second messenger. 5-HT receptors, dependent on the subtype, are linked via G-proteins to either adenylate cyclase (5-HT_{1A}, 5-HT_{1B}), or phospholipase C (5-HT_2, 5-HT_{1C}) which generates two cytoplasmic second messengers, diacylglycerol, and inositol 1,4,5-trisphosphate (IP_3). IP_3 mobilizes intracellular calcium which can serve as a third messenger (for reviews, see Berridge, 1987; Sulser and Sanders-Bush, 1989). The cytoplasmic second and third messengers activate various protein kinases, leading to the phosphorylation of pivotal proteins. Protein kinase-mediated protein phosphorylations most likely repre-sent the final common pathway of signal transduction (Nestler *et al.*, 1984).

The change in sensitivity of the NA receptor-coupled adenylate cyclase system following chronic treatment with antidepressants represents an important step in the regulation and adaptation of a specific biological response as regards the amine hypotheses of affective disorders. Although the changes in receptor number or in the formation of the second messenger cyclic AMP are relatively small, it is important to realize that the receptor-coupled adenylate cyclase system functions, via protein kinase activation, as a highly efficient kinetic amplification system (Walsh and Ashby, 1973). Small changes in NA signal transduction and in the formation of the second messenger cyclic AMP will thus be profoundly amplified.

Adaptive changes also occur in 5-HT$_2$ receptor systems following chronic administration of antidepressants. These changes, i.e. a down-regulation of the density of 5-HT$_2$ receptors and/or a desensitization of the 5-HT$_2$ receptor phosphoinositide signal (Sanders-Bush et al., 1989) are not as consistent, however, as changes which occur in the β-adrenoceptor-coupled adenylate cyclase system. Moreover, ECT, perhaps the most efficacious antidepressant treatment, up-regulates 5-HT$_2$ receptors (Kellar et al., 1981) and enhances 5-HT-induced phosphoinositol hydrolysis (Butler and Barkai, 1987). The possible relationship between the changes in the NA–β-adrenoceptor and the 5-HT–5-HT$_2$ receptor cascades is presently being investigated.

3.7 Glucocorticoids as modulators of aminergic receptor function

Since stressful life events and the vulnerability to stress are believed to be predisposing factors in the precipitation of affective disorders (Paykel, 1979; Anisman and Zackarko, 1982; Akiskal, 1985; see also Chapter 1), it is of interest that alterations in the level of circulating glucocorticoid hormones alter noradrenergic receptor sensitivity in brain. Glucocorticoids represent, in concert with catechol- and indoleamines, the third physiologically important group of regulators of the β-adrenoceptor-coupled adenylate cyclase system in brain (Mobley and Sulser, 1980; Mobley et al., 1983; Roberts et al., 1984; Harrelson et al., 1987). The regulatory role of glucocorticoids has gained in significance as their receptors have been identified immunocytochemically in the nuclei of catecholamine- and 5-HT-containing cell bodies in brain (Harfstrand et al., 1986). Glucocorticoid receptors function as DNA binding proteins which can modify the transcription of specific genes (Burnstein and Cidlowski, 1989). Fuxe and his associates at the Karolinska Institute have shown that chronic treatment with imipramine causes a selective increase of glucocorticoid receptor immunoreactivity in the locus coeruleus and in 5-HT nerve cell groups of the rostral ventromedial medulla (Kitayama et al., 1988). These findings make it tempting to speculate that glucocorticoids may affect the diffusely projecting stress-responsive monoamine systems in brain via changes in transcription of pivotal proteins. It thus becomes imperative to integrate the glucocorticoid receptor system into any modern amine hypothesis of affective disorders.

Considering neuroanatomical, neurochemical, neurophysiological, psycho-pharmacological and endocrine aspects of aminergic receptor systems in brain, and their modification by antidepressant drugs, we have formulated the '5-HT–NA–glucocorticoid link' hypothesis of affective disorders (Sulser and Sanders-Bush, 1987) suggesting that the antidepressant-sensitive, 5-HT-linked and glucocorticoid-responsive β-adrenoceptor system in brain functions as an amplification/adaptation system of vital physiological functions, including mood, sleep, pain and neuroendocrine and central autonomic functions.

3.8 Some clinical aspects of the revised '5-HT–NA–glucorticoid link' hypothesis of affective disorders

Under normal physiological conditions, the '5-HT–NA–glucocorticoid' system is hypothesized to function as a protective adaptive system against excessive oscillations in sensory input. An impairment of this system, occurring at any one of the multiple steps involved in the signal transduction, would result in maladaptation which in turn might trigger changes in pain perception, anhedonia, and produce fully fledged depressive reactions. Successful anti-depressant treatment may work by restoring this 'loss in adaptation', perhaps by a deamplification of the signal input, such that pain is less painful, the anxiety response is more in keeping with the environmental cue, and the like. Conversely, therapeutic resistance to antidepressant treatments could simply reflect our inability to restore the loss of adaptation by failing to correct an impairment in the cascade of signal transduction, most likely at steps beyond the receptors, perhaps at the level of transcriptional activation (Sulser, 1990).

This revised 'NA–5-HT–glucocorticoid link' hypothesis of affective disorders as an *adaptive* hypothesis seems to be relevant with regard to stress-induced depression. A brain area that is important in the aetiology of stress-induced depression is the locus coeruleus (A_6), which is the site of origin of the major noradrenergic projections throughout the neuroaxis. This region is also of importance because of its role as a 'gatekeeper' of information from the spinal cord and lower brain stem autonomic centres which relay information related to autonomic arousal to higher brain areas (Foote et al., 1983). The work of Weiss and colleagues on the function of the NA system in the locus coeruleus in stress-induced depression in laboratory animals is pertinent in this regard (Weiss and Simson, 1988). If animals are exposed to uncontrollable shocks, a behavioural syndrome is observed with many of the characteristics of major depression as defined by DSM-III-R (American Psychiatric Association,

1987), including loss of appetite and weight, decreased spontaneous motor activity, sleep disturbances, decreased responding for 'rewarding brain stimulation', decreased grooming activity, and increased numbers of errors in a 'choice/discrimination stimulation' (Simson and Weiss, 1988; Weiss and Simson, 1988). These behaviours respond to treatment with tricyclic anti-depressants, MAOIs, ECT and atypical antidepressants. It was initially believed, in keeping with the original monoamine hypothesis of depression, that this behavioural depression in animals was produced by a *depletion* of monoamines in the locus coeruleus. However, recent findings indicate the opposite, i.e. that the stress-induced behavioural depression in these animals is due to an *increase* in activity of noradrenergic neurones in the locus coeruleus (Weiss and Simson, 1988). These recent findings are compatible with the suggested therapeutic mode of action of antidepressant treatments causing subsensitivity of the NA–β-adrenoceptor-coupled adenylate cyclase system that would blunt the effects of excessive NA release in noradrenergically-innervated brain regions. Redmond and Huang (1979) have suggested that increased activity in the locus coeruleus–dorsal noradrenergic system is involved in pathological anxiety. It is conceivable that the antidepressant drug-induced subsensitivity of noradrenergic systems is also responsible for the antidepressants' anxiolytic effects.

The role of glucocorticoid receptors in noradrenergic and/or serotonergic cell bodies has yet to be elucidated with regard to affective disorders. However, since disturbances in the hypothalamic–pituitary–adrenal axis play a major role in the pathophysiology of affective disorders (see reviews by Stokes and Jiles, 1987; Owens and Nemeroff 1988), the efforts to unravel the consequences of increased glucocorticoid receptor interactions on transcriptional activity in monoaminergic systems in brain should be rewarding. The findings that chronic imipramine treatment selectively increases glucocorticoid receptor immunoreactivity in the locus coeruleus and in 5-HT nerve cell groups of the rostral ventromedial medulla (Kitayama *et al.*, 1988) provide an important clue on the suggested endocrine regulation of central monoaminergic function.

3.9 New perspectives and future directions

The evolution of the monoamine hypotheses of affective disorders reflects, by and large, the evolution of our understanding of the mode of action of antidepressant drugs. The emergence of molecular neurobiology with its powerful analytical techniques is rapidly changing the traditional focus of neuropharmacological research. The '5-HT–NA–glucocorticoid link' hypothesis of affective disorders evolving from the original 'deficiency hypotheses' now emphasizes the integration of the multiple intracellular signals that regulate neuronal responses. Considering recent results on β-adrenoceptor-mediated gene transcriptions and their synergistic regulation by glucocorticoids (Yoshikawa and Sabol, 1986a, 1986b; Dal Toso *et al.*, 1987), and the evidence that transcriptional activities of DNA binding proteins are regulated by the convergent activities of protein kinase A and protein kinase C (Hoeffler *et al.*, 1989), it is tempting to suggest that the antidepressant-sensitive, 5-HT-linked and glucocorticoid-responsive β-adrenoceptor system may be involved in a much more general way as an amplification–adaptation system of stimulus transcription coupling and the regulation of brain specific gene expression. The recent demonstration that cyclic AMP, phorbol esters and calcium act synergistically to produce high levels of preproenkephalin mRNA from the human proenkephalin enhancer–promoter (Hyman *et al.*, 1989) is compatible with such a view. The pairing of signal transduction pathways is an important mechanism regulating gene trascription. It remains a great challenge to identify phosphoproteins in brain which reflect the changes in the sensitivity of 5-HT and NA receptor systems and to elucidate the function of these phosphoproteins. The question arises whether some of these as yet unidentified protein substrates for protein kinases, stimulated by second and third messengers, could represent DNA binding proteins that interact with regulatory DNA sequences. The recent report that chronic treatment of rats with antidepressants or ECT causes a translocation of the cyclic AMP-dependent protein kinase from the cytosol to the nucleus (Nestler *et al.*, 1989) is of great interest in this regard. The results demonstrate an action of antidepressants beyond the receptors (amplifier system), if given on a clinically relevant time basis, and suggest this action could be protein kinase A-mediated phosphorylation of nuclear proteins.

In view of these recent developments in signal transduction, future neuropharmacological and psychopathological research on affective disorders will have to focus on events beyond the receptor. The pursuit of the revised amine hypothesis of affective disorders at the level of genomic expression appears to be most promising but necessitates the development of novel approaches and a high degree of experimental sophistication. As previously pointed out, 'one can now entertain the possibility that abnormal behaviour patterns—affective, cognitive, somatosensory—might be the consequence of a disarray in the regulation of gene transcription in response to internal (neurohormonal, endocrine), and external (environmental) stimuli which in turn could make an individual vulnerable to psychiatric disorders' (Sulser, 1989). The challenge is considerable, however, as the brain is estimated to express about 30 000 brain-specific genes (Sutcliffe and Milner, 1984).

Acknowledgements

Studies by the authors were supported by USPHS grant MH-29228, a grant from Hoffmann–La Roche and the Tennessee Department of Mental Health and Mental Retardation.

References

Akiskal, H.S. (1985) *Acta Psychiatr. Scand.* **71** (Suppl. 319), 131–139.

American Psychiatric Association (1987) *Diagnostic and Statistical Manual of Mental Disorders*, 3rd edn. (revised), pp 228–230. Washington DC, American Psychiatric Association.

Anisman, H. & Zacharko, R.M. (1982) *Behav. Brain Sci.* **5**, 89–137.

Åsberg, M., Thoren, P., Traskman, L., Bertilsson, L. & Ringberger, V. (1976a) *Science* **191**, 478–480.

Åsberg, M., Traskman, L. & Thoren, P. (1976b) *Arch. Gen. Psychiatry* **33**, 1193–1197.

Ayd, F. (1957) *Am. J. Psychiatry* **114**, 459.

Baker, G.B. & Greenshaw, A.J. (1989) *Cell. Mol. Neurobiol.* **9**, 1–44.

Banerjee, S.P., Kung, L.S., Riggi, S.J. and Chanda, S.K. (1977) *Nature* **268**, 455–456.

Berridge, M.J. (1987) *Ann. Rev. Biochem.* **56**, 159–193.

Brown, G.L., Goodwin, F.K., Ballenger, J.C. *et al.* (1979) *Psychiatry Res.* **1**, 131–139.

Brunello, N., Barbaccia, M.L., Chuang, D.D. & Costa, E. (1982) *Neuropharmacology* **21**, 1145–1149.

Brunello, N., Volterra, A., Cagiano, R., Ianieri, G.C., Cuomo, V. & Racagni, G. (1985) *Naunyn-Schmiedebergs Arch. Pharmacol.* **331**, 20–22.

Bunney, W.E. and Davis, J.M. (1965) *Arch. Gen. Psychiatry* **13**, 483–494.

Burnstein, K.L. & Cidlowski, J.A. (1989) *Ann. Rev. Physiol.* **51**, 683–699.

Butler, P.D. & Barkai, A.I. (1987) *Adv. Exp. Med. Biol.* **221**, 531–547.

Carlsson, A. (1983) In *Discoveries in Pharmacology*, vol. 1 (eds M.J. Parnham, M.J. & Bruinvels, J.), pp 197–206. Amsterdam, Elsevier.

Checkley, S.A. (1988) *Pharmacopsychiatry* **21**, 6–8.

Checkley, S.A., Palazidow, E., Bearn, J. *et al.* (1990) In *30 Years of Imipramine* (eds Leonard, B.E. & Spencer, P.), pp 135–140. London, CNS Publishers.

Coppen, A. & Wood, K. (1982) *Adv. Biochem. Psychopharmacol.* **34**, 249–258.

Dahlstrom, A. & Fuxe, K. (1964) *Acta Physiol. Scand.* **62** (Suppl. 232), 1–55.

Dal Toso, R., Bernardi, M.A., De Costa, E. & Mochetti, I. (1987) *Neuropharmacology* **26**, 1783–1786.

Delay, J., Laine, B. & Buisson, J.F. (1952) *Ann. Med. Psychol.* **110**, 689–692.

de Montigny, C. and Aghajanian, G.K. (1978) *Science* **202**, 1303–1306.

Dumbrille-Ross, A. & Tang, S.W. (1983) *Psychiatry Res.* **9**, 207–215.

Foote, S.L., Bloom, F.E. & Aston-Jones, G. (1983) *Physiol. Rev.* **63**, 844–914.

Friedman, E. & Dallob, A. (1979) *Commun. Psychopharmacol.* **3**, 89–92.

Friedman, E., Yocca, F.D. & Cooper, T.D. (1984) *J. Pharmacol. Exp. Ther.* **228**, 545–550.

Fries, E.D. (1954) *N. Eng. J. Med.* **251**, 1006–1008.

Gillespie, D.D., Manier, D.H. & Sulser, F. (1989) *Neuropsychopharmacology* **2**, 265–271.

Gilman, A.G. (1987) *Ann. Rev. Biochem.* **56**, 615–649.

Goodwin, F.K., Murphy, D.L., Brodie, H.K.H. & Bunney, W.E. (1970) *Biol. Psychiatry* **2**, 341–366.

Gravel, P. & de Montigny, C. (1987) *Synapse* **1**, 233–239.

Green, A.R. & Deakin, J.F.W. (1980) *Nature* **285**, 232–233.

Harfstrand, A., Fuxe, K., Cintra, A. *et al.* (1986) *Proc. Natl. Acad. Sci. USA* **83**, 9779–9783,

Harrelson, A.L., Rosterre, W. & McEwen, B.S. (1987) *J. Neurochem.* **48**, 1648–1655.

Hartig, P.R. (1989) *Trends Pharmacol. Sci.* **10**, 64–69.

Heydorn, W.E., Brunswick, D.J. & Frazer, A. (1982) *J. Pharmacol. Exp. Ther.* **222**, 534–543.

Hoeffler, J.P., Deutsch, P.J., Lin, J. & Habener, L.F. (1989) *Mol. Endocrinol.* **3**, 868–880.

Hyman, S.E., Comb, M.J. & Nguyeu, T.V. (1989) *Soc. Neurosci. Abstr.* **15**, 645.

Jacobsen, E. (1964) in *Depression*. Proceedings of a Symposium, 22–26 September 1959; Cambridge (ed. Davies, E.B.), New York, Cambridge University Press.

Janowsky, A., Okada, F., Manier, D., Applegate, C.D. & Sulser, F. (1982) *Science* **218**, 900–901.

Kellar, K.J., Cascio, C.S., Butler, J.A. & Kurtizke, R.N. (1981) *Eur. J. Pharmacol.* **69**, 515–518.

Kitayama, I., Janson, A.M., Cintra, A. *et al.* (1988) *J. Neural Transm.* **73**, 191–203.

Koslow, S.H., Maas, J.W., Bowden, C.L., Davis, J.M., Hanim, I. & Javaid, J. (1983) *Arch. Gen. Psychiatry* **40**, 999–1010.

Kuhn, R. (1958) *Am. J. Psychiatry* **115**, 459–464.

Lefkowitz, R.J. & Caron, M.G. (1988) *J. Biol. Chem.* **263**, 4993–4996.

Lehmann, H.E. & Kline, N.S. (1983) In *Discoveries in Pharmacology*, vol. 1 (eds Parnham, M.J. & Bruinvels, J.), pp 209–221. Elsevier, Amsterdam.

Linnoila, M., Virkkunen, M., Scheinin, M. *et al.* (1983) *Life Sci.* **33**, 2609–2614.

Loomer, H.P., Saunders, J.C. & Kline, N.S. (1957) *Am. Psychiatr. Assoc. Psychiatr. Res. Rep.* **8**, 129.

Maas, J.W. (1975) *Arch. Gen. Psychiatry* **32**, 1357–1361.

Maas, J.W. (1986) In *Depression: Basic Mechanisms, Diagnosis and Treatment* (eds Rush, A.J. & Altshuler, Z.), pp 72–83. New York, Guilford Press.

Maas, J.W., Fawcett, J.A. & Dekirmenjian, H. (1972) *Arch. Gen. Psychiatry* **26**, 252–262.

Maas, J.W., Hattox, S.E., Green, N.M. & Landis, D.H. (1979) *Science* **205**, 1025–1027.

Maas, J.W., Koslow, S.H., Katz, M.M. *et al.* (1984) *Am. J. Psychiatry* **141**, 1159–1171.

Maj, J., Mogilnicka, E. & Kordeka, A. (1979) *Neurosci. Lett.* **13**, 337–341.

Manier, D.H., Gillespie, D.D., Steranka, L.R. & Sulser, F. (1984) *Experientia* **40**, 1223–1226.

Manier, D.H., Gillespie, D.D. & Sulser, F. (1987) *Biochem. Pharmacol.* **36**, 3308–3310.

Meltzer, H.Y. (ed.) (1987) *Psychopharmacology: The Third Generation of Progress*. Raven Press, New York.

Meltzer, H.Y. & Lowy, M.T. (1987) In *Psychopharmacology: The Third Generation of Progress* (ed Meltzer, H.Y.), pp 513–526. New York, Raven Press.

Mendlewicz, J. & Youdim, M.B.H. (1980) *J. Affective Disord.* **2**, 137–146.

Mobley, P.L. & Sulser, F. (1980) *Nature* **286**, 608–609.

Mobley, P.L., Manier, D.H. & Sulser, F. (1983) *J. Pharmacol. Exp. Ther.* **226**, 71–77.

Muller, J.C., Pryor, W.W., Gibbons, J.E. & Orgain, E.S. (1955) *J.A.M.A.* **159**, 836–839.

Murphy, D.L., Campbell, I. & Costa, J.L. (1978) In *Psychopharmacology: A Generation of Progress* (eds M.A. Lipton, M.A., DiMascio, A. & Killam, K.F.), pp 1235–1247. New York, Raven Press.

Nestler, E.J., Walaas, S.T. & Greengard, P. (1984) *Science* **225**, 1357–1364.

Nestler, E.J., Terwilliger, R.Z. & Duman, R.S. (1989) *J. Neurochem.* **53**, 1644–1647.

Nimgaonkar, V.L., Goodwin, G.M., Davies, C.L. & Green, A.R. (1985) *Neuropharmacology* **24**, 279–283.

Offord, S.J., Ordway, G.A. & Frazer, A. (1988) *J. Pharmacol. Exp. Ther.* **244**, 144–153.

Olpe, H.R. & Schellenberg, A. (1980) *Eur. J. Pharmacol.* **63**, 7–13.

Owens, M.J. & Nemeroff, C.B. (1988) In *The Hypothalamic–Pituitary–Adrenal Axis: Physiology, Pathophysiology, and Psychiatric Implications* (eds Schatzberg, A.F. & Nemeroff, C.B.), pp 1–36. New York, Raven Press.

Paykel, E.S. (1979) In *The Psychobiology of the Depressive Disorders: Implications for the Effects of Stress* (ed Depue, R.A.), pp 245–262. New York, Academic Press.

Redmond, D.E. & Huang, Y.H. (1979) *Life Sci.* **25**, 2149–2162.

Riva, M.A. & Creese, I. (1989a) *Mol. Pharmacol.* **36**, 201–210.

Riva, M.A. & Creese, I. (1989b) *Mol. Pharmacol.* **36**, 211–218.

Roberts, V.J., Singhal, R.L. & Roberts, D.C.S. (1984) *Eur. J. Pharmacol.* **103**, 235–240.

Ross, E.M. (1989) *Neuron* **3**, 141–152.

Roy, A. & Linnoila, M. (1988) *Acta Psychiatr. Scand.* **78**, 529–535.

Sanders-Bush, E., Breeding, M., Knoth, K. & Tsutsuimi, M. (1989) *Psychopharmacology* **99**, 64–69.

Schildkraut, J.J. (1965) *Am. J. Psychiatry* **122**, 509–522.

Schildkraut, J.J. (1978) In *Psychopharmacology: A Generation of Progress* (eds Lipton, M.A., DiMascio, A. & Killam, K.F.), pp 1223–1234. New York, Raven Press.

Schildkraut, J.J. & Kety, S.S. (1967) *Science* **156**, 21–30.

Schultz, J. (1976) *Nature* **261**, 417–418.

Sellinger, M.D., Mendels, J. & Frazer, A. (1980) *Neuropharmacology* **19**, 447–454.

Shopsin, B., Gershon, S., Goldstein, M. *et al.* (1975) *Psychopharmacol. Commun.* **1**, 239–249.

Shopsin, B., Friedman, E. & Gershon, S. (1976) *Arch. Gen. Psychiatry* **3**, 811–819.

Siever, L.J. (1987) In *Psychopharmacology: The Third Generation of Progress* (ed. Meltzer, H.Y.), pp. 493–504. New York, Raven Press.

Siggins, G.R. & Schultz, J.E. (1979) *Proc. Natl. Acad. Sci. USA* **6**, 5987–5991.

Simson, P.E. & Weiss, J.M. (1988) *Neuropsychopharmacology* **1**, 287–295.

Stockmeier, C.A. & Kellar, K.J. (1988) *Eur. J. Pharmacol.* **153**, 135–139.

Stockmeier, C.A. & Kellar, K.J. (1989) *Mol. Pharmacol.* **36**, 903–911.

Stokes, P.E. & Jiles, C.R. (1987) In *Psychopharmacology: The Third Generation of Progress* (ed. Meltzer, H.Y.), pp 589–607. New York, Raven Press.

Sulser, F. (1984) *Neuropharmacology* **23**, 255–261.

Sulser, F. (1989) *Eur. Arch. Psychiatry Neurol. Sci.* **238**, 231–237.

Sulser, F. (1991) In *Refractory Depression-Frontiers in Research and Treatment* (ed. Amsterdam, J.T.). New York, Raven Press (in press).

Sulser, F. & Mishra, R. (1983) In *Discoveries in Pharmacology*, vol. 1 (eds Parnham, M.J. & Bruinvels, J.), pp 233–247. Amsterdam, Elsevier.

Sulser, F. & Sanders-Bush, E. (1987) In *Molecular Basis of Neuronal Responsiveness* (eds Ehrlich, Y.H., Lenox, R.H., Kornecki, E. & Berry, W.O.), pp 489–502. New York, Plenum Press.

Sulser, F. & Sanders-Bush, E. (1989) In *Tribute to B.B. Brodie* (ed. Costa, E.), pp 289–302. New York, Raven Press.

Sutcliffe, J.G. and Milner, R.J. (1984) *Trends Biochem. Sci.* **9**, 95–99.

van Praag, H.M. (1982) *Lancet* **ii**, 1259–1264.

van Praag, H.M. and de Hann, S. (1981) *Acta Psychiatr. Scand.* **63** (Suppl. 290), 191–205.

Vetulani, J. & Sulser, F. (1975) *Nature* **257**, 495–496.

Walsh, D.A. & Ashby, C.S. (1973) *Recent Prog. Horm. Res.* **29**, 329–359.

Weiss, J.M. & Simson, P.E. (1988) In *Mechanisms of Physical and Emotional Stress* (eds Chrousos, G.P., Loriaux, D.L. & Gold, P.W.), pp 425–440. New York, Plenum Press.

Yoshikawa, K. & Sabol, St. (1986a) *Mol. Brain Res.* **1**, 75–83.

Yoshikawa, K. & Sabol, St. (1986b) *Biochem. Biophys. Res. Commun.* **139**, 1–10.

Zeller, E.A. (1982) In *Discoveries in Pharmacology*, vol. 1 (eds Parnham, M.J. & Bruinvels, J.), pp 223–232. Amsterdam, Elsevier.

CHAPTER 4

PERIPHERAL MARKERS
IN AFFECTIVE DISORDERS

J.M. Elliott

Department of Pharmacology and Toxicology,
St Mary's Hospital Medical School, Norfolk Place, London W2 1PG, UK

Table of Contents

BIOLOGICAL ASPECTS OF AFFECTIVE DISORDERS
ISBN 0-12-356510-3

4.1 Background

The development of biochemical tests that can aid in psychiatric diagnosis represents a major goal for research workers. If successful, this may help not only in diagnosis but also in understanding the biochemical aetiology of depressive disorders and hence lead to the development of more precise pharmacological tools for their treatment. Following the establishment of the monoamine theory of depression, numerous studies attempted to correlate depressive status with the levels of monoamines and their metabolites in body fluids, but as indicated below the success of such an approach has been limited. Consequently the search for biochemical parameters which parallel the therapeutic time-course of antidepressant drug action has concentrated attention on the amine receptors rather than the neurotransmitters themselves. Animal models have suggested β-adrenoceptors to be implicated in the action of numerous unrelated antidepressant therapies, based on the actions of drugs, electroconvulsive shock treatment and rapid eye movement (REM) sleep deprivation. Modulation of other receptors and their function, particularly α-adrenoceptors and 5-hydroxytryptamine (5-HT)-related receptors, has also been described following such treatment. However, the extrapolation of such data to man is handicapped by the possibility of species differences and concern that the biochemical changes may reflect responses to toxic rather than therapeutic dose of the drugs. Biochemical investigations in man are primarily limited by the accessibility of suitable tissue. Consequently the majority of studies have concentrated on blood cells, particularly platelets and leucocytes, although the culturing of fibroblasts (and potentially other cells) *in vitro* has extended the range of possibilities. The advantage of such studies is that they overcome the problem of species difference, but at the cost of introducing tissue differences. In addition the *ex vivo* analysis of platelets and leucocytes allows simultaneous comparison between biochemical data and affective status as determined by the psychiatrist, leading to potential state-dependent markers. Furthermore, the biochemical response to antidepressant drug treatment may differ in depressed patients, in whom some biochemical dysfunction is presumed to exist, compared with healthy, normal subjects as exemplified in recent studies (Braddock *et al.*, 1984, 1986). This contrasts with the situation in animal studies where usually 'non-depressed' naïve animals are used to investigate antidepressant drug effects.

The major questions which must be addressed when investigating a peripheral model as a biochemical marker for affective disorders are: (1) Within which particular sub-categories of affective disorder is the model reliable? (2) Does the model represent a state or trait marker and to what extent is it effective in diagnosis? (3) Does the model reflect similar changes within the brain, hence does it represent a primary or secondary biochemical marker? (4) How does the observed difference between healthy and depressed subjects arise and can this information improve our understanding of the biochemical changes associated with affective disorder? In this chapter I will attempt to answer these questions in relation to several proposed peripheral markers of depression, particularly those associated with monoamine receptors and uptake systems.

According to the original monoamine hypothesis of affective disorders (Schildkraut, 1965; Lapin and Oxenkrug, 1969), depression in man is associated with a decrease in noradrenergic and/or serotonergic function. This could result from a change in either presynaptic function (decreased monoamine synthesis, storage or release) or postsynaptic response (decreased receptor number and/or activity). Despite some initial supportive claims, intensive biochemical studies have failed to demonstrate any consistent change in presynaptic function in patients with affective disorders (Sugrue, 1981). Consequently, attempts have been made to subclassify depressive disorders on the basis of increased or decreased levels of noradrenaline and 5-HT and their metabolites, as detected in plasma, urine or cerebrospinal fluid (CSF).

The characterization of hypoadrenergic and hyperadrenergic subgroups based on urinary noradrenaline metabolite levels does not correspond with any of the traditional diagnostic subtypes of affective disorders, although it is claimed that hypoadrenergic patients may respond preferentially to anti-depressants such as desipramine and maprotiline which selectively enhance noradrenaline function (Schildkraut *et al.*, 1978). In relation to serotonergic activity, the level of 5-hydroxyindoleacetic acid (5-HIAA) in CSF is reported to be decreased in depressed patients with a history of attempted suicide (Asberg *et al.*, 1976, 1986; Roy *et al.*, 1989), although the effect has also been associated with more generalized impulsive aggressive behaviour (Brown *et al.*, 1979). The implications of these studies for biochemical aetiology and drug therapy have yet to be determined.

4.2 Peripheral β-adrenoceptors

4.2.1 Characterization of the leucocyte β-adrenoceptor

Investigation of the effects of chronic rather than acute treatment with antidepressant drugs in animals led to the proposal of an alternative hypothesis regarding the aetiology of affective disorders (see Chapter 3) which appears diametrically opposed to the original monoamine hypothesis. Down-regulation and/or desensitization of brain β-adrenoceptor number and function was consistently observed in response to various antidepressant drugs (Vetulani *et al.*, 1976; Banerjee *et al.*, 1977; Wolfe *et al.*, 1978), suggesting that β-adrenoceptor function and hence noradrenergic sensitivity may be enhanced in depressed patients. However, the original monoamine hypothesis proposed a deficit in noradrenergic activity which, in the absence of any presynaptic noradrenaline deficiency, would suggest that β-adrenoceptor function should be decreased in depressed patients. It is therefore important to investigate the human β-adrenoceptor in relation to depression in order to differentiate between these two conflicting hypotheses. Since access to extant neuronal tissue is not ethically feasible in depression, it is important to establish a valid, accessible peripheral model of human β-adrenoceptor function.

The human leucocyte expresses β-adrenoceptors which can be readily characterized by radioligand binding methods and which are positively coupled to adenylate cyclase. Modulation of these receptors has been demonstrated in subjects with bronchial asthma (Parker and Smith, 1973; Alston *et al.*, 1974; Conolly and Greenacre, 1976), hence the leucocyte has become a popular model for the study of human β-adrenoceptors in affective disorders.

4.2.2 Adenylate cyclase activity

Initial studies indicated a decreased sensitivity of leucocytes from depressed patients to synthesize cAMP in response to isoprenaline (Pandey *et al.*, 1979), associated with a decrease in β-adrenoceptor number (Extein *et al.*, 1979). Subsequent studies have in the main confirmed these findings. The decreased cAMP response appears to be specific to β-agonists, since the responses to prostaglandin E_1 (PGE_1) and forskolin are not different from controls (Pandey *et al.*, 1979; Ebstein *et al.*, 1988) and it reflects a decrease in maximal enzyme activity rather than affinity (Halper *et al.*, 1988), commensurate with a reduction in the number of β-adrenoceptors. The effect has been reported in mixed leucocyte (Pandey *et al.*, 1979) and lymphocyte (Mann *et al.*, 1985; Ebstein *et al.*, 1988; Halper *et al.*, 1988) preparations but was not observed in polymorphonuclear leucocytes (Kanof *et al.*, 1989). In one study the response to noradrenaline plus phentolamine was increased in leucocytes from patients with untreated manic-depressive illness compared with euthymic patients, although the response to isoprenaline was not significantly different (Klysner *et al.*, 1987). Comparison between unipolar and bipolar depressed patients revealed no significant difference in isoprenaline-induced cAMP response (Ebstein *et al.*, 1988) and no correlation has been observed between the degree of reduced response and the severity of depression as indicated by the Hamilton depression rating scale (Mann *et al.*, 1985; Ebstein *et al.*, 1988; Halper *et al.*, 1988). In one study a significant negative correlation was reported between the psychomotor agitation score and the isoprenaline-induced cAMP increase (Mann *et al.*, 1985) but this was not replicated in a later study (Halper *et al.*, 1988). The effect of drug treatment on adenylate cyclase activity in depressed patients has not been investigated directly. However, untreated depressed patients who did not subsequently respond to treatment initially displayed weaker isoprenaline sensitivity than those who later responded to treatment (Ebstein *et al.*, 1988). Therefore leucocyte β-adrenoceptor adenylate cyclase activity appears to be diminished in depressed patients, although the extent of this biochemical change does not parallel the severity of the depressive disorder. This biochemical change may, however, be a useful indicator of therapeutic response to antidepressant treatment.

4.2.3 Radioligand binding studies

A reduction in β-adrenoceptor binding capacity on leucocyte membranes from depressed patients has been identified using both tritiated (Carstens *et al.*, 1987) and iodinated (Pandey *et al.*, 1987; Magliozzi *et al.*, 1989) radioligands. Simultaneous assay of both receptor binding and function by

Extein *et al.* (1979) indicated a general correspondence, although Mann *et al.* (1985) observed a significant reduction in cAMP response without a significant decrease in receptor number. The binding in this study, however, was performed on intact cells which may decrease the sensitivity of the assay (Graafsma *et al.*, 1986). Separate analysis of isoprenaline stimulated adenylate cyclase activity (Pandey *et al.*, 1979) and β-adrenoceptor binding (Pandey *et al.*, 1987) have identified concordant decreases in receptor number and function. As with the adenylate cyclase response, the reduction in binding capacity does not correlate with the severity of depression (Mann *et al.*, 1985; Pandey *et al.*, 1987). In one study where lymphocyte β-adrenoceptor capacity was significantly reduced in depressed patients compared with controls, a positive correlation was observed between receptor number and severity of illness as identified by both Hamilton and Beck self-evaluation scales (Carstens *et al.*, 1987). The authors could offer no explanation for this apparently paradoxical observation. The reduction in β-adrenoceptor number does not appear to represent a state-dependent marker for depression, since this effect is apparent in euthymic bipolar depressives receiving lithium (Wood *et al.*, 1986) and was not altered by a course of electroconvulsive therapy which resulted in significant clinical improvement (Cooper *et al.*, 1985). One group has reported a decrease in receptor number following antidepressant drug treatment but their depressed patients initially manifested abnormally high β-adrenoceptor number compared with controls (Healy *et al.*, 1983, 1985). A significant increase in receptor number has also been reported in lymphocytes of post-partum (Butler and Leonard, 1986) and juvenile (Carstens *et al.*, 1988) depressed patients, suggesting that β-adrenoceptor changes may be variable according to specific subtypes of depression.

Hence, leucocyte studies provide some evidence for decreased β-adrenoceptor activity in depressed patients, although several contradictory reports indicate either no change or even increased receptor activity. A decrease in β-adrenoceptor function does not appear to be a general response to psychiatric illness since it is not found in schizophrenic patients (Pandey *et al.*, 1979, 1987; Kanof *et al.*, 1989). Neither is it specific to depression, since similar decreases have been reported in agoraphobic patients when coupled with panic attacks (Brown *et al.*, 1988), and in unipolar depressed patients a significant negative correlation was detected between β-adrenoceptor number and frequency of panic attacks (Magliozzi *et al.*, 1989).

4.2.4 Factors modulating leucocyte β-adrenoceptor activity

Before attempting to interpret these receptor changes, it is necessary to be aware of other factors which may modify β-adrenoceptor activity. As noted above, desensitization and down-regulation of leucocyte β-adrenoceptors in asthmatic patients in response to treatment with β-agonists is well characterized

(Conolly and Greenacre, 1976; Lee *et al.*, 1977) and similar changes have been associated with elevated endogenous plasma catecholamine levels (Fraser *et al.*, 1981; Feldman *et al.*, 1983). Even at physiological catecholamine concentrations, desensitization of lymphocyte β-adrenoceptors has been demonstrated by the increase in receptor number following treatment with β-blockers (Aarons *et al.*, 1980). High levels of plasma catecholamines in depressed patients have been observed in some of the studies mentioned above (Cooper *et al.*, 1985; Buckholtz *et al.*, 1988) and may be anticipated in the situations of psychomotor agitation (Mann *et al.*, 1985) and panic attack (Magliozzi *et al.*, 1989). However, increased monoamine levels are not a consistent feature of depression, therefore it is unlikely that the phenomenon of β-adrenoceptor dysfunction in depression can be ascribed entirely to desensitization following chronic overstimulation.

In addition to the effects of β-agonists, studies in asthmatic patients have demonstrated that treatment with glucocorticoids can restore the sensitivity of the leucocyte β-adrenoceptor after desensitization (Logsdon *et al.*, 1972; Lee *et al.*, 1977) and in normal subjects can directly increase β-adrenoceptor number (Davies and Lefkowitz, 1980). Hypersecretion of cortisol is frequently observed in depressed patients (Gibbons and McHugh, 1962; Halbreich *et al.*, 1985) but is also associated with decreased corticosteroid sensitivity, as indicated by the dexamethasone suppression test (DST) (Carroll *et al.*, 1981; Stokes *et al.*, 1984) and by a decrease in the number of glucocorticoid binding sites in lymphocytes (Gormley *et al.*, 1985; Whalley *et al.*, 1986). If the latter effect predominates, then the observed decrease in β-adrenoceptor activity in lymphocytes from depressed patients may reflect the decreased sustaining effects of glucocorticoids. Support for this hypothesis comes from the observation that lymphocyte β-adrenoceptor activity was found to be lower in DST non-suppressors than suppressors in a range of both depressed and schizophrenic patients (Pandey *et al.*, 1987; Halper *et al.*, 1988), although this was not confirmed in another smaller study (Carstens *et al.*, 1987).

Besides these biochemical effects, some studies have reported cytological changes in leucocyte number and composition in depressed patients (Kronfol *et al.*, 1984, 1985; Murphy *et al.*, 1987), the cause of which is unclear. This would have implications for β-adrenoceptor activity if, as described by some, different subpopulations of leucocytes expressed the receptor to differing degrees (Pochet *et al.*, 1979; Krawietz *et al.*, 1982; Landmann *et al.*, 1984).

4.2.5 β-Adrenoceptor activity in cultured fibroblasts and lymphoblasts

Apart from *ex vivo* studies in leucocytes, β-adrenoceptor function has also been investigated in cultured human fibroblasts and lymphoblasts obtained from depressed and normal subjects. Since these cells are cultured in an artificial environment, any state-dependent effects will be rapidly lost, therefore most studies have concentrated on trait markers within bipolar depressed patients, who demonstrate the strongest hereditary trait amongst the affective disorders (McGuffin and Katz, 1989). The advantage of such studies lies in their avoidance of receptor modulation by plasma catecholamines and hormones, revealing possible differences in intrinsic β-adrenoceptor activity. However, this must be balanced against possible artefactual changes induced by the synthetic media used to nourish the cells and, in the case of lymphoblasts, the viral transformation procedure. Wright *et al.* (1984) reported consistently low binding of [^{125}I]hydroxybenzylpindolol to β-adrenoceptors in four out of six cell lines from bipolar depressed patients but only one out of eight familial controls. However Berrettini *et al.* (1987b) reported no significant difference in β-adrenoceptor binding between cells derived from 17 bipolar depressed patients and 14 unrelated controls. Berrettini *et al.* (1987a) also reported no significant difference in fibroblast adenylate cyclase response to isoprenaline between 12 bipolar patients and 13 unrelated controls, nor in the desensitization observed in such cells following 24-h incubation with isoprenaline. These results suggest that depression may be associated with an hereditary change in β-adrenoceptor activity in some families but clearly not in all cases, and therefore provide further evidence for genetic heterogeneity amongst the depressive disorders.

4.2.6 Summary

Overall these studies suggest that peripheral indicators of human β-adrenoceptor activity are decreased in depressed patients compared with controls. The extent of receptor dysfunction is not related to the severity of the depressive disorder and does not normalize after successful treatment, indicating that it is not a state-dependent marker. The effect is not restricted to any particular subtypes of depressive disorder, although it seems more marked amongst bipolar patients. There appears to be no intrinsic difference in the receptor between depressed patients and controls, as indicated by similar binding affinities. The reduced receptor number in depressed patients therefore probably reflects a difference in regulation either at the synthetic level (transcription and/or translation) or the degradative level (uncoupling, desensitization and down-regulation). Lymphoblast studies provide evidence for distinct genetic differences in β-adrenoceptor number in bipolar depressed patients within some, but by no means all, families. The question of enhanced β-adrenoceptor down-regulation among depressed subjects has not yet been fully assessed. Clearly high plasma catecholamines and reduced glucocorticoid sensitivity, each of which has been identified with depressive disorders, may lead to a decrease in β-adrenoceptor response. A combination of these factors may therefore represent the highest likelihood of a decrease in receptor activity.

However, it is unclear at present whether the reduced receptor function in depressed subjects represents a normal response to abnormal hormonal activity or whether the β-adrenoceptor itself is particularly sensitive to these factors in the depressed patient.

The decreased β-adrenoceptor activity indicated by these peripheral markers corresponds with the prediction of the original monoamine hypothesis (assuming no change in presynaptic adrenergic function) and contradicts the hypothesis of enhanced receptor activity derived from the effect of chronic antidepressant drug treatment in animal models. However, the validity of these peripheral cells as markers for the neuronal β-adrenoceptor is open to question. Notably the receptor located on each of these peripheral cells is the β_2-subtype, whereas that which is modified by antidepressant drugs in rat brain is exclusively the β_1-subtype (Minneman et al., 1979; Heal et al., 1989). Both receptor subtypes are positively linked to adenylate cyclase and can undergo desensitization and down-regulation in response to prolonged agonist stimulation. The selective effect of antidepressants on β_1-adrenoceptors in rat brain may simply reflect differential anatomical location, with the β_2-adrenoceptors being predominantly extrasynaptic. However, the two receptor subtypes derive from different gene products and may therefore differ in their mode of regulation. Secondly, the chemical environment within the synapse and the circulation are different. As indicated above, the leucocyte β-adrenoceptor is modulated by numerous plasma factors; therefore, changes in this receptor may occur as a consequence of some other primary factor(s) whose plasma concentration is closely allied to the subjects' depressive status. This would not discount the β-adrenoceptor as a peripheral marker in depression but may question the relevance of changes on this peripheral cell to that of the neuronal cell, and hence the role of the β-adrenoceptor in the biochemical aetiology of depression.

Comparison with post-mortem studies of the β-adrenoceptor in human brain from depressed and normal subjects is complicated by the diverse findings reported to date (see Chapter 6). However, the parallel between the decreased receptor activity observed in leucocytes of depressed patients and that in cerebral cortical tissue of patients with an identified history of depression (rather than those identified solely on the grounds of suicide) supports the role of these peripheral cells as neuronal markers of β-adrenoceptor activity and the significance of the β-adrenoceptor change to the biochemical mechanism of depression in man.

4.2.7 Future investigations

Having established that a decrease in leucocyte β-adrenoceptor number and/or function is frequently associated with major depressive disorder, future investigations should attempt to identify the mechanism(s) responsible for this change and its relevance to therapeutic outcome. A number of hypotheses can be considered.

Firstly, the β-adrenoceptor itself may be defective, resulting from a modification of the gene code. Such a change should reveal a trait marker evident in all body tissues. Although polymorphism of the human β_2-adrenoceptor DNA has been identified (Lentes et al., 1988), there has been no report associating such an effect with depressive disorder. Furthermore, the affinity of the leucocyte β-adrenoceptor for either radioligands or isoprenaline stimulation of adenylate cyclase revealed no significant difference between depressed and normal subjects, suggesting no intrinsic difference in receptor function.

If the receptor itself is not altered, then the observed effects may result from changes in the regulation of receptor activity. This could derive from either a genetic modification of the mechanisms responsible for the synthesis and/or degradation of the receptor, or from a modification of entirely separate factors which in turn modulate receptor activity. Included within the latter category are plasma catecholamines and corticosteroids and possibly other hormones, including sex steroids and thyroid hormones, which modify β-adrenoceptors in animal tissues. The extent to which receptor regulation is altered in depressive disorders has not been widely investigated. Using cultured fibroblast cells, Berrettini et al. (1987a) found no difference in desensitization sensitivity between normal and bipolar depressed subjects. Additional investigations using other tissues and studying interactions with factors other than catecholamines should clarify the regulatory status of the β-adrenoceptor in depressive disorders. If neither the intrinsic receptor nor its regulatory mechanism is altered in depressed patients, then the β-adrenoceptor modifications noted above may simply reflect changes in some circulatory factor(s) which directly modulate the receptor. In order to differentiate between these various possibilities, future studies should encompass a range of variables, assessing β-adrenoceptor function together with measurements of modulatory factors such as plasma catecholamines and corticosteroid sensitivity.

4.3 Platelet α_2-adrenoceptors

4.3.1 Characterization of the platelet α_2-adrenoceptor

Central neuronal α_2-adrenoceptors are located at both presynaptic and postsynaptic sites. Their implication in the biochemistry of affective disorders derives from animal and human studies. In the rat, chronic treatment with some, but not all, antidepressants reduces α_2-adrenoceptor number in the brain and brings about changes in several associated functional parameters, including motor activity, sedation, hypothermia and regulation of neuro-transmitter release (Green and Nutt, 1985). In man, neuroendocrine and cardiovascular responses to the α_2-adrenoceptor agonist clonidine are attenuated in some depressed patients and may be modified following chronic antidepressant treatment (Katona et al., 1987). The human platelet expresses α_2-adrenoceptors which are qualitatively similar in biochemical terms to those found in human brain and to a slightly lesser degree to those in rat brain (Summers et al., 1983). According to current nomenclature the platelet receptor is of the α_{2A}-subtype whose genomic origin is located on chromosome 10 (Kobilka et al., 1987). The receptor is negatively coupled to adenylate cyclase (Gierschik and Jakobs, 1988), although other postreceptor mechanisms have been proposed (Nunnari et al., 1987), and stimulation of the receptor will initiate or potentiate platelet aggregation. The receptor has been labelled by a variety of agonist, partial agonist and antagonist radioligands, both in intact cells and in membrane preparations. Indeed, as described below, much of the confusion surrounding the status of the platelet α_2-adrenoceptor in affective disorders stems from the diversity of ligands used.

4.3.2 Platelet α_2-adrenoceptors in affective disorders

4.3.2.1 Antagonist radioligand binding studies

In an attempt to monitor human α_2-adrenoceptor activity in relation to affective disorder, several groups have characterized platelet α_2-adrenoceptor in untreated depressed patients compared with matched healthy controls, as summarized in Table 1. Using the selective α_2-adrenoceptor antagonists, [^{3}H]yohimbine or [^{3}H]rauwolscine, there is general agreement that receptor number is not altered in depressed patients compared with healthy controls (Elliott, 1984). Consistent with this finding, no correlation has been observed between receptor number and severity of depression as rated on the Hamilton scale (Pimoule et al., 1983; Stahl et al., 1983a; Braddock et al., 1986; Katona et al., 1989). Most of the patients studied fall within the endogenous category and attempts to distinguish between unipolar and bipolar, endogenous and non-endogenous or DST suppressors and non-suppressors have similarly failed to reveal any differences in receptor number (Braddock et al., 1986; Katona et al., 1989). Using the non-selective α-adrenoceptor antagonist [^{3}H]dihydro-ergocryptine ([^{3}H]DHE), conflicting reports have been made of both increased and decreased binding in depressed patients. In two of these studies (Kafka et al., 1981; Siever et al., 1984) the binding affinity of [^{3}H]DHE was substantially lower than that generally reported, questioning the equivalence

Table 1 Comparison of platelet α_2-adrenoceptor number in control subjects and drug-free depressed patients.

Reference	Radioligand	No. control/depressed	Difference B_{max} depressed versus control (%)
Daiguchi et al. (1981)	[^{3}H]Yohimbine	9/11	NSD
Pimoule et al. (1983)	[^{3}H]Rauwolscine	26/19	NSD
Stahl et al. (1983a)	[^{3}H]Yohimbine	29/16	NSD
Smith et al. (1983)	[^{3}H]Yohimbine	19/5	NSD
Campbell et al. (1985)	[^{3}H]Yohimbine	14/12	NSD
Braddock et al. (1986)	[^{3}H]Yohimbine	39/48	NSD
Wolfe et al. (1987)	[^{3}H]Yohimbine	18/31	NSD
Sevy et al. (1989)	[^{3}H]Yohimbine	14/14	NSD
Katona et al. (1989)	[^{3}H]Yohimbine	44/46	NSD
Garcia-Sevilla et al. (1981a)	[^{3}H]DHE	9/14	−31
Kafka et al. (1981)	[^{3}H]DHE	51/23	+41
Healy et al. (1983)	[^{3}H]DHE	8/19	+52
Siever et al. (1984)	[^{3}H]DHE	51/23	+65
Garcia-Sevilla et al. (1981b)	[^{3}H]Clonidine	21/17	+32
Smith et al. (1983)	[^{3}H]Clonidine	19/5	+38
Doyle et al. (1985)	[^{3}H]Clonidine	10/13	+96
Garcia-Sevilla et al. (1986b)	[^{3}H]Clonidine	20/13	+51
Georgotas et al. (1987)	[^{3}H]Clonidine	10/14	NSD
Pandey et al. (1989)	[^{3}H]Clonidine	33/24	+47
Takeda et al. (1989)	[^{3}H]Clonidine	14/14	+35
Carstens et al. (1986a)	[^{3}H]PAC	22/26	−18
Piletz and Halaris (1988)	[^{3}H]PAC	9/9	NSD
Garcia-Sevilla et al. (1987)	[^{3}H]Adrenaline	23/14	+38
Theodorou et al. (1986)	[^{3}H]UK14304	14/13	NSD

Numerical values for comparison of depressed versus control subjects indicate statistically significant differences.
NSD, non-significant difference.

of the sites labelled to the α_2-adrenoceptor. Indeed, the same workers reported contradictory changes in [^{3}H]DHE binding and noradrenaline-induced inhibition of platelet adenylate cyclase (Siever *et al.*, 1984). Previous studies have identified more sites labelled by [^{3}H]DHE than by the selective α_2-adrenoceptor ligands [^{3}H]yohimbine and [^{3}H]rauwolscine (Motulsky and Insel, 1982; Boon *et al.*, 1983b), although there is no evidence for the existence of α_1-adrenoceptors on the human platelet (Elliott and Grahame-Smith, 1982). The precise nature of these additional sites and their relevance to α_2-adrenoceptor function is not clear at present.

4.3.2.2 Agonist and partial agonist radioligand binding studies

Using the partial agonist [^{3}H]clonidine, several groups have reported increased binding capacity in depressed patients compared with controls. However, one contradictory study found no significant difference between elderly depressed patients and age-matched controls (Georgotas *et al.*, 1987). In earlier studies the increased binding was not related to the severity of the illness (Garcia-Sevilla *et al.*, 1981b, 1986b) but two recent studies report a significant positive correlation between binding capacity assayed before treatment and either the initial depression rating score (Takeda *et al.*, 1989) or the decrease in depression rating after conclusion of treatment (Pandey *et al.*, 1989). Functional significance of the increased binding has been demonstrated by means of increased platelet aggregation response to adrenaline (Garcia-Sevilla *et al.*, 1983, 1986b). Occasionally in these studies the increased binding capacity was associated with a decrease in binding affinity (Garcia-Sevilla *et al.*, 1986a; Takeda *et al.*, 1989). As with other agonists, analysis of the binding data is complicated by the existence of high and low affinity sites, giving rise to curvilinear Scatchard plots. In the case of [^{3}H]clonidine the affinity for these two sites differs by a factor of five or less (Garcia-Sevilla *et al.*, 1981b, 1986a). Hence, accurate determination of the binding characteristics at each site requires data gathered over a wide range of ligand concentrations and analysed by computerized non-linear regression methods. Simple allocation of points on the Scatchard plot to the high or low affinity site and subsequent independent linear regression analysis, as performed in several of the studies indicated in Table 1, is liable to subjective bias and should therefore be avoided. The increased binding of [^{3}H]clonidine in depressed patients is generally associated with the high-affinity site, although equivalent but non-significant increases in the number of low-affinity sites have also been reported (Garcia-Sevilla *et al.*, 1981b, 1986b). We have recently suggested a novel method for distinguishing between binding at the high-affinity GTP-sensitive site and the lower affinity GTP-insensitive site by employing guanine nucleotides to define specific binding of agonist radioligands at α_2-adrenoceptors

(Payvandi *et al.*, 1990b). This method conveys the advantage that estimates for each site can be achieved by independent one-site analysis, thereby improving on the resolving power of two-site analysis.

[^{3}H]PAC (*p*-aminoclonidine) is structurally and biochemically similar to clonidine and although few studies have employed this ligand, the results contrast surprisingly with those using [^{3}H]clonidine. Only one study found increased binding in depressed patients, specifically in adolescent subjects (Carstens *et al.*, 1988), whereas the same authors reported significantly lower binding in adult subjects (Carstens *et al.*, 1986a), and yet another group found no significant difference in binding between depressed patients and healthy controls (Piletz and Halaris, 1988). As with [^{3}H]clonidine, these changes seem to be evident at the high affinity site and, although discrimination between the two sites is somewhat greater for [^{3}H]PAC (approximately 17-fold), analysis using the two-site model is again complex. By contrast, the full agonist [^{3}H]UK14304 displays 50-fold difference in affinity for the two α_2-adrenoceptor states (Neubig *et al.*, 1985; Gibson *et al.*, 1986); therefore, at low nanomolar concentrations binding is predominantly to the high affinity state, resulting in approximately linear Scatchard plots. Using this ligand, Theodorou *et al.* (1986) observed no significant difference in binding capacity between depressed and healthy subjects. The full agonist [^{3}H]adrenaline similarly labels only one site at low concentration (Garcia-Sevilla and Fuster, 1986). Investigations using this ligand identified increased binding capacity in depressed patients with melancholia (Garcia-Sevilla *et al.*, 1987). However, comparison of the absolute binding capacities of [^{3}H]adrenaline (50 fmol/mg protein) and [^{3}H]UK14304 (258 fmol/mg protein) in the control subjects of these studies reveal substantial differences, suggesting that [^{3}H]adrenaline may label a subset of those α_2-adrenoceptors which are linked to guanine nucleotide binding proteins and display high affinity for agonists.

4.3.3 Effect of antidepressant treatment on the platelet α_2-adrenoceptor

The effect of antidepressant treatment on platelet α_2-adrenoceptor binding similarly varies according to the radioligand employed. Using [^{3}H]yohimbine or [^{3}H]rauwolscine, most studies report no significant changes following 1–6 weeks treatment with antidepressant drugs (Pimoule *et al.*, 1983; Stahl *et al.*, 1983a; Campbell *et al.*, 1985; Katona *et al.*, 1989; Wolfe *et al.*, 1989) or electroconvulsive shock (Cooper *et al.*, 1985). Significant clinical improvement occurred in the majority of patients treated. In one study a small but significant decrease (12%) in [^{3}H]yohimbine binding capacity occurred following treatment of depressed patients with amitriptyline for 4–6 weeks, although no significant correlation was observed between the fall in binding and the decrease in Hamilton rating score (Braddock et al., 1986). Administration of amitriptyline at a similar dose to healthy volunteers for 3 weeks did not alter [^{3}H]yohimbine binding (Braddock et al., 1984), suggesting a differential response in depressed and non-depressed subjects, although the relatively shorter duration of treatment in volunteers may also account for this difference.

Using [^{3}H]DHE, Healy et al. (1983) reported a significant reduction in binding in those depressed patients showing clinical improvement, but no change in patients who did not benefit from treatment. Conversely, Wood et al. (1985a) observed no difference in [^{3}H]DHE binding between euthymic bipolar patients receiving lithium and untreated depressed patients, both groups exhibiting significantly lower binding than control subjects.

Garcia-Sevilla and colleagues have frequently reported decreased binding of [^{3}H]clonidine (Garcia-Sevilla et al., 1981b, 1981c, 1986b; Smith et al., 1983) or [^{3}H]adrenaline (Garcia-Sevilla et al., 1987) following antidepressant drug treatment in patients with initially high binding relative to controls. However, the extent of the receptor decrease did not correspond with the degree of clinical improvement, suggesting a direct biochemical response to the presence of the drug rather than a state-dependent change in platelet binding. Indeed, the same group have previously shown that tricyclic antidepressants directly inhibit [^{3}H]clonidine binding in vitro (Garcia-Sevilla et al., 1981a). Recently Pandey et al. (1989) reported no change in [^{3}H]clonidine binding capacity but a significant reduction in affinity following treatment of depressed patients with desipramine. Treatment with lithium, however, caused a significant and substantial decrease in binding capacity. Using [^{3}H]PAC Mooney et al. (1985) observed no significant change in binding following treatment of depressed patients with alprazolam, irrespective of clinical response.

4.3.4 The platelet α_2-adrenoceptor in other psychiatric disorders

Maternity 'blues' is a mild, transient syndrome characterized by crying, depression, irritability and confusion and occurs in approximately 60% of women during the first week post partum (Pitt, 1973). Although it cannot be equated with clinical depression it is representative of a mood disorder. Initial investigations indicated that platelet α_2-adrenoceptor number, as identified by [^{3}H]yohimbine, was significantly greater in those women who experienced the 'blues' than in those who did not, when assayed 7–10 days after birth (Metz et al., 1983). This effect was confirmed by a second, larger study of 108 women (Best et al., 1988). Furthermore, binding in the 'blues' group was significantly greater antepartum than that of an age-matched non-pregnant control group of women, whereas binding in the 'non-blues' group was not significantly different from this control group. Abrupt changes in maternal plasma concentrations of sex-steroids occur following parturition and, as outlined below, platelet α_2-adrenoceptors can be modulated by such steroids. However, no differences were observed in oestrogen and progesterone levels between the 'blues' and 'non-blues' groups before or after parturition. Hence the difference in platelet α_2-adrenoceptor number between the 'blues' and 'non-blues' groups may reflect a difference in sensitivity to steroid-directed regulation of the receptor. Since the sex steroids act by inducing gene transcription, the effects observed in the anucleate platelet must be mediated by changes in the nucleated stem cell, the megakaryocyte. Similar changes may therefore occur in other tissues, hence the phenomenon observed in the platelet may reflect similar disturbances in α_2-adrenoceptor sensitivity in regions of the brain associated with mood and affect. In the rabbit, parallel changes in α_2-adrenoceptor number have been reported in the platelet and hypothalamus following treatment with oestrogen (Bloomfield et al., 1985b). Clearly, further investigation into the regulation of α_2-adrenoceptor activity by sex steroid hormones in women is merited, particularly in relation to the psychological and psychiatric correlates of such activity.

In patients with panic disorder, binding of [^{3}H]yohimbine to platelets was decreased (Cameron et al., 1984; Sevy et al., 1989) or unchanged (Nutt and Fraser, 1987) whereas [^{3}H]clonidine binding was similar to control values (Cameron et al., 1984). Plasma catecholamine levels were higher in these anxious patients, suggesting agonist-induced down-regulation as the mechanism responsible for the decrease in [^{3}H]yohimbine binding. However, the phenomenon of platelet α_2-adrenoceptor desensitization and down-regulation is contentious (see below) and, furthermore, would be expected to have greater impact on agonist than antagonist radioligands, contrary to the observed data.

A significant decrease in plasma noradrenaline concentration, coupled with significantly increased platelet [^{3}H]DHE and [^{3}H]yohimbine binding and adrenaline-induced aggregation response, was observed in young women with anorexia nervosa (Luck et al., 1983). A similar increase in α_2-adrenoceptor number was reported by Heufelder et al. (1985) in anorectic women whose plasma noradrenaline level was not significantly different from controls, although their orthostatic noradrenaline response was lower. Following a 10% increase in body weight, the platelet binding parameters returned to control levels. Substantial loss of body weight in both obese and normal control subjects itself leads to an increase in platelet α_2-adrenoceptor number (Sundaresan et al., 1983, 1985; Goodwin et al., 1987), therefore the changes in receptor activity in patients with anorexia nervosa may be dependent more on metabolic than psychiatric factors.

In schizophrenic patients there is no consensus on platelet α_2-adrenoceptor activity, with reports of increased (Kafka et al., 1981), decreased (Rice et al., 1984) and unchanged (Kafka & van Kammen 1983; Bondy et al., 1984) radioligand binding. Inhibition of PGE_1-stimulated adenylate cyclase by noradrenaline was similar to that of healthy control subjects (Kanof *et al.*, 1988). Recently, increased binding of [^{3}H]clonidine was reported in both schizophrenic and schizoaffective patients and was unaltered by treatment with trifluoperazine (Pandey *et al.*, 1989).

4.3.5 Factors affecting platelet α_2-adrenoceptor activity

As in the case of the leucocyte β-adrenoceptor, the characteristics of the platelet α_2-adrenoceptor can be modified by both endogenous and exogenous compounds within the plasma, which must be taken into account when attempting to rationalize the data presented above. Unlike the leucocyte β-adrenoceptor, however, the mechanism and extent of desensitization and down-regulation of the platelet α_2-adrenoceptor is equivocal. A decrease in receptor number has been demonstrated following prolonged incubation of platelets *in vitro* with high concentrations of agonist (Cooper *et al.*, 1978). Other groups, however, claim that the apparent loss of receptors results from incomplete removal of the agonist during tissue washing procedures prior to the binding assay (Karliner *et al.*, 1982; Motulsky *et al.*, 1986), although they do concede that the receptor appears to be functionally desensitized, as demonstrated by decreased aggregation response. *Ex vivo* studies in subjects receiving chronic treatment with α_2-adrenoceptor agonists, including clonidine and guanfacine, similarly disagree as to whether platelet receptor binding is decreased (Brodde *et al.*, 1982a) or unchanged (Boon *et al.*, 1983a; Motulsky *et al.*, 1983). Likewise, opinion differs as to whether the receptor binding capacity is negatively correlated with plasma catecholamine levels (Davies *et al.*, 1981) or not (Pfeifer *et al.*, 1984).

We have recently demonstrated that chronic treatment of healthy control subjects with the novel α_2-adrenoceptor antagonist idazoxan causes an increase in platelet binding capacity of [^{3}H]UK14304 without affecting binding affinity (Payvandi *et al.*, 1990a). This effect is analogous to the increase in leucocyte β-adrenoceptor number obtained following chronic treatment with β-blockers (Aarons *et al.*, 1980) and probably reflects escape from desensitization normally caused by chronic stimulation of the receptors at physiological concentrations of catecholamines within the plasma. Compared with the leucocyte β-adrenoceptor, however, the sensitivity and/or extent of agonist down-regulation of the platelet α_2-adrenoceptor seems considerably weaker. This may have important ramifications for the interpretation of platelet α_2-adrenoceptor binding in depressed patients, as outlined below.

Besides those which interact directly with the receptor, several other compounds have been shown to modify platelet α_2-adrenoceptor number and function. In women, increased plasma concentrations of oestrogens and progestogens are associated with an increased number of platelet α_2-adreno-ceptors, as labelled by various radioligands, and increased aggregation response to noradrenaline. Such effects have been reported following changes in the concentration of both exogenous synthetic compounds associated with the oral combined contraceptives (Peters *et al.*, 1979) and endogenous hormones associated with pregnancy (Metz *et al.*, 1983; Best *et al.*, 1988) and post-menopausal status of women (Elliott and Grahame-Smith, 1982). The situation with regard to the menstrual cycle is confused, some groups reporting significant changes in receptor activity corresponding to specific phases of the cycle (Jones *et al.*, 1983; Barnett *et al.*, 1984) whereas others report no such differences (Peters *et al.*, 1979; Theodorou *et al.*, 1987). The contrast in steroid concentrations between phases of the menstrual cycle is substantially less than that which occurs following parturition or the onset of the menopause and may therefore be associated with correspondingly smaller changes in α_2-adrenoceptor activity, so accounting for these inconsistent findings. Induction of receptor synthesis by sex steroids is mediated via nuclear promotion of gene transcription. This must occur in the megakaryocyte, the platelet stem cell, since the platelet itself is anucleate. Parallel changes in α_2-adrenoceptor number occur in platelets and uterine tissue obtained from pregnant women at caesarian section (Brodde *et al.*, 1988), therefore it seems likely that receptors may similarly be modulated in other sex steroid-sensitive tissues, including discrete areas of the brain.

Corticosteroids may also regulate platelet α_2-adrenoceptors. Platelets from patients with Cushing's syndrome exhibit increased synthesis and excretion of cortisol and decreased binding capacity for [^{3}H]yohimbine compared with matched controls (Bloomfield *et al.*, 1985a). Hypersecretion of cortisol is commonly associated with depressive disorders, although the hormone concentrations encountered in depression are substantially lower than those in Cushing's syndrome. It might be anticipated, therefore, that platelet α_2-adrenoceptor number would be decreased in depressive disorders but, as reported above, this is contrary to the majority of findings. However, the increased cortisol production in depressed patients may mask a decrease in corticosteroid sensitivity, as discussed in relation to the β-adrenoceptor model. Consequently, a decrease in corticosteroid influence would be anticipated to correspond with an increase in platelet α_2-adrenoceptors.

Chronic heroin abuse is reported to increase platelet binding of [^{3}H]clonidine and potentiate adrenaline-induced platelet aggregation (Garcia-Sevilla *et al.*, 1986b). Withdrawal of heroin further increased agonist binding, the severity of the abstinence syndrome being significantly related to platelet binding capacity (Garcia-Sevilla *et al.*, 1985). Adrenaline-induced platelet aggregation response was correspondingly increased, although binding of the radiolabelled antagonist [^{3}H]yohimbine did not alter throughout withdrawal. On the basis of these data, the authors proposed [³H]clonidine to be a better indicator of platelet α_2-adrenoceptor function than [³H]yohimbine. The opioid and α_2-adrenergic receptor systems are functionally related through their common presynaptic action, and behavioural interactions between the corresponding receptor antagonists have been demonstrated in man (Charney and Heninger, 1986). The mechanism(s) by which chronic administration of opiates increase platelet α_2-adrenoceptor activity and by which withdrawal of the drugs further increase receptor activity are unclear.

As indicated above, metabolic factors implicated in dieting have been shown to increase platelet α_2-adrenoceptor activity (Sundaresan *et al.*, 1983, 1985; Goodwin *et al.*, 1987). Age is claimed to be another modifying factor, but both positive (Yokoyama *et al.*, 1984; Katona *et al.*, 1989) and negative (Brodde *et al.*, 1982b) correlations between age and receptor number have been described, as well as no significant association (Buckley *et al.*, 1986). Seasonal variations in binding parameters have not been ascribed to the α_2-adrenoceptor, with the exception of an effect on binding affinity of [³H]yohimbine (Katona *et al.*, 1989). A strong hereditary element in regulating the platelet α_2-adrenoceptor was demonstrated by a significantly closer correlation between receptor binding capacity in monozygotic than in dizygotic twins (Propping and Friedl, 1983). This finding reinforces the possibility that the platelet may be used as a trait marker for α_2-adrenoceptor dysfunction.

4.3.6 Summary

It is clear from the data summarized above that there is little consistency in the investigations of platelet α_2-adrenoceptor activity in relation to depressive disorders. Segregation of binding data according to individual radioligands achieves some conformity but only at the expense of confusing the precise nature of the binding site(s) involved, since all the ligands employed in these studies are proposed to label the α_2-adrenoceptor.

Technically the 'cleanest' of these radioligands are the selective α_2-adrenoceptor antagonists [³H]yohimbine and [³H]rauwolscine which demonstrate high affinity (K_d 1–4 nM) and low non-specific binding, resulting in a high signal-to-noise ratio. Data obtained using these ligands are unequivocal, indicating no difference in binding to platelets of depressed and healthy subjects. When used at low concentration they are generally accepted as the definitive radioligands for labelling the α_2-adrenoceptor. [³H]DHE is a non-selective α-adrenoceptor antagonist which exhibits high non-specific binding and Kd values ranging between K_d 3 and 35 nM. Consequently, the signal-to-noise ratio is low. Binding in depressed patients has been described as both increased and decreased relative to healthy controls. [³H]DHE was the first radioligand commercially available for labelling α-adrenoceptor, hence its widespread use in the early studies of this type. However, its technical inferiority to [^{3}H]yohimbine and [^{3}H]rauwolscine makes its current use questionable in platelet studies unless the additional sites labelled by [^{3}H]DHE (see above) prove to be functionally significant.

Since their first report in 1981, Garcia-Sevilla and colleagues have consistently observed increased binding of [^{3}H]clonidine at high affinity sites on platelets from depressed patients, whilst [^{3}H]yohimbine binding remains unchanged. Subsequently several groups have independently confirmed this effect. Although an increase in the binding of [^{3}H]adrenaline was also recorded by Garcia-Sevilla et al. (1987), the effect is not common to all agonist radioligands, since it is not demonstrated by [^{3}H]PAC or [^{3}H]UK14304. A major complication in the use of agonist or partial agonist radioligands is the inevitable labelling of two receptor populations with differing affinities. This occurs due to the discrimination by agonists (but not antagonists) between the receptor in its isolated form and that complexed with a guanine nucleotide binding protein (G-protein). The trimeric complex of agonist–receptor–G-protein dissociates slowly in the absence of GTP, resulting in a higher apparent binding affinity for agonists than that of the native receptor (Kim and Neubig, 1987). Appropriate analysis of data in such situations is complex and requires binding to be studied over a wide range of ligand concentrations. Frequently, however, researchers resort to the oversimplified and inaccurate method of bisecting the Scatchard plot into exclusive low and high affinity binding data which are then independently analysed as individual sites. The binding of [^{3}H]clonidine is particularly prone to such misinterpretation since the difference in affinity at the two sites is relatively small. The increased binding in platelets of depressed patients is restricted to the high affinity site, assumed to be that complexed to the G-protein. However, the absolute binding capacity of this site, labelled by either [^{3}H]clonidine or [^{3}H]adrenaline, is substantially lower than that identified by [^{3}H]UK14304, suggesting that the clinically relevant difference may occur within a subset of the receptor–G-protein complexes. This difference in agonist binding capacities has been confirmed in paired assays on individual tissue samples (Rommelspacher et al., 1987) but no functional evidence confirms the existence of such a receptor subset. On balance the binding of agonist radioligands to platelet α_2-adrenoceptors in depressive disorders merits further investigation, paying particular attention to the accurate discrimination between high and low affinity sites.

Assuming that agonist binding to platelet α_2-adrenoceptors is increased in depressed patients, the effect does not appear to be state dependent, since most studies find no correlation between binding capacity and clinical rating of the severity of the illness. Even though treatment with antidepressant drugs is reported to decrease agonist binding, and in some cases antagonist binding, the effect is unrelated to clinical response. Such treatment frequently increases the concentration of plasma catecholamines, which may subsequently desensitize and down-regulate platelet α_2-adrenoceptors. Assuming that the mechanism of desensitization is similar to that elucidated in the case of the β-adrenoceptor, the α_2-adrenoceptor would initially be uncoupled from the G-protein(s) and then eventually be removed from the plasma membrane. In terms of receptor binding, therefore, the number of agonist affinity sites would be reduced before any change in antagonist binding was apparent, corroborating the observed data. As indicated above, however, the phenomenon of agonist desensitization of the platelet α_2-adrenoceptor remains controversial.

Few functional studies have compared platelet α_2-adrenoceptors from depressed and healthy subjects. Platelet aggregation response to adrenaline was reported increased in depressed patients in two studies (Garcia-Sevilla et al., 1983, 1986b) but not different in another (Wood et al., 1985b). Inhibition of adenylate cyclase by adrenaline or noradrenaline was twice reported decreased in depressed patients (Siever et al., 1984; Kafka et al., 1986) and once unchanged (Kanof et al., 1988) relative to controls. Inhibition of adenylate cyclase is more closely coupled to receptor activation than the platelet aggregation response but it, in turn, is dependent on the level of enzyme stimulation which may be altered in depressed subjects (Kanof et al., 1988). Such diversity in functional response does not clarify the situation depicted by the receptor binding data.

Neuroendocrine studies of growth hormone response to clonidine in depressed and healthy subjects suggest decreased α_2-adrenoceptor response in depression (Katona et al., 1987). The hypotensive effect of clonidine and the reduction in plasma 3-methoxy-4-hydroxyphenylethyleneglycol (MHPG) in response to clonidine show no difference between healthy and depressed subjects. In all three functional studies, however, there is evidence of decreased α_2-adrenoceptor response following chronic antidepressant treatment. Consequently, there is little support for the concept derived from platelet studies that α_2-adrenoceptor activity is primarily increased in depression. In contrast, the effect of chronic administration of antidepressant drugs appears to reduce α_2-adrenoceptor activity, as measured by several parameters including centrally-mediated neuroendocrine effects and agonist binding to platelets. A potential mechanism responsible for this effect is increased extracellular noradrenaline inducing desensitization of the α_2-adrenoceptor. In this respect, therefore, the platelet may act as a valid indicator of central α_2-adrenoceptor activity.

4.3.7 Future investigations

As indicated above, the consistent finding of increased [^{3}H]clonidine binding in depressed patients merits further study but appropriate methods should be adopted in order accurately to discriminate binding to high and low affinity sites. Analysis of simultaneous binding to two sites is complex and best avoided. This can, however, be achieved by differentiating specific binding, as classically defined, according to that which is sensitive to guanine nucleotides (high affinity binding to receptor–G-protein complex) and that which is insensitive to guanine nucleotides (low affinity binding to uncoupled receptor). Independent analysis of binding at each site is then simplified without compromising accuracy (Payvandi *et al.*, 1990b). Furthermore, the classification of the high affinity binding site for [^{3}H]clonidine and comparison to that identified by the full agonist [^{3}H]UK14304 may clarify the discrepancy in receptor number which currently exists between them.

Secondly, the effects of antidepressant drug treatment could be extended to include novel compounds which do not inhibit catecholamine reuptake or catabolism. Of particular interest, in this respect, would be selective 5-HT uptake inhibitors and selective α_2-adrenoceptor antagonists. In healthy volunteers, chronic administration of idazoxan, a novel putative antidepressant which selectively blocks α_2-adrenoceptors, resulted in increased platelet α_2-adreno-ceptor number (Payvandi *et al.*, 1990a). A similar study in depressed patients would test the relevance of the decrease in receptor activity observed after tricyclic antidepressants to clinical improvement.

Finally, the acknowledged sensitivity of the platelet α_2-adrenoceptor to modulation by steroid hormones could be utilized by investigating depressive disorders in which hormonal dysfunction is suspected, including postnatal depression and premenstrual syndrome. Evidence of α_2-adrenoceptor dys-regulation in response to hormonal changes may suggest novel therapeutic strategies targeted directly at the α_2-adrenoceptor.

4.4 Platelet 5-HT uptake

4.4.1 Characterization of platelet 5-HT uptake

The biochemical similarities between the platelet and the nerve terminal are best exemplified by the 5-HT transport system (Pletscher, 1978). The kinetics of active 5-HT uptake are qualitatively similar, and competing substrates and inhibitors demonstrate similar affinities at the two sites (Shaskan and Snyder, 1970). In both tissues 5-HT is stored in membrane-bound vesicles and is released by exocytotic secretion. The platelet, however, unlike the nerve terminal does not express tryptophan hydroxylase and therefore cannot synthesize 5-HT. Peripheral 5-HT originates mainly from the enterochromaffin cells. Whole blood 5-HT comprises almost exclusively platelet 5-HT, indicating the efficiency of the platelet 5-HT uptake mechanism in normal circumstances. Administration of tricyclic antidepressants (Todrick and Tait, 1969) or selective 5-HT uptake blockers (Ross and Aberg-Wistedt, 1983; Beving *et al.*, 1985) significantly inhibits 5-HT uptake into rat brain synaptosomes and human platelets and presumably into human brain serotonergic nerve terminals. Hence, the platelet has been utilized as a popular tool to investigate 5-HT uptake in affective disorders and as a pharmacodynamic measure of anti-depressant drug action.

4.4.2 Platelet 5-HT uptake in affective disorders

Altered 5-HT transport into platelets of depressed patients was first reported by Tuomisto and Tukainen (1976), who described a decrease in the maximal rate of transport (V_{max}) compared with healthy control subjects. The affinity of uptake was not significantly different between the two groups, indicating that the decreased uptake did not result from treatment with antidepressant drugs. Subsequently, several other groups reported similar findings (Coppen *et al.*, 1978; Scott *et al.*, 1979; Meltzer *et al.*, 1981). Recent work has generally confirmed this effect (Rausch *et al.*, 1986, 1988; Butler and Leonard, 1988; Pecknold *et al.*, 1988), although comparison of absolute uptake characteristics has been confused by the identification of both circadian and seasonal variations, as discussed below. Corresponding studies of platelet 5-HT content indicate a decrease in unipolar endogenous (Muck-Seler *et al.*, 1983; Le Quan-Bui *et al.*, 1984; Healy *et al.*, 1985) but not in non-endogenous or bipolar depressed patients (Stahl *et al.*, 1983b; Healy *et al.*, 1985). Attempts to differentiate between depressive subtypes according to 5-HT uptake indicate no differences (Stahl *et al.*, 1983b; Arora *et al.*, 1984; Rausch *et al.*, 1986). Classification of depressed patients as suppressors or non-suppressors on the dexamethasone suppression test also reveal no difference in 5-HT uptake characteristics (Meltzer *et al.*, 1983).

4.4.3 Factors affecting platelet 5-HT uptake

Treatment with the potent 5-HT uptake blockers chlorimipramine, imipramine or citalopram substantially reduces 5-HT uptake in both depressed patients (Arora and Meltzer, 1983; Beving *et al.*, 1985) and healthy volunteers (Poirier *et al.*, 1985, 1987), leading to an acute decrease in platelet 5-HT content (Sarrias *et al.*, 1987). Treatment with drugs which demonstrate weaker serotonergic effects, such as nomifensine (Butler and Leonard, 1986), mapro-tiline and amineptine (Poirier *et al.*, 1987), do not reduce 5-HT uptake. Paradoxically, 5-HT content is often increased following chronic treatment with antidepressant drugs, including those which directly inhibit uptake (Coppen *et al.*, 1976; Banki, 1978). Clinical improvement in patients is frequently (Tuomisto *et al.*, 1979; Born *et al.*, 1980; Healy *et al.*, 1985) but not always (Suranyi-Cadotte *et al.*, 1985b) accompanied by normalization of platelet 5-HT uptake, suggesting this to be a state-dependent marker. It is not, however, specific to major depressive disorder, since significant reduction in platelet 5-HT uptake has also been identified in schizophrenia (Rotman *et al.*, 1979; Arora and Meltzer, 1982), panic disorder (Pecknold *et al.*, 1988), migraine (Coppen *et al.*, 1979; Malmgren *et al.*, 1980), hypertension (Kamal *et al.*, 1984) and asthma (Malmgren *et al.*, 1980).

Cyclical variation in platelet 5-HT uptake kinetics has been described with both diurnal and seasonal periodicity in healthy subjects. The reports vary, however, regarding the period of maximal uptake between autumn/winter (Arora *et al.*, 1984), summer/autumn (Egrise *et al.*, 1986) and summer/winter (Malmgren *et al.*, 1989). Patients with major depressive disorder also exhibit seasonal variation but the rate of uptake is generally lower than controls and may peak at a different time of year (Malmgren *et al.*, 1989). A circadian pattern has also been detected in healthy subjects, with minimal uptake occurring during the night (Modai *et al.*, 1986). In depressed patients this pattern was not discernable (Humphries *et al.*, 1985), although it could be restored following effective treatment (Healy *et al.*, 1986). Disruption of circadian and seasonal biorhythms as a potential cause of depressive disorders is discussed more fully in Chapter 7.

4.4.4 Summary and future investigations

In summary, 5-HT uptake appears to be lower in platelets of depressed patients compared with healthy controls, particularly at specific times of the day/year. This decrease results from a reduction in the maximal uptake rate without change in affinity and therefore represents a decrease in the number of membrane pump sites and/or a decrease in pump efficiency. The effect is usually not apparent in euthymic patients and therefore appears to act as a state-dependent marker. However measurement of $[^3H]$5-HT uptake into isolated platelets *in vitro* is usually performed in autologous plasma and is therefore liable to modulation by plasma factors, including hormones and antidepressant drugs, many of which directly inhibit such uptake. Since the effect of these drugs can persist for weeks after dosing has stopped (Ross and Aberg-Wistedt, 1983; Poirier *et al.*, 1985), it is essential to establish a sufficiently long drug-free interval (at least 4 weeks) before testing. The decrease in platelet 5-HT uptake is not specific to depressive disorders but may provide an interesting biochemical model for the study of circadian and seasonal cycles, particularly in relation to affective disorders.

4.5 [³H]Imipramine binding

4.5.1 Characterization of the [³H]imipramine binding site

At low nanomolar concentration [³H]imipramine labels a site in human platelets (Briley *et al.*, 1979; Paul *et al.*, 1980) and in human (Rehavi *et al.*, 1980) and rat (Raisman *et al.*, 1979) brain that appears to be closely associated with the 5-HT active transport site. A good correlation exists between the potency of various drugs to inhibit both [³H]5-HT uptake and specific [³H]imipramine binding (Hrdina, 1986), and lesion of serotonergic cell bodies in rat brain causes a parallel regional reduction in 5-HT uptake and [³H]imipramine binding (Sette *et al.*, 1981). Both [³H]5-HT uptake and [³H]imipramine binding are sodium-dependent (Rudnick, 1977; Moret and Briley, 1986), although secondary low affinity binding sites for [³H]imipramine which are not sodium-dependent have also been described (Moret and Briley, 1986; Hrdina, 1987). The function of these alternative sites is not clear. Kinetic analysis of displacement of [³H]imipramine binding in brain tissue by 5-HT and non-tricyclic uptake blockers suggests that [³H]imipramine may label a site closely associated with but distinct from the 5-HT uptake pump which functions to regulate the uptake process (Sette *et al.*, 1983). Other groups, however, find no difference between these two sites (Marcusson *et al.*, 1986; Hrdina, 1988). This discussion is presented in greater detail elsewhere (Langer and Schoemaker, 1988; Hrdina, 1989).

4.5.2 Platelet [³H]imipramine binding in affective disorders

Shortly after the initial identification of [³H]imipramine binding sites on human platelets, Briley *et al.* (1980) reported that the binding capacity was significantly lower (57%) in depressed female patients than in age-matched healthy female controls. Binding affinity was not significantly different between the two groups, suggesting that the effect was not caused by persistence of antidepressant drugs inhibiting binding of [³H]imipramine in the patient samples. The previously observed deficit in platelet 5-HT uptake could therefore be explained on the basis of a reduced number of 5-HT transport sites.

Subsequently, many groups have repeated this investigation, as summarized in Table 2, of which only half have described a significant decrease in [³H]imipramine binding capacity in platelets from depressed patients. Consequently, the validity of the platelet [³H]imipramine binding site as a consistent biochemical marker for depressive disorder has come under close scrutiny. Even where significant differences have been observed, considerable overlap occurs between the patient and control groups, suggesting that

Table 2 Platelet [³H]imipramine binding capacity in depressed patients and control subjects.

Reference	B_{max} (fmol/mg protein)		Difference depressed versus control (%)
	Control (n)	Depressed (n)	
Briley et al. (1980)	604 (21)	257 (16)	−57
Asarch et al. (1980)			
male	764 (7)	608 (11)	−20
female	650 (9)	519 (12)	−20
Paul et al. (1981)	450 (28)	318 (14)	−29
Raisman et al. (1981)	581 (39)	300 (37)	−48
Raisman et al. (1982)	539 (27)	368 (14)	−32
Mellerup et al. (1982)	1010 (33)	1190 (31)	+18
Baron et al. (1983)	991 (15)	776 (15)	NSD
P.L. Wood et al. (1983a)			
unipolar	658 (17)	519 (25)	−21
bipolar	764 (17)	467 (7)	−29
Suranyi-Cadotte et al. (1983)		372 (6)	−43
Whitaker et al. (1984)		798 (16)	NSD
Wagner et al. (1985)	1123 (53)	1012 (63)	−10
Tang and Morris (1985)	1025 (45)	1057 (20)	NSD
Lewis and McChesney (1985)			
unipolar	1238 (20)	870 (11)	−30
bipolar		754 (6)	−40
Hrdina et al. (1985)	1000 (10)	894 (20)	NSD
Arora et al. (1985)	920 (80)	803 (50)	−13
Suranyi-Cadotte et al. (1985b)	767 (8)	569 (10)	−26
Gentsch et al. (1985)	1590 (16)	1510 (55)	NSD

Muscettola et al. (1986)	1030 (31)		
bipolar depressed		885 (9)	NSD
bipolar hypomanic		924 (10)	NSD
Poirier et al. (1986)			
male	1060 (5)	574 (6)	−46
female	1381 (10)	736 (11)	−47
Egrise et al. (1986)	463/935† (9)	495/907† (7)	NSD
Baron et al. (1986)	945 (58)		
unipolar		821 (34)	NSD
bipolar		754 (33)	−20
Braddock et al. (1986)	120* (37)	122* (28)	NSD
Nankai et al. (1986)	1361 (28)	1076 (28)	−22
Carstens et al. (1986b)	1300 (20)	1200 (29)	NSD
Georgotas et al. (1987)	669 (9)	585 (23)	NSD
Innis et al. (1987)	1075 (22)	737 (9)	−31
Desmedt et al. (1987)	788 (34)		
unipolar		756 (21)	NSD
bipolar		846 (16)	NSD
Kanof et al. (1987)	1070 (30)	1025 (38)	NSD
Roy et al. (1987)			
male	567 (18)	571 (11)	NSD
female	613 (25)	541 (32)	−12
Schneider et al. (1987b)	2103 (14)	1560 (18)	−26
Plenge et al. (1988)	1240 (21)		
endogenous		1210 (34)	NSD
non-endogenous		1330 (12)	NSD
Nemeroff et al. (1988)			
age < 50	908 (25)	525 (29)	−42
age > 60	943 (18)	547 (19)	−42

Table 2 *continued.*

Reference	B_{max} (fmol/mg protein)		Difference depressed versus control (%)
	Control (*n*)	Depressed (*n*)	
Maj *et al.* (1988)	625 (19)	497 (37)	−20
Gentsch *et al.* (1989)			
08.00	1240 (11)	1270 (19)	NSD
15.00	1300 (11)	1200 (19)	NSD
Takeda *et al.* (1989)	634 (16)	545 (14)	−14
Theodorou *et al.* (1989)			
male	1503 (14)	1571 (13)	NSD
female	1758 (32)	1510 (34)	−14
Healy *et al.* (1990)			
male	1113 (18)	1092 (12)	NSD
female	1050 (26)	1084 (27)	NSD

Numerical values for comparison of depressed versus control subjects indicate statistically significant differences.

NSD, non-significant difference.

* B_{max} expressed as fmol/10^8 cells.

† Values expressed as nadir/peak during 12-month study.

decreased [^{3}H]imipramine binding may be restricted to a particular subgroup of depressed patients. Attempts to distinguish such a subgroup have not been successful. Comparison of unipolar and bipolar depressed patients have indicated decreased binding in both groups (P.L. Wood *et al.*, 1983a), in bipolar only (Baron *et al.*, 1986) and in neither group (Desmedt *et al.*, 1987). No differences were apparent between endogenous and non-endogenous depressed patients (Braddock *et al.*, 1986; Roy *et al.*, 1987; Plenge *et al.*, 1988; Theodorou *et al.*, 1989; Healy *et al.*, 1990) or between DST suppressors and non-suppressors (Braddock *et al.*, 1986; Carstens *et al.*, 1986b; Desmedt *et al.*, 1987; Nemeroff *et al.*, 1988; Theodorou *et al.*, 1989). A positive family history of depressive disorder was associated with low binding in some studies (Lewis and McChesney, 1985; Suranyi-Cadotte *et al.*, 1985b; Schneider *et al.*, 1986) but could not be confirmed in others (Carstens *et al.*, 1986b; Theodorou *et al.*, 1989). Individual reports of abnormal binding associated with psychomotor retardation (Carstens *et al.*, 1986b), psychotic depression (Arora *et al.*, 1985) and suicidal intent (Wagner *et al.*, 1985) have yet to be substantiated. Apart from two studies (Tanimoto *et al.*, 1985; Nankai *et al.*, 1986), the majority have found no correlation between [^{3}H]imipramine binding and the severity of depression (Raisman *et al.*, 1981; Braddock *et al.*, 1986; Georgotas *et al.*, 1987; Kanof *et al.*, 1987; Takeda *et al.*, 1989; Theodorou *et al.*, 1989).

In an attempt to clarify this situation a multicentre investigation of platelet [^{3}H]imipramine binding in depression was set up under the auspices of the World Health Organization (WHO). One hundred and fifty-four depressed patients (drug free for at least 4 weeks) and 130 matched controls were recruited from nine areas (Athens, Basel, Brussels, Copenhagen, Irvine, Milan/Naples, Moscow, Munich and Tokyo) and platelet [^{3}H]imipramine binding was analysed locally in Basel, Brussels and Irvine. The remainder were all sent to Copenhagen for assay. A standardized protocol was used at all centres. Substantial variation in binding capacity of control subjects was noted between the different centres, even when assayed within the same laboratory. Consequently, data from each centre were analysed individually and then normalized according to the local control value before global comparison. No significant differences in binding capacity or affinity were observed between depressed patients and controls from any individual centre or for the sample population overall (Mellerup and Langer, 1990). Binding was higher in men than women, but when divided according to sex the only significant difference was that of increased binding amongst male depressed patients in the Copenhagen group compared with local male controls. The age of the patient group was significantly higher than control but no significant correlation was found between age and binding capacity. Unipolar endogenous ($n = 109$) and bipolar endogenous ($n = 21$) depressed patients did not differ from each other or controls in terms of [^{3}H]imipramine binding but demonstrated significantly lower binding capacity, both separately and together, than non-endogenous depressed patients ($n = 24$). The latter were not significantly different from controls and within the four centres from which they originated were not significantly different from the endogenous groups. It seems likely, therefore, that the apparent distinction between endogenous and non-endogenous subtypes in fact reflects the disparity in absolute binding capacity between centres. Within the patient group, distinction between those who had received antidepressant medication prior to the washout period and those who had received no treatment during the current depressive episode revealed no further differences, except from one centre in which binding was significantly lower in the fully untreated group compared with controls. Binding affinity in the two groups of depressed patients was the same, indicating no contamination of the binding assay by persistent previous medication.

These data, therefore, do not support the platelet [³H]imipramine binding site as a reliable marker for endogenous depression but do not exclude the possibility that valid differences may occur within other subgroups of depressive disorders.

4.5.3 Platelet [³H]imipramine binding following drug treatment and clinical response

The effect of drug treatment on [³H]imipramine binding varies according to the drug employed. Following acute (Schneider *et al.*, 1986) or chronic (Poirier *et al.*, 1987) administration of chlorimipramine, binding was substantially decreased and remained low for up to 4 weeks following withdrawal. Chronic administration of amitripyline to depressed patients produced no change in binding (Braddock *et al.*, 1986), whereas in healthy volunteers binding affinity was decreased and capacity increased (Braddock *et al.*, 1984). After discontinuation of treatment the affinity rapidly returned to normal, whereas the capacity change persisted for some weeks. Desmethylimipramine, zimeldine and alaproclate administered to healthy or depressed subjects similarly caused an increase in binding capacity (Cowen *et al.*, 1986; Wagner *et al.*, 1987; Arora and Meltzer, 1988). No change in [³H]imipramine binding occurred following short-term treatment with nortriptyline, minaprine, imipramine or maprotiline in depressed patients (Wagner *et al.*, 1987; Maj *et al.*, 1988; Theodorou *et al.*, 1989) or amineptine, maprotiline or imipramine in healthy volunteers (Suranyi-Cadotte *et al.*, 1985b; Poirier *et al.*, 1987). Hence the varied response to drugs which directly inhibit 5-HT uptake provides little indication as to their therapeutic mode of action.

Lithium is widely used in the prophylactic management of bipolar depression and is reported to modify platelet 5-HT uptake following chronic administration, although it has no direct effect *in vitro* (Poirier *et al.*, 1988).

Administration of lithium to healthy volunteers for 3 weeks produced no change in [³H]imipramine binding to platelets either during or after treatment (Glue *et al.*, 1986; Poirier *et al.*, 1988). Treatment of bipolar depressed patients with lithium also had no effect (P.L. Wood *et al.*, 1983b). Similarly, a course of six electroconvulsive shocks in depressed patients did not alter platelet [³H]imipramine binding during or shortly after treatment (Langer *et al.*, 1986).

Amongst those groups reporting significantly lower binding in depressed patients, clinical recovery was eventually (Suranyi-Cadotte *et al.*, 1985b; Langer *et al.*, 1986), but rarely immediately, accompanied by normalization of binding (Raisman *et al.*, 1981; Schneider *et al.*, 1986; Maj *et al.*, 1988). Consequently, platelet [³H]imipramine binding may be interpreted as a slow-responding state-dependent marker. Low binding in euthymic depressive patients has been interpreted as indicative of a trait marker (Suranyi-Cadotte *et al.*, 1983; Baron *et al.*, 1986; Wagner *et al.*, 1987) but this may reflect premature re-evaluation of [³H]imipramine binding following a depressive episode. Alternatively, some patients may appear in remission but may retain some biochemical dysfunction which increases the likelihood of relapse. In support of this hypothesis, two studies identified low [³H]imipramine binding as predicting poor clinical outcome (Hrdina *et al.*, 1985; Wagner *et al.*, 1987).

A further confusing factor in the attempts to re-evaluate platelet [³H]imipramine binding some months after initial analysis is the presence of seasonal variation (Egrise *et al.*, 1983; Whitaker *et al.*, 1984; Hrdina *et al.*, 1985), similar to that of platelet 5-HT uptake (Egrise *et al.*, 1986; Malmgren *et al.*, 1989). However, this effect has not been confirmed in all long-term studies (Tang and Morris, 1985; Galzin *et al.*, 1986; Baron *et al.*, 1988) and even when apparent does not appear consistent. Hence, winter coincided with maximal binding in one study (Hrdina *et al.*, 1985) and minimal binding in another (Kanof *et al.*, 1987), whilst summer represented peak effect in two studies (Egrise *et al.*, 1986; Arora and Meltzer, 1988) and the nadir in another (Whitaker *et al.*, 1984). Recently two studies carried out by the same laboratory on different patients both identified significant seasonal variation in platelet [³H]imipramine binding capacity but summer coincided with maximum binding in one study (Theodorou *et al.*, 1989) and minimum binding in the other (Healy *et al.*, 1990).

4.5.4 Specificity of platelet [³H]imipramine binding as a marker for affective disorders

Although major depressive disorder represents the most intensely studied illness in relation to platelet [³H]imipramine binding, it is not the only situation in which significant changes in binding have been reported. Schizophrenia has been associated with increased (Desmedt et al., 1987), decreased (Arora et al., 1986) and unchanged (Kanof et al., 1987) binding capacity. Panic disorder was initially identified with low binding (Lewis et al., 1985) but all subsequent studies have reported no difference from controls (Innis et al., 1987; Nutt and Fraser, 1987; Peckhold et al., 1987; Schneider et al., 1987a; Uhde et al., 1987). A reduction in binding in anorexia nervosa (Weizman et al., 1986) contrasts with the finding of no change following substantial weight loss in healthy volunteers (Goodwin et al., 1987). Decreased binding has been reported in patients with obsessive compulsive disorder (Weizman et al., 1986) and confirmed within a subgroup of depressed patients with obsessional features (Theodorou et al., 1989). This is particularly interesting in view of current reports of favourable clinical response of such patients to treatment with selective 5-HT uptake blocking drugs (Flament et al., 1987; Price et al., 1987; Murphy et al., 1989). No change in platelet [^{3}H]imipramine binding was observed in Alzheimer's disease or Parkinson's disease (Suranyi-Cadotte et al., 1985a; Nemeroff et al., 1988). In migraine, reports of decreased platelet 5-HT uptake have been paralleled by reduced [^{3}H]imipramine binding (Geaney et al., 1984a). Binding was also reduced in patients with chronic psychogenic pain in two studies (Magni et al., 1987; Mellerup et al., 1988), although in the latter the patients also exhibited depressive symptoms.

4.5.5 Comparison of 5-HT uptake and [^{3}H]imipramine binding on human platelets

Decreased 5-HT uptake and [^{3}H]imipramine binding in platelets of depressed patients have been independently reported by many groups but few have analysed the two processes simultaneously. Raisman et al. (1982) observed a similar decrease in both maximal rate of 5-HT uptake and [^{3}H]imipramine binding capacity in 14 depressed patients drug free for at least 7 days prior to assay, compared with 27 control subjects. However, they found no individual correlation between the uptake and binding parameters in either depressed or healthy subjects. P.L. Wood et al. (1983a) also reported parallel decreases in platelet 5-HT uptake and [^{3}H]imipramine binding in depressed patients. In schizophrenic patients, however, 5-HT uptake was significantly decreased by 48% relative to controls, whereas [^{3}H]imipramine binding showed no difference. Similarly platelet 5-HT uptake was significantly lower in patients with depression, Alzheimer's disease, Parkinson's disease and cirrhosis of the liver compared with controls, whereas [^{3}H]imipramine binding was decreased only in the depressed patients (Ahtee et al., 1981; Suranyi-Cadotte et al., 1985a). Conversely, platelet [^{3}H]imipramine binding was decreased in female patients with anorexia nervosa, without any change in 5-HT uptake (Weizman et al., 1986). In a similar manner, administration of chlorimipramine to healthy volunteers reduced both 5-HT uptake and [³H]imipramine binding of platelets during treatment but within 14 days of drug withdrawal the 5-HT uptake had returned to normal, whereas [³H]imipramine binding remained significantly depressed (Poirier *et al.*, 1987).

Compared to the simple bimolecular interaction of [³H]imipramine with its binding site, the active transport of 5-HT into the platelet is a complex process dependent on binding of substrate (5-HT) and cofactor (sodium ions), translocation across the lipid bilayer utilizing energy in the form of ATP and release of substrate into the cytosol. Interruption of any of these processes, except substrate binding, would therefore inhibit 5-HT uptake without necessarily affecting [³H]imipramine binding. If, however, the [³H]imipramine binding site is the same as the substrate site on the 5-HT transport protein, then any change in [³H]imipramine binding capacity ought to be reflected in a parallel shift in maximal 5-HT transport rate. The incongruent changes reported above, together with the complex kinetic interaction between 5-HT and [³H]imipramine (Sette *et al.*, 1983), question the precise nature of the [³H]imipramine binding site.

Paroxetine is a non-tricyclic, highly selective 5-HT uptake blocker which, in its tritiated form, labels the 5-HT transport protein in rat and human brain and platelets with high affinity (Mellerup *et al.*, 1983; Habert *et al.*, 1985). As with [³H]imipramine, the potency of compounds to block [³H]5-HT uptake correlates closely with their potency to inhibit [³H]paroxetine binding, and lesion of serotonergic cell bodies in rat brain causes substantial and similar reductions in cortical [³H]5-HT uptake and [³H]paroxetine binding (Habert *et al.*, 1985). Although the binding capacities of [³H]paroxetine and [³H]imipramine in human platelet membranes appear equivalent (Mellerup *et al.*, 1983), their sensitivity to radiation inactivation (Mellerup *et al.*, 1985) and temperature (Plenge and Mellerup, 1984) differ, suggesting that the two sites exist on different proteins. It is highly pertinent to the current issue, therefore, that two studies of platelet [³H]paroxetine binding found no significant difference between depressed patients and healthy controls (D'haenen *et al.*, 1988; Galzin *et al.*, 1988), even though the latter group have consistently identified low [³H]imipramine binding in depressed subjects.

4.5.6 Summary

The major outstanding question in this area concerns the validity of platelet [³H]imipramine binding as a marker for major depressive disorder in man. The recent WHO-sponsored survey concluded that no consistent association exists between platelet [³H]imipramine binding and endogenous depression, although leaving open the possibility that such an association may exist for other subtypes (Mellerup *et al.*, 1990). Conversely, some laboratories consistently report decreased [^{3}H]imipramine binding in platelets from depressed subjects. This discrepancy may result from three potential sources. Firstly, at the clinical level, groups in different countries may differ in terms of their definition of depressive disorder. This would appear unlikely in view of the general application of diagnostic criteria such as DSM-III and ICD-9. Secondly, methodological differences in binding protocol may be responsible. As indicated in Table 2, the variation in absolute [^{3}H]imipramine binding capacity between different laboratories over the past 10 years is substantial. Even when assayed in the same laboratory, control platelet samples from different geographical sources varied almost fourfold in [^{3}H]imipramine binding capacity, between 360 and 1300 fmol/mg protein, whilst that from a different laboratory analysed by the same protocol resulted in a capacity of 2514 fmol/mg protein (Mellerup et al., 1990). Such differences probably result from variable contamination of the isolated platelets with leucocytes and erythrocytes which increase the protein content and hence reduce the apparent binding capacity when expressed in terms of femtomoles per milligram of protein. Relevant to this is the finding that platelet [^{3}H]imipramine binding capacity is negatively correlated with membrane protein concentration (Friedl et al., 1983; Arora et al., 1985; Theodorou et al., 1989). In addition, some binding sites may be lost during freezing and storage, as demonstrated by Healy et al. (1990). Although such effects may account for differences between laboratories, they are unlikely to apply within a single laboratory where a consistent protocol is employed, and therefore are unlikely to generate the apparent difference between depressed and control subjects. Finally, there is the possibility that low binding in some depressed patients results from blockade of [^{3}H]imipramine sites by antidepressant drugs retained within the platelet membrane. Withdrawal of all antidepressant drugs for at least 4 weeks prior to assay appears to minimize this interference, as determined by the similarity in [^{3}H]imipramine binding affinity from control and depressed subjects, but this does not discount the possibility of persistent non-competitive inhibition.

If platelet [^{3}H]imipramine binding does represent a reliable marker for general or specific subgroups of depressive disorders, it is not clear whether this represents a trait or state-dependent effect. The low binding observed in euthymic depressive subjects suggests a trait marker, and a genetic influence on platelet [^{3}H]imipramine binding has been demonstrated in twin studies compared with unrelated paired samples (Friedl and Propping, 1984). However, the intraclass correlation between monozygotic and dizygotic twins was not significantly different, suggesting that other non-genetic factors may substantially influence binding capacity. The eventual normalization in platelet [^{3}H]imipramine binding observed in several studies following complete rather than partial recovery in depressed patients would suggest it to be a slowly-adapting state-dependent marker, in which case some mechanism must exist to modify the number of [^{3}H]imipramine binding sites on extant platelets. Potential candidates for such peripheral modulators include the sex steroid and glucocorticoid hormones, both of which have been shown to influence platelet [^{3}H]imipramine binding capacity in man (Best *et al.*, 1985; Bloomfield *et al.*, 1985a). However, the lack of correspondence between [^{3}H]imipramine binding and the menstrual cycle (Poirier *et al.*, 1986) or the dexamethasone suppression test indicates that additional factors must be involved.

The relevance of the [^{3}H]imipramine binding site to the biochemical aetiology of depression depends on the role of this site in neuronal tissue and evidence of abnormalities in depressed patients. [^{3}H]Imipramine binding sites in human brain appear to be closely associated with 5-HT transport (Rehavi *et al.*, 1980), although, as indicated above, the site labelled by [^{3}H]imipramine may not correspond exactly with the 5-HT uptake site. In the brains of suicide victims, however, there are conflicting reports that [^{3}H]imipramine binding is increased, decreased or unchanged, as discussed in detail elsewhere in this volume. Clearly this does not illuminate the situation with regard to the platelet binding site. However, the absence of a parallel change in [^{3}H]imipramine binding within platelet and brain would not nullify the platelet site as a valuable marker in depression but would suggest that modulation of the platelet site represents a secondary response to peripheral mediators regulated within the brain. This situation would, however, rule out the possibility that [^{3}H]imipramine binding may act as a trait marker. The effects of antidepressant drug treatment on [^{3}H]imipramine sites in human brain have not been identified. In the rat, treatment with imipramine or desipramine reduced [^{3}H]imipramine binding in the brain (Kinnier *et al.*, 1980; Raisman *et al.*, 1980), although this effect has been challenged on the grounds of persistent drug interfering with the assay (Plenge and Mellerup, 1982). In the cat, decreased [^{3}H]imipramine binding was observed in both platelet and brain following imipramine treatment (Briley *et al.*, 1982), reinforcing the validity of the platelet as a biochemical marker for central [^{3}H]imipramine sites.

4.5.7 Future investigations

When assessing future progress in this field, a prime objective should be to compare the binding characteristics of cells obtained from a centre which regularly observes decreased binding in depressed patients with one which consistently does not find such a difference, using the protocol of the former. This should maximize the likelihood of confirming the effect and detailed methodological comparison may then identify the source of the discrepancy. Secondly, [^{3}H]imipramine binding should be carried out in parallel with [^{3}H]paroxetine binding and [^{3}H]5-HT uptake in an attempt to characterize the nature of the $[^3H]$imipramine binding site in depressed patients in relation to the 5-HT transport protein. Finally, it may be revealing to investigate sodium-independent binding of $[^3H]$imipramine in platelets of depressed and normal subjects. In those groups reporting significantly reduced binding in depression, specific binding of $[^3H]$imipramine is generally defined by 100 μmol/l desipramine, a concentration sufficiently high to displace $[^3H]$imipramine from its low affinity sites which are sodium-independent. It is possible, therefore, that these sites, whose identity and function are at present unknown, may represent the clinically relevant marker sites.

4.6 Platelet 5-HT receptors

4.6.1 Studies of the platelet 5-HT receptor in affective disorders

5-HT receptors have been implicated in depression by virtue of the action of antidepressant drugs in modifying 5-HT reuptake and catabolism, the decrease in number and/or response of such receptors in rat brain following chronic antidepressant treatment and the changes in 5-HT receptor binding in post-mortem brain from suicides. The human platelet expresses a functional 5-HT receptor which, on the basis of radioligand binding, resembles the 5-HT$_2$ subtype (Geaney et al., 1984b; McBride et al., 1987; Elliott and Kent, 1989) and appears similar to that identified by the same ligands in human brain tissue (Cross, 1982; Elliott and Kent, 1989). Stimulation of the receptor initiates phosphatidylinositol turnover (de Chaffoy de Courcelles et al., 1985), also characteristic of the 5-HT$_2$ receptor, and activates platelet shape-change (Laubscher and Pletscher, 1979) and, at higher concentration, platelet aggregation (Mitchell and Sharp, 1964).

Comparison of 5-HT-induced aggregation response in platelets from depressed and healthy subjects by Wood et al. (1984) indicated no significant difference, but studies by Healy et al. (1983) and Butler and Leonard (1988) demonstrated a significantly lower response in depressed patients, which was normalized following successful treatment. Radioligand binding studies do not, however, support the functional subsensitivity revealed by the aggregation studies. Using ^{125}I-labelled iodolysergic acid diethylamide $[^{125}I]$iodoLSD, Cowen et al. (1987) and McBride et al. (1987) found no significant difference in receptor number on platelets from depressed and healthy subjects. Using $[^3H]$LSD (Arora and Meltzer, 1989) or $[^3H]$ketanserin (Biegon et al., 1987; Butler and Leonard, 1988), binding capacity was greater in depressed patients than matched controls. In the latter study, increased receptor number was associated with decreased aggregation response (Butler and Leonard, 1988).

Treatment with tricyclic antidepressants caused an increase in binding capacity of [^{3}H]LSD in healthy volunteers (Cowen *et al.*, 1986) and of [^{125}I]iodoLSD in depressed patients (Cowen *et al.*, 1987) but a decrease in [^{3}H]ketanserin binding in depressed patients (Biegon *et al.*, 1987). Aggregation response in unipolar and bipolar depressed patients receiving lithium was enhanced relative to normal controls but this effect was not related to psychiatric morbidity (Wood *et al.*, 1985a).

4.6.2 Summary and future investigations

The confusing changes in platelet 5-HT receptor number and aggregation response in depressed patients parallels the situation with regard to 5-HT$_2$ receptors in human post-mortem brain studies. The lack of any consistent effect in platelets may reflect technical difficulties associated with these assays. Platelet aggregation is a complex phenomenon involving not only the 5-HT receptor but also numerous post-receptor events, including morphological and biochemical changes within and between platelets. Furthermore, the maximal aggregation response to 5-HT is small relative to that induced by potent platelet aggregators such as ADP or thrombin. Concomitant with this fact, the density of 5-HT receptors identified by radioligand binding is low, resulting in relatively high non-specific binding and a low signal-to-noise ratio. Consequently, large blood samples are necessary to perform such assays and, even then, the accuracy is not as great as that achieved at other platelet receptors. This problem can be obviated by using ligands of high specific activity, such as [^{125}I]iodoLSD. Interestingly, both studies employing this ligand found no significant difference between platelets from depressed patients and controls (Cowen *et al.*, 1987; McBride *et al.*, 1987).

Further investigation may clarify the situation regarding platelet 5-HT receptor number and response in depressive disorders. In particular the novel radioligand 1-(2,5-dimethoxy-4-^{125}I-iodophenyl)-2-aminopropane ([^{125}I]DOI) possesses high affinity for 5-HT$_2$ receptors and high specific activity. As an agonist, this molecule may provide additional information on the functional nature of the platelet 5-HT$_2$ receptor in depression. Such investigation would be particularly interesting if paired with analysis of 5-HT-induced phosphatidylinositol turnover, which is more closely coupled to 5-HT$_2$ receptor stimulation than platelet aggregation.

4.7 Peripheral histamine studies

The role of histamine in depression and antidepressant drug action has received little attention. Several tricyclic antidepressants possess significant histamine receptor blocking activity (Kanof and Greengard, 1978) but this is thought to contribute more to their side-effects than their prime therapeutic mode of action (Coupet and Szuchs-Myers, 1981).

4.7.1 Leucocyte histamine H_2 receptors

Specific peripheral markers for histamine receptors or uptake sites are few. Leucocytes express a functional H_2 histamine receptor which is positively linked to adenylate cyclase (Sadava and Wilmington, 1984). Accumulation of cAMP in response to $10 \mu mol/l$ histamine was significantly greater in leucocytes from untreated depressed patients compared with healthy controls or euthymic patients, whether currently receiving treatment or not (Klysner et al., 1987). In a more recent study, however, no significant differences were observed between depressed patients, schizophrenic patients and controls in relation to histamine-stimulated adenylate cyclase activity (Kanof et al., 1989). The status of the leucocyte histamine H_2 receptor in depression therefore remains equivocal.

4.7.2 Platelet accumulation of histamine

Although human platelets do not possess a specific histamine transport mechanism, K. Wood et al. (1983) reported significantly slower accumulation of histamine in vitro by cells from depressed female patients than by healthy female controls. The patients were receiving a variety of antidepressant treatments at the time of assay, including tricyclics and monoamine oxidase (MAO) inhibitors. A follow-up study, including both male and female depressed patients, supported the initial finding (Wood et al., 1984). However, no significant difference was seen between control and patients receiving lithium. In vitro lithium was shown directly to enhance histamine uptake within the $0.5-1.0 \mu mol/l$ concentration range (Wood, 1989). The significance of these findings to the activity of histamine-related neuronal activity is uncertain. The rate of histamine accumulation by platelets is approximately 1000-fold slower than that of 5-HT (Wood, 1989), suggesting that it occurs either by passive diffusion through the membrane or via the 5-HT transport site, at much lower affinity and rate than 5-HT itself. If the latter proved to be correct, then any antidepressants which block 5-HT uptake would also reduce the rate of histamine accumulation, since the platelets used in such assays are suspended in autologous plasma. This would not, however, explain the enhancement of histamine transport by lithium.

4.8 Platelet monoamine oxidase activity

In man, MAO exists in two forms, type A and type B, both of which are found in the brain but only type B in platelets. These enzymes are responsible for the catabolism of 5-HT, noradrenaline and dopamine. Since the introduction of MAO inhibitors as antidepressant drugs, much work has concentrated on the investigation of platelet MAO activity in psychiatric disorders. This body of work has recently been comprehensively reviewed (Sandler *et al.*, 1981; Fowler *et al.*, 1982; Wirz-Justice, 1988; Youdim, 1988). Although not unanimous in their findings, many studies find that platelet MAO activity is decreased in bipolar compared with unipolar depressed patients or controls, and may be higher in endogenous than in non-endogenous or reactive depression. Differences in MAO activity may also be related to particular syndromes such as suicidal behaviour (low activity) and anxiety (high activity). They are not specific to affective illness, since changes have also been reported in schizophrenia, alcoholism and Alzheimer's disease. Platelet MAO activity is particularly useful as an indicator of the pharmacodynamic effect of MAO inhibitors, although restricted to effects on MAO-B. This is particularly relevant in view of the recent revival of interest in the use of MAO inhibitors and the introduction of new reversible enzyme inhibitors (Nutt and Glue, 1989).

4.9 Peripheral acetylcholine receptors

Several antidepressants possess significant antimuscarinic activity, giving rise to the common parasympathetic side-effects of dry mouth and constipation. Rather than being an unwelcome side-effect, however, some investigators have proposed that this cholinergic activity plays an important therapeutic role in the action of antidepressants by restoring an imbalance between central adrenergic and cholinergic neurotransmission (Janowsky *et al.*, 1972; Davis and Berger, 1978). In an attempt to monitor the activity of muscarinic acetylcholine receptors, peripheral models have been established using lymphocytes (Dulis *et al.*, 1979; Bering *et al.*, 1987) and cultured fibroblasts (Nadi *et al.*, 1984). Comparison of [^{3}H]quinuclidyl benzilate ([^{3}H]QNB) binding to fibroblast membranes obtained from 18 patients with major depressive disorder (17 bipolar; 1 unipolar) and 12 normal controls indicated significantly more receptors in tissue from the depressed patients (Nadi *et al.*, 1984). Binding capacity in 18 relatives of the depressed patients who themselves had a history of minor or major depressive disorder was higher than that in five unaffected relatives or in the controls. The authors concluded that increased muscarinic receptor number may be a trait marker associated with familial vulnerability to depressive disorders. However, attempts by Lin and Richelson (1986) to repeat this study were unsuccessful. They observed much lower receptor densities than Nadi *et al.* (1984), even in identical cell lines, and could find no evidence of functional association between the receptors and either cAMP or cGMP synthesis. The significance of cholinergic receptors to depression and antidepressant drug mechanisms therefore remains equivocal.

4.10 Peripheral PGE$_1$ receptors

Both platelets and leucocytes express prostaglandin PGE$_1$ receptors which are positively linked to adenylate cyclase. Studies of leucocyte cAMP response to PGE$_1$ show no significant difference between cells from depressed patients and those from healthy controls (Pandey *et al.*, 1979; Kanof *et al.*, 1986, 1989; Ebstein *et al.*, 1988). In platelets the cAMP response to PGE$_1$ is reported to be unchanged (Wang *et al.*, 1974; Kafka *et al.*, 1981) or decreased (Kanof *et al.*, 1986) in depressed patients compared with healthy controls. However, this decrease is not specific to depressive disorders and is not related to symptom severity (Kanof *et al.*, 1986).

4.11 Leucocyte glucocorticoid receptors

Increased cortisol secretion is frequently observed in depressed patients, and sensitivity to exogenous corticosteroids appears to be decreased, as demonstrated by the dexamethasone suppression test (Carroll *et al.*, 1981; Halbreich *et al.*, 1985; and see Chapter 5). Quantification of corticosteroid receptors on lymphocytes using [^{3}H]dexamethasone indicates significantly fewer receptors on cells from depressed patients compared with healthy controls (Gormley *et al.*, 1985; Whalley *et al.*, 1986). After administration of dexamethasone (1 mg) the binding capacity was significantly reduced in patients whose endogenous cortisol secretion was suppressed but was unchanged in patients classed as non-suppressors (Gormley *et al.*, 1985). In euthymic patients, the density of glucocorticoid receptors was not significantly different from healthy controls, suggesting that this acts as a state-dependent marker for depressive disorders

(Hunter *et al.*, 1988). However, others have reported no difference in corticosteroid receptor number between healthy controls and depressed patients, irrespective of their sensitivity to dexamethasone (Schlechte and Sherman, 1985).

4.12 General conclusions

The general consensus of the data presented above is that none of the peripheral models proposed to date can be considered reliable enough to act as a biochemical marker for affective disorder. Considerable debate surrounds each of the potential models and even in those which are strongly supported there is considerable overlap between values observed in healthy and depressed subjects on assay. The trend in recent years has been to subcategorize the patient group in order to identify localized markers, such as β-adrenoceptor changes in depressed patients with psychomotor agitation and $[^3H]$imipramine binding decrease in depressed patients with obsessive compulsive symptoms. Also, some studies have simultaneously analysed several parameters in order to establish a biochemical profile of each subgroup. Although such protocols inevitably increase the size of each study and the complexity of the statistical analysis employed, the chances of success are likely to be improved. Exhaustive analysis of individual parameters has produced little reward, indicating, as many have suspected, that depression is not the result of a single biochemical defect. Future progress in understanding the biochemical basis of affective disorders will depend upon parallel developments in studies using animal models, in categorization of the disorder by means of psychiatric assessment and in the gradual amalgamation of biochemical, physiological and genetic studies carried out in man.

References

Aarons, R.D., Nies, A.S., Gal, J., Hegstrand, L.R. & Molinoff, P.B. (1980) *J. Clin. Invest.* **65**, 949–957.

Ahtee, L., Briley, M., Raisman, R., Lebrec, D. & Langer, S.Z. (1981) *Life Sci.* **29**, 2323–2329.

Alston, W.C., Patel, K.R. & Kerr, J.W. (1974) *Br. Med. J.* **1**, 90–93.

Arora, R.C. & Meltzer, H.Y. (1982) *Psychiatry Res.* **6**, 327–333.

Arora, R.C. & Meltzer, H.Y. (1983) *Psychiatry Res.* **9**, 29–36.

Arora, R.C. & Meltzer, H.Y. (1988) *Biol. Psychiatry* **23**, 397–404.

Arora, R.C. & Meltzer, H.Y. (1989) *Life Sci* **44**, 725–734.

Arora, R.C., Kregel, L. & Meltzer, H.Y. (1984) *Biol. Psychiatry* **19**, 795–804.

Arora, R.C., Wunnicke, V. & Meltzer, H.Y. (1985) *Biol. Psychiatry* **20**, 116–119.

Arora, R.C., Locascio, J.J. & Meltzer, H.Y. (1986) *Psychiatry Res.* **19**, 215–224.

Asarch, K.B., Shic, J.C. & Kulcsar, A. (1980) *Commun. Psychopharmacol.* **4**, 425–432.

Asberg, M., Traskman, L. & Thoren, P. (1976) *Arch. Gen. Psychiatry* **33**, 1193–1197.

Asberg, M., Nordstrom, P. & Traskman-Bendz, L. (1986) In *Suicide* (ed. Roy, A.), pp 47–71. Baltimore, Williams & Wilkins.

Banerjee, S.P., Kung, L.S., Riggi, S.J. & Chandra, S.K. (1977) *Nature* **268**, 455–456.

Banki, C.M. (1978) *Acta Psychiatr. Scand.* **57**, 232–238.

Barnett, D.B., Nahorski, S.R. & Richardson, A. (1984) *Br. J. Pharmacol.* **81**, 159P.

Baron, M., Barkai, A., Gruen, R., Kowalik, S. & Quitkin, F. (1983) *Biol. Psychiatry* **18**, 1403–1409.

Baron, M., Barkai, A., Gruen, R., Peselow, E., Fieve, R.R. & Quitkin, F. (1986) *Am. J. Psychiatry* **143**, 711–717.

Baron, M., Barkai, A., Kowalik, S., Fieve, R.R., Quitkin, F. & Gruen, R. (1988) *Neuropsychobiology* **19**, 9–11.

Bering, B., Moises, H.W. & Muller, W.E. (1987) *Biol. Psychiatry* **22**, 1451–1458.

Berrettini, W.H., Bardakjian, J., Cappellari, C.B. *et al.* (1987a) *Biol. Psychiatry* **22**, 1439–1443.

Berrettini, W.H., Cappellari, C.B., Nurnberger, J.I. & Gershon, E.S. (1987b) *Neuropsychobiology* **17**, 15–18.

Best, N.R., Cowen, P.J., Elliott, J.M., Fraser, S., Gosden, B. & Stump, K. (1985) *Br. J. Clin. Pharmacol.* **19**, 555P.

Best, N.R., Wiley, M., Stump, K., Elliott, J.M. & Cowen, P.J. (1988) *Psychol. Med.* **18**, 837–842.

Beving, H., Bjerkenstedt, L., Malmgren, R., Olsson, P. & Unge, G. (1985) *J. Neural Transm.* **61**, 95–104.

Biegon, A., Weizman, A., Karp, L., Ram, A., Tiano, S. & Wolff, M. (1987) *Life Sci.* **41**, 2485–2492.

Bloomfield, J.G., Elliott, J.M. & Evans, D.J. (1985a) *Br. J. Pharmacol.* **86**, 402P.

Bloomfield, J.G., Elliott, J.M. & Rutterford, M.G. (1985b) *Br. J. Pharmacol.* **85**, 323P.

Bondy, B.V., Ackenheil, M., Birzle, W., Elbers, R. & Frohler, M. (1984) *Biol. Psychiatry* **19**, 1377–1393.

Boon, N.A., Elliott, J.M., Davies, C.L. *et al.* (1983a) *Clin. Sci.* **65**, 207–208.

Boon, N.A., Elliott, J.M., Grahame-Smith, D.G., St John-Green, T. & Stump, K. (1983b) *J. Auton. Pharmacol.* **3**, 89–95.

Born, G.V.R., Grignani, G. & Martin, K. (1980) *Br. J. Clin. Pharmacol.* **9**, 321–325.

Braddock, L., Cowen, P.J., Elliott, J.M., Fraser, S. & Stump, K. (1984) *Neuropharmacology* **23**, 285–286.

Braddock, L., Cowen, P.J., Elliott, J.M., Fraser, S. & Stump, K. (1986) *Psychol. Med.* **16**, 765–773.

Briley, M., Raisman, R. & Langer, S.Z. (1979) *Eur. J. Pharmacol.* **58**, 347–348.

Briley, M., Langer, S.Z., Raisman, R., Sechter, D. & Zarifian, E. (1980) *Science* **209**, 303–305.

Briley, M., Raisman, R., Arbilla, S., Casadamont, M. & Langer, S.Z. (1982) *Eur. J. Pharmacol.* **81**, 309–314.

Brodde, O.-E., Anlauf, E., Graben, N. & Bock, K.D. (1982a) *Eur. J. Clin. Pharmacol.* **23**, 403–409.

Brodde, O.-E., Anlauf, M., Graben, N. & Bock, K.D. (1982b) *Eur. J. Pharmacol.* **81**, 345–347.

Brodde, O.-E., Seher, U., Nohlen, M., Fischer, W.M. & Michel, M.C. (1988) *Eur. J. Pharmacol.* **150**, 403–404.

Brown, G.L., Goodwin, F.K., Ballenger, J.C., Goyer, P.J. & Major, L.F. (1979) *Psychiatry Res.* **1**, 131–139.

Brown, S.L., Charney, D.S., Woods, S.W., Heninger, G.R. & Tallman, J. (1988) *Psychopharmacol.* **94**, 24–28.

Buckholtz, N.S., Davies, A.O., Rudorfer, M.V., Golden, R.N. & Potter, W.Z. (1988) *Biol. Psychiatry* **24**, 451–457.

Buckley, C., Curtin, D., Walsh, T. & O'Malley, K. (1986) *Br. J. Clin. Pharmacol.* **21**, 721–722.

Butler, J. & Leonard, B.E. (1986) *Int. Clin. Psychopharmacol.* **1**, 244–252.

Butler, J. & Leonard, B.E. (1988) *Int. Clin. Psychopharmacol.* **3**, 343–347.

Cameron, O.G., Smith, C.B., Hollingsworth, P.J. Nesse, R.M. & Curtis, G.C. (1984) *Arch. Gen. Psychhiatry* **41**, 1144–1148.

Campbell, I.C., McKernan, R.M., Checkley, S.A., Glass, I.B., Thompson, C. & Shur, E. (1985) *Psychiatry Res.* **14**, 17–31.

Carroll, B.J., Feinberg, M., Greden, J.F. *et al.* (1981) *Arch. Gen. Psychiatry* **38**, 15–22.

Carstens, M.E., Engelbrecht, A.H., Russell, V.A. *et al.* (1986a) *Psychiatry Res.* **18**, 321–331.

Carstens, M.E., Engelbrecht, A.H., Russell, V.A. *et al.* (1986b) *Psychiatry Res.* **18**, 333–342.

Carstens, M.E., Engelbrecht, A.H., Russell, V.A. *et al.* (1987) *Psychiatry Res.* **20**, 239–248.

Carstens, M.E., Engelbrecht, A.H., Russell, V.A., van Zyl, A.M. & Taljaard, J.J. (1988) *Psychiatry Res.* **23**, 77–88.

Charney, D.S. & Heninger, G.R. (1986) *Arch. Gen. Psychiatry* **43**, 1037–1041.

Conolly, M.E. & Greenacre, J.K. (1976) *J. Clin. Invest.* **58**, 1307–1316.

Cooper, B., Handin, R.I., Young, L.H. & Alexander, R.W. (1978) *Nature* **274**, 703–706.

Cooper, S.J., Kelly, J.G. & King, D.J. (1985) *Br. J. Psychiatry* **147**, 23–29.

Coppen, A., Turner, P., Rowsell, A.R. & Padgham, C. (1976) *Postgrad. Med. J.* **52**, 156–158.

Coppen, A., Swade, C. & Wood, K. (1978) *Clin. Chim. Acta* **87**, 165–168.

Coppen, A., Swade, C., Wood, K. & Carroll, J.D. (1979) *Lancet* **ii**, 914.

Coupet, J. & Szuchs-Myers, V.A. (1981) *Eur. J. Pharmacol.* **74**, 149–153.

Cowen, P.J., Geaney, D.P., Schachter, M., Green, A.R. & Elliott, J.M. (1986) *Arch. Gen. Psychiatry* **43**, 61–67.

Cowen, P.J., Charig, E.M., Fraser, S. & Elliott, J.M. (1987) *J. Affective Disord.* **13**, 45–50.

Cross, A.J. (1982) *Eur. J. Pharmacol.* **82**, 77–80.

Daiguchi, M., Meltzer, H.Y., Tong, C., U'Prichard, D.C., Young, M. & Kravitz, H. (1981) *Life Sci.* **29**, 2059–2064.

Davies, A.O. & Lefkowitz, R.J. (1980) *J. Clin. Endocrinol. Metab.* **51**, 599–605.

Davies, I.B., Sudera, D. & Sever, P.S. (1981) *Clin. Sci.* **61**, 207s–210s.

Davis, K.L. & Berger, P.A. (1978) *Biol. Psychiatry* **13**, 23–49.

de Chaffoy de Courcelles, D., Leysen, J.E., de Clerk, F., van Belle, H. & Janssen, P.A.J. (1985) *J. Biol. Chem.* **260**, 7603–7608.

Desmedt, D.H., Egrise, D. & Mendlewicz, J. (1987) *J. Affective Disord.* **12**, 193–198.

D'haenen, H., De Waele, M. & Leysen, J.E. (1988) *Psychiatry Res.* **26**, 11–17.

Doyle, M.C., George, A.J., Ravindran, A.V. & Philpott, R. (1985) *Am. J. Psychiatry* **142**, 1489–1490.

Dulis, B.H., Gordon, M.A. & Wilson, I.B. (1979) *Mol. Pharmacol.* **15**, 28–34.

Ebstein, R.P., Lerer, B., Shapira, B., Shemesh, Z., Moscovich, D.G. & Kindler, S. (1988) *Br. J. Psychiatry* **152**, 665–669.

Egrise, D., Desmedt, D., Schoutens, A. & Mendlewicz, J. (1983) *Neuropsychobiology* **10**, 101–102.

Egrise, D., Rubinstein, M., Schoutens, A., Cantraine, F. & Mendlewicz, J. (1986) *Biol. Psychiatry* **21**, 283–292.

Elliott, J.M. (1984) *J. Affective Disord.* **6**, 219–239.

Elliott, J.M. & Grahame-Smith, D.G. (1982) *Br. J. Pharmacol.* **76**, 121–130.

Elliott, J.M. & Kent, A. (1989) *J. Neurochem.* **53**, 191–196.

Extein, I., Tallman, J., Smith, C.C. & Goodwin, F.K. (1979) *Psychiatry Res.* **1**, 191–197.

Feldman, R.D., Limbird, L.E., Nadeau, J., Fitzgerald, G.A., Robertson, D. & Wood, A.J.J. (1983) *J. Clin. Invest.* **72**, 164–170.

Flament, M.F., Rapoport, J.L., Murphy, D.L., Berg, C.J. & Lake, C.R. (1987) *Arch. Gen. Psychiatry* **44**, 219–225.

Fowler, C.J., Tipton, K.F., MacKay, A.V.P. & Youdim, M.B.H. (1982) *Neuroscience* **7**, 1577–1594.

Fraser, J., Nadeau, J., Robertson, D. & Wood, A.J.J. (1981) *J. Clin. Invest.* **67**, 1777–1784.

Friedl, W. & Propping, P. (1984) *Psychiatry Res.* **11**, 279–285.

Friedl, W., Propping, P. & Weck, B. (1983) *Psychopharmacology* **80**, 96–99.

Galzin, A.M., Loo, H., Sechter, D. & Langer, S.Z. (1986) *Biol. Psychiatry* **21**, 876–882.

Galzin, A.M., Poirier, M.F., Loo, H., Sechter, D., Zarifian, E. & Langer, S.Z. (1988) *Br. J. Pharmacol.* **93**, 12P.

Garcia-Sevilla, J.A. & Fuster, M.J. (1986) *Eur. J. Pharmacol.* **124**, 31–41.

Garcia-Sevilla, J.A., Hollingsworth, P.J. & Smith, C.B. (1981a) *Eur. J. Pharmacol.* **74**, 329–341.

Garcia-Sevilla, J.A., Zis, A.P., Hollingsworth, P.J., Greden, J.F. & Smith, C.B. (1981b) *Arch. Gen. Psychiatry* **38**, 1327–1333.

Garcia-Sevilla, J.A., Zis, A.P., Zelnik, T.C. & Smith, C.B. (1981c) *Eur. J. Pharmacol.* **69**, 121–123.

Garcia-Sevilla, J.A., Garcia-Vallejo, P. & Guimon, J. (1983) *Eur. J. Pharmacol.* **94**, 359–360.

Garcia-Sevilla, J.A., Ugedo, L., Ulibari, I. & Gutierrez, M. (1985) *Eur. J. Pharmacol.* **114**, 365–374.

Garcia-Sevilla, J.A., Guimon, J., Garcia-Vallejo, P. & Fuster, M.J. (1986a) *Arch. Gen. Psychiatry* **43**, 51–57.

Garcia-Sevilla, J.A., Ugedo, L., Ulibari, I. & Gutierrez, M. (1986b) *Psychopharmacology* **88**, 489–492.

Garcia-Sevilla, J.A., Udina, C., Fuster, M.J., Alvarez, E. & Casas, M. (1987) *Acta Psychiatr. Scand.* **75**, 150–157.

Geaney, D.P., Rutterford, M.G., Elliott, J.M., Schachter, M., Peet, K.M.S. & Grahame-Smith, D.G. (1984a) *J. Neurol. Neurosurg. Psychiatry* **47**, 720–723.

Geaney, D.P., Schachter, M., Elliott, J.M. & Grahame-Smith, D.G. (1984b) *Eur. J. Pharmacol.* **97**, 87–93.

Gentsch, C., Lichtsteiner, M., Gastpar, M., Gastpar, G. & Feer, H. (1985) *Psychiatry Res.* **14**, 177–187.

Gentsch, C., Lichtsteiner, M., Gastpar, M., Gastpar, G. & Feer, H. (1989) *J. Affective Disord.* **16**, 65–70.

Georgotas, A., Schweitzer, J., McCue, R.E., Armour, M. & Friedhoff, A.J. (1987) *Life Sci.* **40**, 2137–2143.

Gibbons, F.L. & McHugh, P.R. (1962) *J. Psychiatr. Res.* **1**, 162–171.

Gibson, J.M., Horton, R.W., Theodorou, A.E. & Yamaguchi, Y. (1986) *Br. J. Pharmacol.* **87**, 89P.

Gierschik, P. & Jakobs, K.H. (1988) In *The Alpha-2 Adrenergic Receptors* (ed. Limbird, L.E.), pp 75–113. Clifton, Humana Press.

Glue, P.W., Cowen, P.J., Nutt, D.J., Kolakowska, T. & Grahame-Smith, D.G. (1986) *Psychopharmacology* **90**, 398–402.

Goodwin, G.M., Fraser, S., Stump, K., Fairburn, C.G., Elliott, J.M. & Cowen, P.J. (1987) *J. Affective Disord.* **12**, 267–274.

Gormley, G.J., Lowy, M.T., Reder, A.T., Hospelhorn, V.D., Antel, J.P. & Meltzer, H.Y. (1985) *Am. J. Psychiatry* **142**, 1278–1284.

Graafsma, S., Rodrigues-de Miranda, J. & Thien, T. (1986) *N. Engl. J. Med.* **314**, 924.

Green, A.R. & Nutt, D.J. (1985) In *Preclinical Psychopharmacology* (eds Grahame-Smith, D.G. & Cowen, P.J.), pp 1–34. Amsterdam, Elsevier.

Habert, E., Graham, D., Tahraoui, L., Claustre, Y. & Langer, S.Z. (1985) *Eur. J. Pharmacol.* **118**, 107–114.

Halbreich, U., Asnis, G.M., Shindledecker, R., Zumoff, B. & Nathan, S.N. (1985) *Arch. Gen. Psychiatry* **42**, 904–908.

Halper, J.P., Brown, R.P., Sweeney, J.A., Kocsis, J.H., Peters, A. & Mann, J.J. (1988) *Arch. Gen. Psychiatry* **45**, 241–244.

Heal, D.J., Butler, S.A., Hurst, E.M. & Buckett, W.R. (1989) *J. Neurochem.* **53**, 1019–1025.

Healy, D., Carney, P.A. & Leonard, B.E. (1983) *J. Psychiatr. Res.* **17**, 251–260.

Healy, D., Carney, P.A., O'Halloran, A. & Leonard, B.E. (1985) *J. Affective Disord.* **9**, 285–296.

Healy, D., O'Halloran, A., Carney, P.A. & Leonard, B.E. (1986) *J. Psychiatr. Res.* **20**, 345–353.

Healy, D., Theodorou, A.E., Whitehouse, A.M. *et al.* (1990) *Br. J. Psychiatry* **157**, 208–215

Heufelder, A., Warnhoff, M. & Pirke, K.M. (1985) *J. Clin. Endocrinol. Metab.* **61**, 1053–1060.

Hrdina, P.D. (1986) In *Neuromethods. 4: Receptor Binding* (eds Boulton, A.A., Baker, G.B. & Hrdina, P.D.), pp 455–438. Clifton, Humana Press.

Hrdina, P.D. (1987) *Can. J. Physiol. Pharmacol.* **65**, 2422–2426.

Hrdina, P.D. (1988) *Eur. J. Pharmacol.* **148**, 279–283.

Hrdina, P.D. (1989) *Int. J. Clin. Pharm. Res.* **9**, 119–122.

Hrdina, P.D., Lapierre, Y.D., Horn, E.R. & Bakish, D. (1985) *Prog. Neuropsychopharmacol. Biol. Psychiatry* **9**, 619–623.

Humphries, L.L., Shirley, P., Allen, M., Codd, E.E. & Walker, R.F. (1985) *Biol. Psychiatry* **20**, 1073–1081.

Hunter, R., Dick, H., Christie, J.E., Goodwin, G.M. & Fink, G. (1988) *J. Affective Disord.* **14**, 155–159.

Innis, R.B., Charney, D.S. & Heninger, G.R. (1987) *Psychiatry Res.* **21**, 33–41.

Janowsky, D.S., El-Yousef, M.K., Davis, J.M. & Sekerke, H.J. (1972) *Lancet* **ii**, 632–635.

Jones, S.B., Bylund, D.B., Reiser, C.A., Shekim, W.O., Byer, J.A. & Carr, G.W. (1983) *Clin. Pharmacol. Ther.* **34**, 90–96.

Kafka, M.S. & van Kammen, D.P. (1983) *Arch. Gen. Psychiatry* **40**, 264–270.

Kafka, M.S., van Kammen, D.P., Kleinmann, J.E. *et al.* (1981) *Commun. Psychopharmacol.* **4**, 477–486.

Kafka, M.S., Nurnberger, J.I., Siever, L., Targum, S., Uhde, T.W. & Gershon, E.S. (1986) *J. Affective Disord.* **10**, 163–169.

Kamal, D., Le Quan-Bui, K.M. & Meyer, P. (1984) *Hypertension* **6**, 568–573.

Kanof, P.D. & Greengard, P. (1978) *Nature* **272**, 329–333.

Kanof, P.D., Johns, C., Davidson, M., Siever, L.J., Coccaro, E.F. & Davis, K.L. (1986) *Arch. Gen. Psychiatry* **43**, 987–993.

Kanof, P.D., Coccaro, E.F., Johns, C.A., Siever, L.J. & Davis, K.L. (1987) *Biol. Psychiatry* **22**, 278–286.

Kanof, P.D., Johns, C.A., Davidson, M., Siever, L.J., Coccaro, E.F. & Davis, K.L. (1988) *Psychiatry Res.* **23**, 11–22.

Kanof, P.D., Coccaro, E.F., Johns, C.A., Davidson, M., Siever, L.J. & Davis, K.L. (1989) *Biol. Psychiatry* **25**, 413–420.

Karliner, J.S., Motulsky, H.J. & Insel, P.A. (1982) *Mol. Pharmacol.* **21**, 36–43.

Katona, C.L.E., Theodorou, A.E. & Horton, R.W. (1987) *Psychiat. Dev.* **2**, 129–149.

Katona, C.L.E., Theodorou, A.E., Davies, S.L. *et al.* (1989) *J. Affective Disord.* **17**, 219–228.

Kim, M.H. & Neubig, R.R. (1987) *Biochemistry* **26**, 3664–3672.

Kinnier, W.J., Chuang, D.M. & Costa, E. (1980) *Eur. J. Pharmacol.* **67**, 289–294.

Klysner, R., Geisler, A. & Rosenberg, R. (1987) *J. Affective Disord.* **13**, 227–232.

Kobilka, B.K., Matsui, J., Kobilka, T.S. *et al.* (1987) *Science* **238**, 650–656.

Krawietz, W., Werdan, K., Schober, M., Erdmann, E., Rindfleisch, G.E. & Hannig, K. (1982) *Biochem. Pharmacol.* **31**, 133–136.

Kronfol, Z., Turner, R., Nasrallah, H. & Winokur, G. (1984) *Psychiatry Res.* **13**, 13–18.

Kronfol, Z., Nasrallah, H.A., Chapman, S. & House, J.D. (1985) *J. Affective Disord.* **9**, 169–173.

Landmann, R.M.A., Burgisser, E., Wesp, M. & Buhler, F.R. (1984) *J. Receptor Res.* **4**, 37–50.

Langer, S.Z. & Schoemaker, H. (1988) *Prog. Neuro-Psychopharmacol. Biol. Psychiatry* **12**, 193–216.

Langer, S.Z., Sechter, D., Loo, H., Raisman, R. & Zarifian, E. (1986) *Arch. Gen. Psychiatry* **43**, 949–952.

Lapin, I.P. & Oxenkrug, G.F. (1969) *Lancet* **i**, 132–134.

Laubscher, A. & Pletscher, A. (1979) *Life Sci.* **24**, 1833–1840.

Lee, T.P., Busse, W.W. & Reed, C.E. (1977) *J. Allergy Clin. Immunol.* **59**, 408–418.

Lentes, K.U., Berrettini, W.H., Hoehe, M.R., Chung, F.Z. & Gershon, E.S. (1988) *Nucleic Acids Res.* **16**, 2359.

Le Quan-Bui, K.H., Plaisant, O., Leboyer, M. *et al.* (1984) *Psychiatry Res.* **13**, 129–139.

Lewis, D.A. & McChesney, C. (1985) *Arch. Gen. Psychiatry* **42**, 485–488.

Lewis, D.A., Noyes, R., Coryell, W. & Clancy, J. (1985) *Psychiatry Res.* **16**, 1–9.

Lin, S.-C. & Richelson, E. (1986) *Am. J. Psychiatry* **143**, 658–660.

Logsdon, P.J., Middleton, E. & Coffey, R.G. (1972) *J. Allergy Clin. Immunol.* **50**, 45–56.

Luck, P., Mikhailidis, D.P., Dashwood, M.R. *et al.* (1983) *J. Clin. Endocrinol. Metab.* **57**, 911–914.

McBride, P.A., Mann, J.J., Polley, M.J., Wiley, A.J. & Sweeney, J.A. (1987) *Life Sci.* **40**, 1799–1809.

McGuffin, P. & Katz, R. (1989) *Br. J. Psychiatry* **155**, 294–304.

Magliozzi, J.R., Gietzen, D., Maddock, R.J. *et al.* (1989) *Biol. Psychiatry* **26**, 15–25.

Magni, G., Andreoli, F., Arduino, C. *et al.* (1987) *Pain* **30**, 311–320.

Maj, M., Mastronardi, P., Palomba, U., Romano, M., Ventra, C. & Kemali, D. (1988) *Pharmacopsychiatry* **21**, 101–103.

Malmgren, E., Olsson, P., Tornling, G. & Unge, G. (1980) *Thromb. Res.* **18**, 733–741.

Malmgren, R., Aberg-Wistedt, A. & Martensson, B. (1989) *Biol. Psychiatry* **25**, 393–402.

Mann, J.J., Brown, R.P., Halper, J.P. *et al.* (1985) *N. Engl. J. Med.* **313**, 715–720.

Marcusson, J.O., Backstrom, I.T. & Ross, S.B. (1986) *Mol. Pharmacol.* **30**, 121–129.

Mellerup, E.T., Plenge, P. & Rosenberg, R. (1982) *Psychiatry Res.* **7**, 221–227.

Mellerup, E.T., Plenge, P. & Engelstoft, M. (1983) *Eur. J. Pharmacol.* **96**, 303–309.

Mellerup, E.T., Plenge, P. & Nielsen, M. (1985) *Eur. J. Pharmacol.* **106**, 411–413.

Mellerup, E.T., Bech, P., Hansen, H.J., Langemark, M., Loldrup, D. & Plenge, P. (1988) *Psychiatry Res.* **26**, 149–156.

Mellerup, E.T. & Langer, S.Z. (1990) *Pharmacopsychiatry* **23**, 113–117.

Meltzer, H.Y., Arora, R.C., Baber, R. & Tricou, B.J. (1981) *Arch. Gen. Psychiatry* **38**, 1322–1326.

Meltzer, H.Y., Arora, R.C., Tricou, B.J. & Fang, V.S. (1983) *Psychiatry Res.* **8**, 41–47.

Metz, A., Stump, K., Cowen, P.J., Elliott, J.M., Gelder, M.G. & Grahame-Smith, D.G. (1983) *Lancet* **i**, 495–498.

Minneman, K.P., Dibner, M.D., Wolfe, B.B. & Molinoff, P.B. (1979) *Science* **204**, 866–868.

Mitchell, J.R.A. & Sharp, A.A. (1964) *Br. J. Haematol.* **10**, 78–92.

Modai, I., Malmgren, R., Asberg, M. & Beving, H. (1986) *Psychopharmacology* **88**, 493–495.

Mooney, J.J., Schatzberg, A.F., Cole, J.O., Kizuka, P.P. & Schildkraut, J.J. (1985) *J. Psychiat. Res.* **19**, 65.

Moret, C. & Briley, M. (1986) *J. Neurochem.* **47**, 1609–1612.

Motulsky, H.J. & Insel, P.A. (1982) *Biochem. Pharmacol.* **31**, 2591–2597.

Motulsky, H.J., O'Connor, D.T. & Insel, P.A. (1983) *Clin. Sci.* **64**, 265–272.

Motulsky, H.J., Shattil, S.J., Ferry, N., Rozansky, D. & Insel, P.A. (1986) *Mol. Pharmacol.* **29**, 1–6.

Muck-Seler, D., Deanovic, Z., Jamnicky, B., Jakupcevic, M. & Mihovilovic, M. (1983) *Psychopharmacology* **79**, 262–265.

Murphy, D., Gardner, R., Greden, J.F. & Carroll, B.J. (1987) *Psychol. Med.* **17**, 381–385.

Murphy, D.L., Zohar, J., Benkelfat, C., Pato, M.T., Pigott, T.A. & Insel, P.A. (1989) *Br. J. Psychiatry* **155** (Suppl. 8), 15–24.

Muscettola, G., Lauro, A.D. & Giannini, C.P. (1986) *Psychiatry Res.* **18**, 343–353.

Nadi, N.S., Nurnberger, J.I. & Gershon, E.S. (1984) *N. Engl. J. Med.* **311**, 225–230.

Nankai, M., Yoshimoto, S., Narita, K. & Takahashi, R. (1986) *J. Affective Disord.* **11**, 207–212.

Nemeroff C.B., Knight, D.L., Krishnan, R.R. *et al.* (1988) *Arch. Gen. Psychiatry* **45**, 919–923.

Neubig, R.R., Gantzos, R.D. & Brasier, R.S. (1985) *Mol. Pharmacol.* **28**, 475–486.

Nunnari, J.M., Repaske, M.G., Brandon, S., Cragoe, E.J. & Limbird, L.E. (1987) *J. Biol. Chem.* **262**, 12387–12392.

Nutt, D.J. & Fraser, S. (1987) *J. Affective Disord.* **12**, 7–11.

Nutt, D.J. & Glue, P. (1989) *Br. J. Psychiatry* **154**, 287–291.

Pandey, G.N., Dysken, M.W., Garrer, D.L. & Davis, J.M. (1979) *Am. J. Psychiatry* **136**, 675–678.

Pandey, G.N., Janicak, P.G. & Davis, J.M. (1987) *Psychiatry Res.* **22**, 265–273.

Pandey, G.N., Janicak, P.G., Javaid, J.I. & Davis, J.M. (1989) *Psychiatry Res.* **28**, 73–88.

Parker, C.W. & Smith, J.W. (1973) *J. Clin. Invest.* **52**, 48–59.

Paul, S.M., Rehavi, M., Skolnick, P. & Goodwin, F.K. (1980) *Life Sci.* **26**, 953–960.

Paul, S.M., Rehavi, M., Skolnick, P., Ballenger, J. & Goodwin, F.K. (1981) *Arch. Gen. Psychiatry* **38**, 1315–1317.

Payvandi, N., Kay, G., Elliott, J.M., Wilson, S., Glue, P. & Nutt, D.J. (1990a) *J. Psychopharmacol.* **4**, 274.

Payvandi, N., Elliott, J.M. & Heal, D.J. (1990b) *Eur. J. Pharmacol.* **183**, 740–741.

Pecknold, J.C., Chang, H., Fleury, D. *et al.* (1987) *J. Psychiatr. Res.* **21**, 319–326.

Pecknold, J.C., Suranyi-Cadotte, B., Chang, H. & Nair, N.P. (1988) *Neuropsychopharmacology* **1**, 173–176.

Peters, J.R., Elliott, J.M. & Grahame-Smith, D.G. (1979) *Lancet* ii, 933–936.

Pfeifer, M.A., Ward, K., Malpass, T. *et al.* (1984) *J. Clin. Invest.* **74**, 1063–1072.

Piletz, J.E. & Halaris, A. (1988) *Prog. Neuropsychopharmacol. Biol. Psychiatry* **12**, 541–553.

Pimoule, C., Briley, M.S., Gay, C. *et al.* (1983) *Psychopharmacology* **79**, 308–312.

Pitt, B. (1973) *Br. J. Psychiatry* **122**, 431–433.

Plenge, P. & Mellerup, E.T. (1982) *Psychopharmacology* **77**, 94–99.

Plenge, P. & Mellerup, E.T. (1984) *Biochim. Biophys. Acta* **770**, 22–28.

Plenge, P., Mellerup, E.T. & Gjerris, A. (1988) *Acta Psychiatr. Scand.* **78**, 156–161.

Pletscher, A. (1978) *Essays Neurochem. Neuropharmacol.* **3**, 49–101.

Pochet, R., Delespese, G., Gausset, P.W. & Collet, H. (1979) *Clin. Exp. Immunol.* **38**, 578–584.

Poirier, M.F., Le Quan-Bui, K.H., Loo, H. & Meyer, P. (1985) *Psychopharmacology* **86**, 194–196.

Poirier, M.F., Benkelfat, C., Galzin, A.M. & Langer, S.Z. (1986) *Psychopharmacology* **88**, 86–89.

Poirier, M.F., Galzin, A.M., Loo, H. *et al.* (1987) *Biol. Psychiatry* **22**, 287–302.

Poirier, M.F., Galzin, A.M., Pimoule, C. *et al.* (1988) *Psychopharmacology* **94**, 521–526.

Price, L.H., Goodman, W.K., Charney, D.S. & Heninger, G.R. (1987) *Am. J. Psychiatry* **144**, 1059–1061.

Propping, P. & Friedl, W. (1983) *Hum. Genet.* **64**, 105–109.

Raisman, R., Briley, M. & Langer, S.Z. (1979) *Eur. J. Pharmacol.* **54**, 307–314.

Raisman, R., Briley, M. & Langer, S.Z. (1980) *Eur. J. Pharmacol.* **61**, 373–380.

Raisman, R., Sechter, C., Briley, M., Zarifian, E. & Langer, S.Z. (1981) *Psychopharmacology* **75**, 368–371.

Raisman, R., Briley, M., Bouchami, F., Sechter, C., Zarifian, E. & Langer, S.Z. (1982) *Psychopharmacology* **77**, 332–335.

Rausch, J.L., Janowsky, D.S., Risch, S.C. & Huey, L.Y. (1986) *Psychiatry Res.* **19**, 105–112.

Rausch, J.L., Rich, C.L. & Risch, S.C. (1988) *Psychopharmacology* **95**, 139–141.

Rehavi, M., Paul, S.M., Skolnick, P. & Goodwin, F.K. (1980) *Life Sci.* **26**, 2273–2279.

Rice, H.E., Smith, C.B., Silk, K.R. & Rosen, J. (1984) *Psychiatry Res.* **12**, 69–77.

Rommelspacher, H., Strauss, S., Fahndrich, E. & Hargh, H.J. (1987) *J. Neural Transm.* **69**, 85–96.

Ross, S.B. & Aberg-Wistedt, A. (1983) *Psychopharmacology* **79**, 298–303.

Rotman, A., Modai, I., Munitz, H. & Wijsenbeek, H. (1979) *FEBS Lett.* **101**, 134–136.

Roy, A., Everett, D., Pickar, D. & Paul, S.M. (1987) *Arch. Gen. Psychiatry* **44**, 320–327.

Roy, A., De Jong, J. & Linnoila, M. (1989) *Arch. Gen. Psychiatry* **46**, 609–612.

Rudnick, G. (1977) *J. Biol. Chem.* **252**, 2170–2175.

Sadava, D. & Wilmington, K. (1984) *Life Sci.* **35**, 2545–2548.

Sandler, M., Reveley, M.A. & Glover, V. (1981) *J. Clin. Pathol.* **34**, 292–302.

Sarrias, M.J., Artigas, F., Martinez, E. *et al.* (1987) *Biol. Psychiatry* **22**, 1429–1438.

Schildkraut, J.J. (1965) *Am. J. Psychiatry* **122**, 509–517.

Schildkraut, J.J., Orsulak, P.J. & LaBrie, R.A. (1978) *Arch. Gen. Psychiatry* **35**, 1436–1439.

Schlechte, J.A. & Sherman, B. (1985) *Psychoneuroendocrinology* **10**, 469–474.

Schneider, L.S., Fredrickson, E.R., Severson, J.A. & Sloane, R.B. (1986) *Psychiatry Res.* **19**, 257–266.

Schneider, L.S., Munjack, D., Severson, J.A. & Palmer, R. (1987a) *Biol. Psychiatry* **22**, 59–66.

Schneider, L.S., Severson, J.A., Sloane, R.B. & Fredrickson, E.R. (1987b) *J. Affective Disord.* **15**, 195–200.

Scott, M., Reading, H. & Loudon, J. (1979) *Psychopharmacology* **60**, 131–135.

Sette, M., Briley, M.S. & Langer, S.Z. (1981) *J. Neurochem.* **37**, 40–42.

Sette, M., Briley, M.S. & Langer, S.Z. (1983) *J. Neurochem.* **40**, 622–629.

Sevy, S., Papadimitriou, G.N., Surmont, D.W., Goldman, S. & Mendlewicz, J. (1989) *Biol. Psychiatry* **25**, 141–152.

Shaskan, E.G. & Snyder, S.J. (1970) *J. Pharmacol. Exp. Ther.* **175**, 404–418.

Siever, L.J., Kafka, M.S., Targum, S. & Lake, C.R. (1984) *Psychiatry Res.* **11**, 287–302.

Smith, C.B., Hollingsworth, P.J., Garcia-Sevilla, J.A. & Zis, A.P. (1983) *Prog. Neuropsychopharmacol. Biol. Psychiatry* **7**, 241–247.

Stahl, S.M., Lemoine, P.M., Ciaranello, R.D. & Berger, P.A. (1983a) *Psychiat. Res.* **10**, 157–164.

Stahl, S.M., Woo, D.J., Mefford, I.N., Berger, P.A. & Ciaranello, R.D. (1983b) *Am. J. Psychiat.* **140**, 26–30.

Stokes, P.E., Stoll, P.M., Doslow, S.H. *et al.* (1984) *Arch. Gen. Psychiatry* **41**, 257–266.

Sugrue, M.F. (1981) *Pharm. Ther.* **13**, 219–247.

Summers, R.J., Barnett, D.B. & Nahorski, S.R. (1983) *Life Sci.* **33**, 1105–1112.

Sundaresan, P.R., Weintraub, M., Hershey, L.A., Kroening, B.H., Hasday, J.D. & Banerjee, S.P. (1983) *Clin. Pharmacol. Ther.* **33**, 777–785.

Sundaresan, P.R., Madan, M.K., Kelvie, S.L. & Weintraub, M. (1985) *Clin. Pharmacol. Ther.* **37**, 337–342.

Suranyi-Cadotte, B.E., Wood, P.L., Schwartz, G. & Nair, N.P. (1983) *Biol. Psychiatry* **18**, 923–927.

Suranyi-Cadotte, B.E., Gauthier, S., Lafaille, F. *et al.* (1985a) *Life Sci.* **37**, 2305–2311.

Suranyi-Cadotte, B.E., Quirion, R., Nair, N.P., Lafaille, F. & Schwartz, G. (1985b) *Life Sci.* **36**, 795–799.

Takeda, T., Harada, T. & Otsuki, S. (1989) *Biol. Psychiatry* **26**, 52–60.

Tang, S.W. & Morris, J.M. (1985) *Psychiatry Res.* **16**, 141–146.

Tanimoto, K., Maeda, K. & Terada, T. (1985) *Biol. Psychiatry* **20**, 340–343.

Theodorou, A.E., Hale, A.S., Davies, S.L. *et al.* (1986) *Eur. J. Pharmacol.* **126**, 329–332.

Theodorou, A.E., Mistry, H., Davies, S.L., Yamaguchi, Y. & Horton, R.W. (1987) *J. Psychiatr. Res.* **21**, 163–169.

Theodorou, A.E., Katona, C.L.E., Davies, S.L. *et al.* (1989) *Psychiatry Res.* **29**, 87–103.

Todrick, A. & Tait, A.C. (1969) *J. Pharm. Pharmacol.* **21**, 751–762.

Tuomisto, J. & Tukainen, E. (1976) *Nature* **262**, 596–598.

Tuomisto, J., Tukainen, E. & Ahlfors, U.G. (1979) *Psychopharmacology* **65**, 141–147.

Uhde, T.W., Berrettini, W.H., Roy-Byrne, P.P., Boulenger, J.P. & Post, R.M. (1987) *Biol. Psychiatry* **22**, 52–58.

Vetulani, J., Stawarz, R.J., Dingell, J.V. & Sulser, F. (1976) *Naunyn-Schmiedebergs Arch. Pharmacol.* **293**, 109–114.

Wagner, A., Aberg-Wistedt, A., Asberg, M., Ekqvist, B., Martensson, B. & Montero, D. (1985) *Psychiatry Res.* **16**, 131–139.

Wagner, A., Aberg-Wistedt, A., Asberg, M., Bertilsson, L., Martensson, B. & Montero, D. (1987) *Arch. Gen. Psychiatry* **44**, 870–877.

Wang, Y.C., Pandey, G.N., Mendels, J. & Frazer, A. (1974) *Psychopharmacology* **36**, 291–300.

Weizman, R., Carmi, M., Tyano, S., Apter, A. & Rehavi, M. (1986) *Life Sci.* **38**, 1235–1242.

Whalley, L.J., Borthwick, N., Copolov, D., Dick, H., Christie, J.E. & Fink, G. (1986) *Br. Med. J.* **292**, 859–861.

Whitaker, P.M., Warsh, J.J., Stancer, H.C., Persad, E. & Vint, C.K. (1984) *Psychiatry Res.* **11**, 127–131.

Wirz-Justice, W. (1988) *Experientia* **44**, 145–152.

Wolfe, B.B., Harden, T.K., Sporn, J.R. & Molinoff, P.B. (1978) *J. Pharmacol. Exp. Ther.* **207**, 446–457.

Wolfe, N., Cohen, B.M. & Gelenberg, A.J. (1987) *Psychiatry Res.* **20**, 107–116.

Wolfe, N., Gelenberg, A.J. & Lydiard, R.B. (1989) *Biol. Psychiatry* **25**, 389–392.

Wood, K. (1989) In *Biochemical and Pharmacological Aspects of Depression* (eds Tipton, K.F. & Youdim, M.B.H.), pp 51–68. London, Taylor & Francis.

Wood, K., Harwood, J. & Coppen, A. (1983) *Lancet* ii, 519–520.

Wood, K., Harwood, J. & Coppen, A. (1984) *J. Affective Disord.* **7**, 149–158.

Wood, K., Swade, C., Abou-Saleh, M.T. & Coppen, A. (1985a) *J. Affective Disord.* **8**, 69–72.

Wood, K., Swade, C. & Coppen, A. (1985b) *Acta Pharmacol. Toxicol.* **56** (Suppl. 1), 203–211.

Wood, K., Whiting, K. & Coppen, A. (1986) *J. Affective Disord.* **10**, 3–8.

Wood, P.L., Suranyi-Cadotte, B.E., Nair, N.P., LaFaille, F. & Schwartz, G. (1983a) *Neuropharmacology* **22**, 1211–1214.

Wood, P.L., Suranyi-Cadotte, B.E., Schwartz, G. & Nair, N.P. (1983b) *Biol. Psychiatry* **18**, 715–719.

Wright, A.F., Crichton, D.N., Loudon, J.B., Morten, J.E. & Steel, C.M. (1984) *Ann. Hum. Genet.* **48**, 201–214.

Yokoyama, M., Kusui, A., Sakamoto, S. & Fukuzaki, H. (1984) *Thromb. Res.* **34**, 287–295.

Youdim, M.B.H. (1988) *Experientia* **44**, 137–141.

CHAPTER 5

NEUROENDOCRINE CHALLENGE TESTS IN AFFECTIVE DISORDERS: IMPLICATIONS FOR FUTURE PATHOPHYSIOLOGICAL INVESTIGATIONS

Pedro L. Delgado and Dennis S. Charney

Department of Veterans Affairs Medical Center & Department of Psychiatry, Yale University School of Medicine, West Haven, Connecticut 06515, USA

Table of Contents

BIOLOGICAL ASPECTS OF AFFECTIVE DISORDERS
ISBN 0-12-356510-3

5.1 Introduction

A wide variety of clinical and preclinical data currently exists supporting a significant role for dysfunction of catecholamine and indoleamine neurotransmission in the pathophysiology of depression and the mechanism of antidepressant action. These data come from a broad spectrum of experimental designs in both laboratory animals and human subjects. Catecholamine and indoleamine hypotheses of antidepressant action and depression have been only partially supported (Heninger et al., 1990) and as increased understanding of the complex regulation of neurotransmitter synthesis, release, presynaptic and postsynaptic receptors, the interaction of receptors with second messenger systems, and ultimately the effects of these receptor interactions on gene expression has emerged, the early hypotheses have been modified (Charney et al., 1990). The purpose of this chapter is to review one paradigm used to assess the role of catecholamine and indoleamine neurotransmission in depression and the mechanism of antidepressant action: neuroendocrine challenge strategies.

The use of neuroendocrine challenge tests in the investigation of the neurobiology of depression and the mechanism of antidepressant action has paralleled the growth in the understanding of the regulation of pituitary hormones by central nervous system catecholamine and indoleamine neurotransmitters and technological advances in the ability to measure small amounts of various drugs, hormones, and neurotransmitters and their metabolites.

Initial investigations of neuroendocrine abnormalities in depression resulted from the observations of the increased occurrence of depression in disorders of endocrine dysfunction such as Cushing's disease and hypothyroidism (Sachar, 1973). These data suggested that while endocrinopathies probably were not directly responsible for major psychiatric disorders, abnormal function of the hypothalamus and other limbic areas might be involved (Sachar, 1973). As a result of these observations, the basal and stimulated release of pituitary and adrenal hormones began to be investigated in depressed patients as compared with healthy subjects.

The cortisol response to stress was one of the first neuroendocrine responses investigated in humans (Selye, 1936; Mason *et al.*, 1965). Investigations of basal cortisol excretion in depressed patients demonstrated that these patients maintained abnormally elevated corticosteroid secretion (Gibbons, 1964). Shortly thereafter, the growth hormone response to insulin-induced hypoglycaemia was reported to be blunted in patients with endogenous depression (Sachar *et al.*, 1971).

In parallel to the development of the catecholamine hypotheses of depression (Bunney and Davis, 1965; Schildkraut, 1965), the regulation of the pituitary hormone secretion by catecholamine and indoleamine neurotransmitters was being discovered (Wurtman, 1970). Consequently the suggestion was made that pharmacological probes which cause the secretion of pituitary hormones might be used to 'open a window' into central nervous system function (Wurtman, 1970; Sachar, 1973). Stated simply, if a drug's mechanism of action is understood, and the factors which influence the release of a hormone are understood, then a drug which influences a neurotransmitter system involved in the release of a hormone can be used as a 'probe' of the state of the regulating neurotransmitter system by measuring the change in the secretion of the hormone. This model was extremely useful, since the route of administration of a drug or probe could be controlled and the measurement of the hormone response could be derived easily from plasma.

The critical factors in this reasoning are the specificity of a drug and the completeness with which the factors (including other neurotransmitter systems) influencing the release of the hormone are understood. Other variables which can affect the amount of a hormone released in response to a specific probe include individual differences in age and gender, pharmacokinetic factors relating to drug metabolism, differences in uptake or transport of the drug into the central nervous system, and the effects of differing pretreatment or drug-induced levels of stress, anxiety or arousal.

In *in vitro* pharmacological dose–response relationships the specificity of the interaction between the drug or probe and the response being measured can be controlled by the use of specific agonists and antagonists at varying doses in order to test mathematical models which would be predicted by specific kinds of interactions with neurotransmitter receptors (Furchgott, 1972). In humans, these types of procedures are extremely difficult to achieve in a given subject because of the time, inconvenience and possible risks involved.

However, probably the most significant limitation of the neuroendocrine challenge strategy is the uncertainty involved in extrapolating from a neuroendocrine measure of the responsiveness of a particular neurotransmitter system to the presumed responsiveness of that system in other brain areas.

Because of the significant shortcomings of the neuroendocrine challenge approach, the results of these studies must be assessed in the context of data derived from other paradigms, such as behavioural and electrophysiological studies in laboratory animals, human cerebrospinal fluid (CSF) measurements of neurotransmitters and their metabolites, human receptor binding studies at autopsy, brain imaging studies and clinical studies assessing treatment response to specific antidepressant medications. When this is done, an enhanced understanding of the probable neuroregulatory factors involved in depression and the mechanism of antidepressant action can evolve (Heninger et al., 1990). Moreover, neuroendocrine challenge strategies do have the distinct advantages of being carried out in the living person, being related to dynamic, functional responses which are regulated by central nervous system (CNS) activity, and of being relatively easy and safe to perform (Price et al., 1990).

5.2 Biological hypotheses of depression and antidepressant action

The catecholamine deficiency hypothesis of depression was based on the observation that antidepressant drugs increased synaptic concentrations of noradrenaline (NA) while the catecholamine depleting drug, reserpine, seemed to cause depression-like symptoms (Bunney and Davis, 1965; Schildkraut, 1965). This hypothesis postulated that depression was due to a deficiency and that mania was due to an excess of brain NA. Likewise, the indoleamine hypothesis postulated that a deficit of brain serotonin (5-HT) was responsible for depression, while drugs which increased synaptic 5-HT, such as monoamine oxidase (MAO) inhibitors or 5-HT precursors such as 5-hydroxytryptophan (5-HTP) and L-tryptophan (TRP), relieved depression (Coppen, 1967; Murphy et al., 1978).

However, these hypotheses have not accounted for the lack of immediate efficacy of antidepressant treatments, given the rapid effect of various antidepressants on increasing synaptic NA and 5-HT concentrations. Moreover, deficiencies of NA or 5-HT or their metabolites in CSF, blood or urine have not been consistently demonstrated in depressed patients despite intensive efforts to do so (Charney *et al.*, 1981b), although a subgroup of depressed patients with a history of impulsivity or suicide appear to have decreased CSF levels of the primary metabolite of 5-HT, 5-hydroxyindoleacetic acid (5-HIAA) (Asberg *et al.*, 1987).

However, all of the effective antidepressant medications (except bupropion) and electroconvulsive therapy (ECT) do appear to have profound effects on the catecholamine and indoleamine neurotransmitter systems (Carlsson and Lindqvist, 1978; Charney *et al.*, 1981b). As new data emerged that alterations in the function of CNS neurotransmitter systems could occur by changes in the sensitivity of postsynaptic receptors, without an alteration in the content of the neurotransmitter itself, the deficiency hypotheses were modified and the 'receptor sensitivity hypothesis' of antidepressant action was proposed. This hypothesis stated that the delayed therapeutic effects of antidepressant treatment were related to time-dependent alterations in monoamine and indoleamine receptor sensitivity and implied that the pathophysiology of depression may be more related to abnormal regulation of receptor sensitivity than to deficiencies of a neurotransmitter (Charney *et al.*, 1981b).

A similar view, the 'dysregulation hypothesis', was subsequently expressed by Siever and Davis. The dysregulation hypothesis proposed that in affective disorders regulatory or homeostatic mechanisms controlling neurotransmitter function were dysregulated and that effective pharmacological agents restore normal regulation to these systems (Siever and Davis, 1985). Figure 1, utilizing a 5-HT neurone as an example, depicts the possible sites of dysfunction in affective disorder patients and the possible sites of action of antidepressant drugs.

Neuroendocrine challenge tests have been used to test both of these hypotheses. In theory, if abnormal sensitivity of CNS neurotransmitter receptors or abnormal regulation of CNS neurotransmitter systems exist in affective disorders, then these abnormalities may be identified by investigating the hormonal responses elicited by pharmacologically altering these neurotransmitter systems. Likewise, if antidepressant medications work by causing functional alterations in one or more neurotransmitter systems, then these alterations might also be measurable.

5.3 Assessment of 5-HT function

5-HT neurones innervate large portions of the CNS and appear to modulate intrinsic activity in many brain regions, leading to a general modulatory effect on various behaviours (Aghajanian, 1981; Aghajanian *et al.*, 1987). While 5-HT nerve terminals are found in most brain regions, the cell bodies from

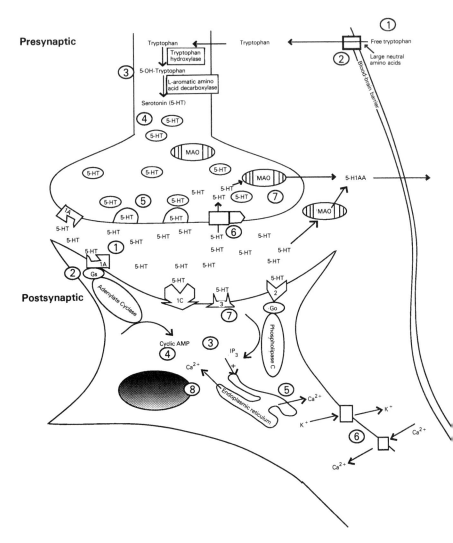

Figure 1 Schematic representation of serotonergic neurone and possible sites of biological abnormalities in affective disorder patients and sites of antidepressant action. Presynaptic factors: 1, plasma level of precursor; 2, uptake of precursor; 3, transmitter synthesis; 4, transmitter storage; 5, transmitter release; 6, transmitter reuptake; 7. transmitter degradation. Postsynaptic factors: 1, receptor binding; 2, receptor–G-protein coupling; 3, second messenger system; 4, protein phosphorylation; 5, calcium release; 6, ion channels; 7, regulation of receptor function; 8, gene expression. Shapes containing 1A, 1C, 2 and 3 represent subtypes of 5-HT receptor. Gs: stimulatory subtype of guanylate triphosphate binding protein (G-protein). Go: other subtype of G-protein.

which these nerve terminals originate come from a relatively localized area of the brain stem located within the raphe nuclei (Dahlstrom and Fuxe, 1964). The 5-HT cell bodies within the raphe nuclei are subdivided into nine groups (B1–B9). Most of the ascending projections of these 5-HT nuclei come from the dorsal raphe (B7), median raphe (B8), and the B9 cell groups (Kuhar *et al.*, 1971; Parent *et al.*, 1981). Ascending 5-HT cell bodies project to distinct and separate brain regions and are organized in a topographical fashion which appears to be functionally significant. Not only is the pattern of innervation of the cortex by 5-HT neurones complex, but 5-HT nerve terminals appear to be composed of two distinct classes of nerve terminals with different pharmacological and probably functional properties (Molliver, 1987). Adding even another layer of data is the fact that there are at least five distinct subtypes of 5-HT receptors in humans. These receptor subtypes have been designated 5-HT_{1A}, 5-HT_{1C}, 5-HT_{1D}, 5-HT_2 and 5-HT_3 (Gonzalez-Heydrich and Peroutka, 1990). The anatomical localization of 5-HT receptor subtypes is also complex and appears to follow a pattern which is closely related to the pattern of differing types of nerve terminals and most likely also has functional significance (Molliver, 1987).

The 5-HT system has been one of the most intensively studied neuro-transmitter systems in relation to the biology of depression and the mechanism of antidepressant action. The emphasis on 5-HT has been maintained primarily because of results from studies investigating the mechanism of antidepressant action (Heninger and Charney, 1987). The most intriguing of these have been electrophysiological studies in laboratory animals suggesting that most antidepressant drugs and ECT enhance neurotransmission across 5-HT synapses after chronic but not acute administration (de Montigny and Blier, 1984; Fuxe *et al.*, 1984; Blier *et al.*, 1990). Interestingly, antidepressants appear to cause an enhancement of 5-HT function through different mechanisms. Tricyclic antidepressant drugs and ECT appear to sensitize postsynaptic neurones to the effects of 5-HT, while MAO inhibitors enhance availability of 5-HT and 5-HT reuptake inhibitors desensitize presynaptic inhibitory 5-HT autoreceptors (Blier *et al.*, 1990).

Other evidence for the involvement of the 5-HT system in depression comes from preclinical studies in laboratory animals investigating the relationship of 5-HT function to various behaviours. These studies demonstrate that the 5-HT system is involved in the regulation of many of the types of physiological processes which form the core of the symptoms of depression. The behaviours regulated by the 5-HT system in laboratory animals include a wide variety of physiological processes, including appetite, sleep, sexual function, pain sensitivity, body temperature and circadian rhythms (Meltzer and Lowy, 1987).

Clinical studies have also contributed to the evidence supporting an involvement of 5-HT in depression. Several studies have demonstrated that some depressed patients, especially those prone to impulsive acts and suicide, have decreased CSF levels of the 5-HT metabolite, 5-HIAA (Asberg et al., 1987). Also, 5-HT reuptake sites, as labelled by imipramine, have been found to be reduced in the brains of suicide victims (Stanley et al., 1982) and on platelets of depressed patients (Briley et al., 1980), and 5-HT$_2$ receptors may be increased in the brains of some suicide victims (Stanley and Mann, 1983; Mann et al., 1986; and see Chapter 6). Further evidence from clinical studies comes from the recent studies demonstrating that highly selective 5-HT reuptake inhibitors (Chouinard, 1985) and selective 5-HT$_{1A}$ partial agonists (Robinson et al., 1990) are effective antidepressants.

Two important clinical studies published in the 1970s reported that the 5-HT synthesis inhibitor, p-chlorophenylalanine (PCPA), appeared to reverse the antidepressant effects of both imipramine (Shopsin et al., 1975) and tranylcypromine (Shopsin et al., 1976) within 24 h in patients with major depression. Further, rapid depletion of plasma TRP (discussed in detail below), a procedure which briefly lowers CNS 5-HT content, temporarily reverses antidepressant response in 67% of recently remitted depressed patients (Delgado et al., 1990a).

Within this context, neuroendocrine measures of CNS 5-HT function have been utilized to test the 5-HT hypothesis of depression and antidepressant action. Increased 5-HT activity leads to an enhanced release of several hormones, including the pituitary hormones prolactin, adrenocorticotropic hormone (ACTH) and growth hormone, as well as the peripherally released hormones cortisol and renin. The neuroendocrine responses to various precursors of 5-HT synthesis (5-HTP, TRP), 5-HT releasers (fenfluramine), 5-HT reuptake inhibitors (clomipramine), and direct acting 5-HT receptor agonists (m-chlorophenylpiperazine (MCPP), MK-212, gepirone, ipsapirone, tandospirone) and antagonists (ritanserin, ketanserin, metergoline) have been used to assess 5-HT function in depression.

5.3.1 L-TRP

One of the most extensively studied of the neuroendocrine challenge tests has been the neuroendocrine response to intravenous administration of the 5-HT precursor, TRP. The synthesis of 5-HT is dependent on dietary intake of its precursor, the essential amino acid TRP (Gal and Dreses, 1962; Culley et al., 1963; Fernstrom et al., 1973; Tagliamonte et al., 1973; Curzon, 1979). TRP enters the brain through a transport mechanism for which it competes with large neutral amino acids (LNAA). Both increases (Moir and Eccleston, 1968; Fernstrom and Hirsch, 1975) and decreases

(Curzon, 1981) in dietary TRP intake lead to corresponding changes in brain TRP and 5-HT levels in laboratory animals.

Intravenous TRP reliably enhances the release of prolactin and less reliably increases the release of growth hormone and ACTH in humans (Charney *et al.*, 1982a; Winokur *et al.*, 1986). In rhesus monkeys, the prolactin response to TRP infusion is blocked by the non-selective 5-HT antagonist, metergoline, whereas the selective $5-HT_2$ receptor antagonist, ritanserin, causes only an 18% attenuation of the prolactin response (Heninger *et al.*, 1989). The prolactin response to TRP in humans is attenuated by the concomitant administration of the nonselective 5-HT antagonists methysergide (MacIndoe and Turkington, 1973), cyproheptidine (Cowen *et al.*, 1985a) and metergoline (McCance *et al.*, 1987).

The prolactin response to TRP in humans is not blocked by the concomitant, short-term administration of the selective $5-HT_2$ antagonists ritanserin (Charig *et al.*, 1986) or ketanserin (Cowen and Anderson, 1986). More surprising is the finding that acute pretreatment with ritanserin further enhances the prolactin response to TRP (Charig *et al.*, 1986), while administration of ritanserin for two weeks has no effect on the prolactin response (Idzikowski *et al.*, 1987). These data have been interpreted as supporting a primary role for $5-HT_1$ receptors in the regulation of prolactin release by TRP, although the nature of the contribution from $5-HT_2$ receptors remains controversial (Heninger *et al.*, 1989; Price *et al.*, 1990).

The prolactin (Heninger *et al.*, 1984; Cowen and Charig, 1987; Deakin *et al.*, 1990) and growth hormone (Cowen and Charig, 1987; Deakin *et al.*, 1990) responses to intravenous TRP infusion are blunted in depressed patients when compared with healthy controls. Moreover, melancholic patients have been reported to be more likely to have a blunted response, an effect which is masked by significant weight loss and exaggerated by elevated plasma cortisol levels (Deakin *et al.*, 1990). The issue of the blunting of the prolactin responses to TRP in melancholic versus non-melancholic patients is controversial however, since Price *et al.* have found a blunted prolactin response to TRP infusion in non-melancholic but not in melancholic patients (L.H. Price *et al.*, unpublished data). As suggested by Deakin *et al.* and Cowen and Charig, the relationship of plasma cortisol and weight loss to the blunted prolactin response may explain the discrepant findings (Cowen and Charig, 1987; Deakin *et al.*, 1990).

Long-term treatment with the antidepressant drugs desipramine, amitriptyline, fluvoxamine, MAO inhibitors, clomipramine, carbamazepine and lithium enhance the prolactin response to intravenous TRP infusion (Charney *et al.*, 1984a; Price *et al.*, 1985, 1989a, 1989b; Anderson and Cowen, 1986; Cowen, 1988; Cowen *et al.*, 1989; Elphick *et al.*, 1990) but the atypical antidepressants bupropion, mianserin, and trazodone have no effect

(Cowen *et al.*, 1989; Price *et al.*, 1989b). However, in none of the above studies is the degree of enhancement of the prolactin response correlated with treatment outcome.

While cortisol responds poorly to TRP infusion when administered in the morning (Winokur *et al.*, 1986), afternoon infusion of TRP gives more consistent ACTH and cortisol responses and these responses are blunted in drug-free, euthymic bipolar patients when compared to healthy subjects, although no differences in prolactin or growth hormone were observed (Nurnberger *et al.*, 1989).

5.3.2 5-HTP

Neuroendocrine responses to another 5-HT precursor, 5-HTP, have also been studied in depression but the results are difficult to interpret because 5-HTP is metabolized into 5-HT both intraneuronally and extraneuronally and may act as a false transmitter in non-serotonergic neurones (Fuxe *et al.*, 1971; Ng *et al.*, 1972). Further, 5-HTP may have direct actions on cortisol release at the level of the adrenal gland (Van de Kar *et al.*, 1985).

5-HTP leads to an increase in plasma ACTH and cortisol but has no effect on prolactin (Meltzer *et al.*, 1984). This is in contrast to the neuroendocrine profile seen with most other 5-HT agonists which cause the release of prolactin. The cortisol response is increased in depressed patients compared with controls (Meltzer *et al.*, 1984). The increased cortisol response to 5-HTP is attenuated after tricyclic antidepressant treatment (nortriptyline, imipramine, desipramine) but increased further by lithium when compared with the drug-free state (Meltzer and Lowy, 1987).

5.3.3 Fenfluramine

Fenfluramine administration causes release and blocks the reuptake of 5-HT resulting in an increase in the secretion of prolactin and cortisol (Quattrone *et al.*, 1983; Muhlbauer and Muller-Oerlinghausen, 1985) but not growth hormone (Mitchell and Smythe, 1990). The prolactin response to fenfluramine is blocked by metergoline (Quattrone *et al.*, 1983).

Prolactin responses to oral fenfluramine have been found blunted in some depressed patients when compared with healthy subjects (Siever *et al.*, 1984; Coccaro *et al.*, 1989), although these responses have been inconsistent and some studies have found no difference between healthy subjects and depressed patients (Asnis *et al.*, 1988; Weizman *et al.*, 1988). Mitchell and Smythe have recently reported that, while the peak increase in prolactin was decreased in endogenous depressed patients following fenfluramine, this apparent 'blunting' was accounted for by covarying for both baseline prolactin and cortisol levels (Mitchell and Smythe, 1990).

The cortisol response to fenfluramine in depressed patients has been reported as no different (Asnis *et al.*, 1988; Mitchell and Smythe, 1990) or reduced (Weizman *et al.*, 1988) when compared with controls. In the Mitchell and Smythe study, while there was a significantly different peak–base change in cortisol following fenfluramine, there was only a trend towards significance when baseline cortisol levels were taken into account, as was the case for the prolactin response (Mitchell and Smythe, 1990).

The prolactin response to fenfluramine is enhanced after chronic anti-depressant treatment with lithium (Muhlbauer, 1984) and imipramine (Shapira *et al.*, 1989, 1990). These data are similar to those obtained for the enhanced prolactin response to TRP infusion (Price *et al.*, 1990). Further, the prolactin response to fenfluramine has been reported to be enhanced after ECT treatment (Shapira *et al.*, 1990).

5.3.4 Clomipramine

5-HT reuptake inhibitors have also been used to assess neuroendocrine responses in depression. Clomipramine has been one of the most studied of these agents. It is a highly potent and selective 5-HT reuptake inhibitor but is metabolized into a demethylated metabolite which has significant effects on blocking the reuptake of NA. By using an intravenous infusion of clomipramine, investigators have hoped to diminish the metabolism into the demethylated metabolite and thus increase the selectivity of this test towards the 5-HT system (Golden *et al.*, 1989). Intravenous infusion of clomipramine leads to an increased release of prolactin, growth hormone, ACTH and cortisol in healthy subjects (Golden *et al.*, 1989, 1990). The prolactin response to intravenous clomipramine is blunted and the growth hormone response exaggerated in depressed patients compared with healthy subjects (Golden *et al.*, 1990). In healthy subjects the prolactin response to intravenous clomipramine is enhanced after 3–4 days of lithium treatment, while the cortisol response is unchanged (McCance *et al.*, 1989).

5.3.5 5-HT receptor agonists

Direct 5-HT receptor agonists have only recently begun to be studied in depression. The non-selective 5-HT agonist, MCPP, a metabolite of the antidepressant trazodone, causes an increase in the release of prolactin, cortisol and growth hormone in healthy humans (Mueller *et al.*, 1985; Charney *et al.*, 1987; Murphy *et al.*, 1989; Kahn *et al.*, 1990). Price *et al.* have recently studied the neuroendocrine profile of MCPP in depressed patients and preliminary results suggest that there is no difference between depressed patients and healthy subjects (L.H. Price *et al.*, unpublished data).

MK 212, a purported 5-HT$_2$ receptor agonist, causes an increase in ACTH and cortisol in healthy subjects (Meltzer and Lowy, 1987). The neuroendocrine profile of MK 212 has not been studied in depression.

Recently, a novel group of drugs belonging to the azaspirodecanedione family have been developed, demonstrating high partial agonist affinity for the 5-HT$_{1A}$ receptor. These compounds are currently being investigated as possible anxiolytics and antidepressants. The hormone responses to 5-HT agonists are thought to be related to partial agonist activity of these drugs on postsynaptic 5-HT$_{1A}$ receptors and the hypothermic response is thought to be mediated through presynaptic 5-HT$_{1A}$ activity (Cowen *et al.*, 1990). The neuroendocrine activity of four of these drugs (buspirone, ipsapirone, tandospirone (SM-3997) and gepirone) has been studied in humans.

Buspirone was the first of this class of drug to be used clinically in the treatment of anxiety and whose neuroendocrine profile has been studied in humans (Meltzer *et al.*, 1983). Buspirone (up to 30 mg/subject) administered orally leads to increases in growth hormone, prolactin and cortisol, and decreases in mean body temperature (Meltzer *et al.*, 1983; Cowen *et al.*, 1990). However, the neuroendocrine responses to buspirone have been controversial because of the dopamine antagonist activity associated with this compound (Peroutka, 1988).

Unlike buspirone, ipsapirone, gepirone and tandospirone possess less intrinsic activity for dopamine receptors in radioligand binding studies (Peroutka, 1988). Ipsapirone (up to 3 mg/kg) leads to an increase in the secretion of cortisol and a decrease in body temperature, but no significant effect on prolactin or growth hormone (Lesch *et al.*, 1989). Gepirone (up to 20 mg/subject), another closely related and relatively selective 5-HT$_{1A}$ agonist, causes robust increases in ACTH, cortisol, β-endorphin, prolactin and growth hormone, as well as causing a significant decrease in body temperature (Anderson *et al.*, 1990). Tandospirone (up to 50 mg/subject), likewise causes increases in growth hormone and cortisol, but no change in prolactin (Delgado *et al.*, 1990b). It is unclear whether the differences in neuroendocrine profile between the compounds in humans is due to differences in intrinsic agonist activity, selectivity or metabolites. It is known that these 5-HT$_{1A}$ agonists are metabolized into a pharmacologically active compound, 1-phenylpiperazine, with significant α_2-adrenergic antagonist activity (Bianchi *et al.*, 1988).

Ipsapirone is the only drug in this class whose neuroendocrine profile has been studied in depressed patients. It causes a decrease in body temperature in healthy subjects and this response is blunted in depressed patients (Lesch *et al.*, 1990a). Chronic treatment with amitriptyline further impaired the ipsapirone-mediated hypothermic response in depressed patients (Lesch et al., 1990b). These findings suggest that depressed patients may have abnormalities of presynaptic 5-HT$_{1A}$ receptor function or of presynaptic 5-HT function apart from the sensitivity of 5-HT$_{1A}$ receptors. This could involve mechanisms regulating cell firing, transmitter release or synthesis. The effects of chronic antidepressant treatment on the temperature response are consistent with the preclinical studies suggesting that 5-HT$_{1A}$ agonists decrease presynaptic 5-HT$_{1A}$ receptor sensitivity in laboratory animals (Blier and de Montigny, 1990).

It is worth noting that in none of the above studies with indirect acting 5-HT agonists such as TRP, 5-HTP or fenfluramine, or 5-HT reuptake inhibitors such as intravenous clomipramine, or direct acting 5-HT agonists such as MCPP and ipsapirone have there been any significant changes in mood in unmedicated depressed patients. Likewise, there have been no significant changes in mood with any of these direct and indirect 5-HT agonists in acute or chronically antidepressant-treated patients.

5.3.6 Other challenge tests of 5-HT function

One of the greatest limitations of neuroendocrine challenge studies has been the possibility that the physiological responsiveness of the hypothalamic–pituitary 5-HT system may differ significantly from that of the 5-HT systems in other brain areas. Therefore, any other response measure which can help validate the neuroendocrine response data becomes invaluable. Behavioural responses to pharmacological challenge agents are some of the most helpful of the response measures because they directly reflect the condition being investigated. Ultimately, if one cannot induce behavioural changes in the manner in which the hypothesis being tested predicts, then there is something wrong with the model. In most neuroendocrine challenge tests, the behavioural responses to the various agonists and antagonists which should be having significant effects on the CNS systems involved in depression are very seldom significant or related to the illness being studied.

Based on the dependence of brain 5-HT on plasma levels of TRP, numerous studies have investigated the behavioural and biochemical effects of plasma TRP depletion in laboratory animals, and recently we have been investigating the neuroendocrine and behavioural effects of dietary TRP depletion in depressed patients and healthy subjects as a method with which to evaluate the 5-HT hypothesis of depression and antidepressant action.

Dietary TRP depletion may specifically reduce brain 5-HT function (Fernstrom, 1977; Curzon, 1981; Moja et al., 1989; Young et al., 1989). Ingestion of TRP-free amino acid mixtures in vervet monkeys decreases plasma TRP and CSF TRP and 5-HIAA, with no change in CSF tyrosine, homovanillic acid (HVA) or 3-methoxy-4-hydroxyphenylethylene glycol (MHPG) (Young *et al.*, 1989). Moreover, ingestion of TRP-free amino acid mixtures in laboratory animals leads to extremely rapid changes in both plasma TRP and brain 5-HT, with maximal reductions of brain 5-HT occurring within 2 h of ingestion of the TRP-free mixture (Moja *et al.*, 1989; Young *et al.*, 1989). TRP-free or low-TRP diets administered to healthy humans cause reductions of plasma TRP levels (Young *et al.*, 1969, 1971; Delgado *et al.*, 1989). Maintenance on such diets for up to 1 month without serious medical or psychological consequences has been reported (Rose *et al.*, 1954).

Dietary TRP depletion alters behavioural indices of 5-HT function, increasing pain sensitivity (Lytle *et al.*, 1975; Messing *et al.*, 1976), acoustic startle (Walters *et al.*, 1979) and muricidal behaviour (Gibbons *et al.*, 1979; Vergnes and Kempf, 1981), reducing rapid eye movement (REM) sleep (Moja *et al.*, 1979) and enhancing the prolactin (PRL) response to 5-hydroxytryptophan (5-HTP) infusion (Clemens *et al.*, 1980) in laboratory animals. The effects of TRP depletion on pain sensitivity, acoustic startle, muricidal behaviour and REM sleep are reversed by TRP repletion, probably through alterations in central 5-HT function.

Utilizing the prolactin response to infused L-TRP as a measure of CNS 5-HT functional activity we found that dietary TRP restriction (diet 13% of usual daily TRP intake) for an 8-day period in healthy humans reduced plasma TRP levels by 15–20% and led to an enhancement of the prolactin response to TRP infusion, suggesting the development of supersensitivity (Delgado *et al.*, 1989). However, no significant behavioural effects were noted and the degree of reduction of plasma TRP was modest. Subsequent studies with a 10-day low-TRP diet in seven depressed patients in clinical remission revealed no consistent effects on mood (P.L. Delgado, unpublished data).

Studies of mammalian protein metabolism have demonstrated that ingestion of a large bolus of amino acids deficient in one essential amino acid leads to a rapid reduction in the plasma levels of the deficient amino acid (Harper *et al.*, 1970). This is thought to be due to the anabolic effects of amino acid ingestion leading to depletion of plasma reserves of the deficient amino acid in the synthesis of new protein by the liver (Harper *et al.*, 1970). This method has been studied in healthy male subjects by Young *et al.* and been shown rapidly to reduce plasma TRP by 70–80% within 5 h following ingestion of the TRP-free amino acid load (Young *et al.*, 1985; Smith *et al.*, 1987).

We have studied a combination of a 1-day low-TRP diet followed by a TRP-depleting amino acid drink in depressed patients. Each patient receives two tests, each consisting of a 24-h, 160 mg/day, low-TRP diet followed the next morning by administration of a 15-amino acid drink, in a double-blind, placebo-controlled (TRP depletion or control testing), balanced cross-over fashion. On one test the diet is supplemented with 500 mg L-TRP t.i.d. and the amino acid drink contained 2.3 g L-TRP (control); on the other test the diet and amino acid drink are not supplemented with TRP (TRP depletion). Total and free TRP decreased by approximately 90% 5 h following the TRP-free, 15-amino acid drink in drug-free, symptomatic depressed patients and depressed patients in clinical remission after antidepressant treatment (Delgado *et al.*, 1988, 1990a).

In 69 drug-free, symptomatic depressed patients, ratings of mood did not change the day of the TRP-free, 15-amino acid drink, but 30% of these patients demonstrated a clinically apparent decrease in Hamilton Depression Scale (HDRS) score (25–74% decrease) on return to normal TRP intake, *the day after* the TRP-free amino acid drink. This clinical improvement was transient, lasting from 24 h to 7 days. All patients who improved eventually returned to their previously depressed state. There were no consistent behavioural effects *during* the TRP-depleted state. Control testing produced no significant behavioural changes.

Of the first 21 remitted depressive patients studied (Delgado *et al.*, 1990a), 67% experienced a 300% increase in HDRS score on the day of the TRP-free, 15-amino acid drink (12 within 3–7 hours after the TFD and three by the next day) with gradual (48–72 h) return to remitted state (below). Analysis of variance with repeated measures of the individual items on the HDRS during the 3-day TRP depletion test revealed that depressed mood, anxiety, terminal insomnia, decreased appetite, loss of energy, loss of interest, loss of pleasure, decreased concentration, ruminative thinking and worthlessness/failure were significantly altered.

Table 1 depicts the relationship of antidepressant type to depressive relapse in the 38 remitted patients studied with the TRP depletion to date. While 13/14 patients responding to fluvoxamine, fluoxetine or a MAO inhibitor relapsed, only 2/11 patients responding to desipramine relapsed. However, these data should be interpreted with caution because patients were not randomly assigned to antidepressant medication and the patients assigned to desipramine were less refractory and less frequently melancholic (Delgado *et al.*, 1990a). Further, plasma free TRP levels during the TRP depletion test were correlated with HDRS score at 7 h following the TRP-free amino acid drink.

These data suggest that some antidepressant treatments (fluvoxamine and MAO inhibitors) may be dependent on CNS 5-HT availability for their therapeutic effects to be evident, while other antidepressant treatments such as desipramine may be relatively less dependent on 5-HT availability. Furthermore, for the behavioural effects of TRP depletion to be evident in remitted depressed patients on antidepressant medication it appears that depletion of plasma free TRP has to reach some threshold value.

Table 1 Depressive relapse during tryptophan depletion as a function of antidepressant type.

Antidepressant	No. relapses / total patients
Desipramine	2/11
Fluoxetine	2/2
Fluvoxamine	5/6
Monoamine oxidase inhibitors	6/6
Desipramine + lithium	1/3
Fluvoxamine + lithium	2/3
Fluoxetine + thioridazine	0/1
Amphetamine	1/1
Bupropion	0/2
Nortriptyline	1/2
Imipramine	1/1
Total	22/38

What is perhaps even more intriguing is that the drug-free depressed patients did not worsen during the TRP-depleted state as predicted, but rather improved on the day following the test, a totally unexpected result. This implies that while enhancement of 5-HT function is necessary for maintaining an antidepressant response, the 5-HT system may be modulating some other neurotransmitter system or brain region which is centrally important in the pathophysiology of depression, rather than directly modulating mood itself.

5.3.7 Summary

The data reviewed above suggests that presynaptic 5-HT dysfunction may be present in some depressed patients and that antidepressant medications reverse that defect. This data is summarized in Table 2. The blunting of the prolactin response to TRP and fenfluramine, as well as the preliminary reports of a blunted hypothermic response to the 5-HT$_{1A}$ partial agonist, ipsapirone, support this. That the blunted prolactin response to TRP and fenfluramine is due to presynaptic dysfunction is suggested by the preliminary results demonstrating normal prolactin responses to MCPP. Further, lowering 5-HT content does not seem to worsen a depressed state, suggesting either that the functional state of the 5-HT system is already inhibited or that lowered 5-HT function is not directly involved in the state of depression.

The above neuroendocrine data with both TRP and fenfluramine assessing the effects of antidepressants on 5-HT function also strongly suggest that many

Table 2 Neuroendocrine abnormalities of the serotonergic system in depressed patients and effects of antidepressant treatments.

Receptor subtype/location	Stimulus	Response	Type of abnormality in patients	Effect of ADT	Type of ADT
Presynaptic and postsynaptic 5-HT$_1$	Tryptophan	⇑ Prolactin	Blunted response	Increase response	Desipramine Amitriptyline Fluvoxamine Clomipramine MAOI Lithium Carbamazepine
				No effect	Mianserin Bupropion Trazodone
	Fenfluramine	⇑ Prolactin	Blunted response	Increase response	TCA ECT
Presynaptic 5-HT$_{1A}$	Ipsapirone	⇓ Temperature	Blunted response	Further blunting	Amitriptyline
Postsynaptic 5-HT$_1$/5-HT$_2$	MCPP	⇑ Prolactin ⇑ Cortisol	None Increased response	Not tested 'Normalize'	TCA
	5-HTP			Increase further	MAOI

ADT, antidepressant treatment; MAOI, monoamine oxidase inhibitors; TCA, tricyclic antidepressants; ECT, electroconvulsive therapy; MCPP, *m*-clorophenylpiperazine; 5-HTP, 5-hydroxytryptophan.

antidepressants, but not all, enhance 5-HT function, and that interfering with that by lowering 5-HT content transiently reverses the antidepressant response.

The question as to why neither TRP, 5-HTP, fenfluramine or direct acting 5-HT agonists cause an immediate improvement in mood remains unanswered. Explanations suggesting that the degree of activation of the 5-HT system is not sufficient to cause a change in mood do not seem satisfactory, given the robust neuroendocrine response to these precursors and agonists. Other explanations have suggested that the initial response to many of these agents is not an activation because of negative feedback mechanisms via inhibitory presynaptic receptors. However, massive increases in 5-HT release, as caused by the combination of TRP and an MAO inhibitor, do not rapidly alleviate depression, rather the acute response (as is often the case with fenfluramine and potent 5-HT reuptake inhibitors) is nausea and clonic movements (Price et al., 1985).

The data from neuroendocrine studies suggest that an enhanced synaptic transmission through the 5-HT system may initiate a series of events which lead to an antidepressant response in some patients and that interfering with 5-HT synthesis once the antidepressant response has commenced will immediately reverse the antidepressant response. However, the fact that drugs which rapidly increase 5-HT transmission do not lead to even a transient mood improvement acutely would suggest that, while enhanced 5-HT neurotransmission may set into motion a series of events which results in an antidepressant response, the functional activity of this system itself is not directly causing the depressed mood or reversing the depressed mood, but rather regulating some other system or brain area which is.

5.4 Assessment of NA function

Noradrenergic cell bodies primarily originate from the locus coeruleus in the dorsal pons (Redmond, 1987). These cell bodies project to most brain regions and, like 5-HT neurones, seem to exert a modulatory effect on their target site. Interestingly, not all NA-containing nerve terminals in the cortex make synaptic contact with the local cortical neurones, rather these neurones release NA akin to the manner in which hormones are secreted, and thus appear to have generalized effects on other neuromodulatory systems (Woodward et al., 1979). Locus coeruleus neurones are not uniform and demonstrate a laminar distribution and at least four distinct cell types exist (Chan-Palay and Asan, 1989). There is a natural loss of locus coeruleus neurones with ageing and recent morphological studies suggest that this loss of cell bodies can range from 30 to 40%. Interestingly, in one morphological study of locus coeruleus neuronal loss with ageing it was noted that the subject with the greatest loss of locus coeruleus neurones (55% loss) was a woman with a history of chronic depression without dementia (Chan-Palay and Asan, 1989).

The locus coeruleus is exquisitely sensitive to novel stimuli; it appears to modulate levels of arousal and has been postulated to be involved in opiate and alcohol withdrawal states, anxiety disorders, and depression (Charney and Redmond, 1983; Redmond, 1987). Locus coeruleus neurones receive inputs from many different neurotransmitter systems and the firing rate and sensitivity to other incoming stimuli is regulated by these other neurotransmitter systems. These modulating systems include inhibitory input from the 5-HT, opioid, γ-aminobutyric acid (GABA), dopamine and glycine systems and excitatory input from the corticotrophin releasing hormone (CRH), purinergic, glutamate, substance P and muscarinic cholinergic systems (see Redmond, 1987, for review). Another regulatory mechanism is through an inhibitory presynaptic α_2-adrenoreceptor which, when stimulated, decreases the firing rate of locus coeruleus neurones.

Abnormalities of noradrenergic function have long been suspected in affective disorders (Bunney and Davis, 1965; Schildkraut, 1965). The NA deficiency hypothesis of depression was based on the observation that the catecholamine depleting drug, reserpine, caused symptoms similar to depression in some individuals and MAO inhibitors and tricyclic antidepressants led to an enhanced synaptic availability of NA. As with the 5-HT hypothesis of depression, as new knowledge regarding the processes regulating neuro-transmitter synthesis, release and receptor activation have emerged, the original deficiency hypothesis has been replaced by the previously described receptor sensitivity (Charney et al., 1981b) and dysregulation (Siever and Davis, 1985) hypotheses.

The primary evidence for an involvement of the noradrenergic system in depression involves investigations into the mechanism of action of antidepressant drugs. Long-term treatment with tricyclic antidepressants, MAO inhibitors, trazodone, iprindole, and ECT, but not selective 5-HT reuptake inhibitors, bupropion, mianserin and nomifensine, decrease β-adrenoreceptor binding in laboratory animals (Charney et al., 1981b). Increases in α_1-adrenoreceptor binding have been reported for many antidepressants and decreases in α_2-adrenoreceptor binding have been reported for some antidepressants, but these findings have been much less consistent than for β-adrenoreceptors (see Charney et al., 1981b, for review).

Electrophysiological studies in laboratory animals suggest that these changes compensate for the acute effects of antidepressants on NA release and restore the overall transmission of noradrenergic neurones to their pretreatment level (Blier et al., 1986).

Moreover, antidepressants which have no effect on noradrenergic function are effective at relieving depression (Heninger and Charney, 1987) and interfering with the synthesis of NA with the tryrosine hydroxylase inhibitor, α-methyl-p-tyrosine (AMPT), did not disturb the antidepressant response to imipramine in recently remitted depressed patients (Shopsin et al., 1975). The vast majority of neuroendocrine challenge studies of the noradrenergic system in depression have involved investigations of α_2-adrenergic receptor responsiveness. Both presynaptic and postsynaptic α_2-adrenergic receptors are present in the CNS. Stimulation of postsynaptic α_2-adrenergic receptors causes an increased release of growth hormone (Lal et al., 1975). The release of growth hormone by α_2-adrenergic receptor agonists is thought to be mediated by the postsynaptic activation of α_2-adrenergic receptors within the brain exerting a stimulatory effect on the secretion of growth hormone releasing hormone in the hypothalamus (Frohman and Jansson, 1986). However, factors other than adrenergic receptor activation exert an effect on the growth hormone response to clonidine, such that depletion of both 5-HT and NA leads to a weaker growth hormone response to clonidine than depletion of NA alone in rats (Soderpalm et al., 1987).

5.4.1 Clonidine

Stimulation of presynaptic α_2-adrenergic receptors causes a decrease in the firing rate of the locus coeruleus and a decrease in sympathetic outflow (Leckman et al., 1981). The decrease in sympathetic outflow through the inhibition of the locus coeruleus firing rate is thought to be significantly reflected by a decrease in plasma levels of the primary metabolite of NA, MHPG (Leckman et al., 1981).

Clonidine is an α_2-adrenergic receptor agonist which causes an increase in the secretion of growth hormone, and increased subjective reporting of sedation, a decrease in the secretion of MHPG and a decrease in blood pressure in humans (Lal et al., 1975; Matussek et al., 1980). The growth hormone response to both oral and intravenous clonidine has been consistently found to be blunted in endogenous depressed patients compared with healthy controls (Matussek et al., 1980; Checkley et al., 1981, 1984; Boyer et al., 1982; Charney et al., 1982b; Siever et al., 1982a; Ansseau et al., 1984, 1988). However, studies with low-dose oral clonidine (Dolan and Calloway, 1986) and low-dose intravenous clonidine (Katona et al., 1986) have not found a difference in the growth hormone response between patients and controls. The blood pressure and MHPG changes have been more variable, with most studies failing to find significant differences (Heninger et al., 1990).

Antidepressant treatment with desipramine, amitriptyline, clorgyline, trazodone or mianserin (Charney et al., 1981c, 1982c, 1983, 1984b;

Siever *et al.*, 1982b; Price *et al.*, 1986) have no effect on the growth hormone response to clonidine, while short-term treatment with lithium tends to normalize a blunted growth hormone response to clonidine in both depressives and controls while causing a blunted response in those healthy controls who had normal responses prior to lithium (Brambilla *et al.*, 1988).

Long-term treatment with desipramine and amitriptyline (Charney *et al.*, 1981a, 1981b, 1981c, 1982c), but not trazodone or mianserin (Charney *et al.*, 1984b; Price *et al.*, 1986), blocked the decrease in plasma MHPG and blood pressure caused by clonidine. This effect of some antidepressants is thought to be due to decreased presynaptic α_2-adrenergic receptor sensitivity.

Questions regarding technical aspects of the growth hormone response to clonidine have been raised. For example, the relationship of the blunted growth hormone response to clonidine to recent antidepressant treatment (within 2 weeks) has been questioned. Depressed patients having had antidepressant treatment within a 2-week period of the test have been reported to be more likely to demonstrate a blunted growth hormone response to clonidine when compared with depressed patients who have never had had antidepressant treatment (Schittecatte *et al.*, 1989). However, these findings contrast with the data cited above demonstrating the lack of effect of chronic antidepressant treatment on the growth hormone response to clonidine.

Further complicating the issue is the report of temporal instability in the growth hormone response to clonidine in healthy subjects (this issue also exists for most other neuroendocrine probes). Only 5 of 12 healthy subjects tested at four times over a 3-week period maintained a growth hormone response > 5 ng/ml (Matussek, 1988). Repeated testing to assess the stability of the test has not been done in depressed patients.

5.4.2 Guanfacine

Another α_2-adrenergic receptor agonist, guanfacine, has been studied in depressed patients (Eriksson *et al.*, 1988). Guanfacine is a slightly more selective α_2-adrenergic receptor agonist than clonidine and causes an increase in the secretion of growth hormone which is not different in depressed patients compared with healthy controls (Eriksson *et al.*, 1988). The reasons for this inconsistency between the growth hormone response to clonidine and guanfacine is not clear, although the possibility that clonidine, as a partial agonist, may be more likely to uncover a functional defect in α_2-adrenergic receptor responsiveness than the full agonist, guanfacine, was cited as a possible explanation (Eriksson *et al.*, 1988). Further, issues of endogenous versus non-endogenous subtype and dose may confound the interpretation.

In the above study, Eriksson *et al.* measured the growth hormone response to guanfacine as well as to growth hormone releasing hormone in the same subjects. They found that there was a significant correlation between the growth hormone responses to these two agents, suggesting that the variability of the growth hormone response might be due to factors other than α_2-adrenergic receptor responsiveness (Eriksson *et al.*, 1988).

5.4.3 Yohimbine

Yohimbine is an α_2-adrenergic receptor antagonist and increases the firing rate of the locus coeruleus with a resultant increase in sympathetic outflow (Redmond, 1987). Oral and intravenous yohimbine causes an increase in MHPG and blood pressure in healthy human subjects (Charney *et al.*, 1982d; Goldberg *et al.*, 1986). Depressed patients demonstrate an increased cortisol and blood pressure response to intravenous yohimbine compared with healthy subjects, while plasma MHPG is not significantly different between the two groups of subjects (Heninger *et al.*, 1988). The effects of acute or chronic antidepressant treatments on the neuroendocrine or behavioural responses to yohimbine in depressed patients have not been studied.

5.4.4 Amphetamine

Amphetamine causes release and blocks reuptake of both NA and dopamine. It has been used as a neuroendocrine challenge probe of both of these neurotransmitter systems, with growth hormone and cortisol primarily being used to assess the response. The growth hormone response is thought to be due to dopaminergic stimulation of dopamine-2-receptors and NA stimulation of postsynaptic α_2-adrenergic receptors. The cortisol response is thought to be mediated by NA stimulation of postsynaptic α-adrenergic receptors, possibly of the α_1-adrenergic type.

Studies assessing both the dopaminergic and noradrenergic systems have reported a blunted growth hormone response to amphetamine in depressed patients compared with healthy subjects (Langer *et al.*, 1975, 1976; Arato *et al.*, 1983). In these studies (Langer *et al.*, 1975, 1976) the blunted growth hormone response was only seen in endogenous depressives and not in non-endogenous depressives. However, questions regarding the interpretations of the blunted growth hormone response have been raised because of the 'normal' blunting of the growth hormone response seen after menopause and the presence of more postmenopausal women in the patient groups than in the control groups in the above cited studies (Matussek, 1988). Subsequent studies investigating the growth hormone response to amphetamine in postmenopausal endogenous depressed patients (and two male endogenous depressive patients) and matched controls have reported no difference in this hormone response (Halbreich *et al.*, 1982).

Nurnberger *et al.* (1982) have studied the neuroendocrine effects of amphetamine in 'well state' bipolar twins and matched healthy twins in an effort to distinguish state and trait variables in the neuroendocrine, biochemical, physiological and behavioural responses to amphetamine. While there were no patient–control differences in any of the measures, the behavioural 'excitation' and pretreatment levels of plasma MHPG, prolactin and growth hormone were significantly correlated between the twins, while plasma amphetamine level, cortisol and blood pressure and heart rate were discordant.

The cortisol response to methylamphetamine and dextroamphetamine has also been used as a measure of noradrenergic function. Interestingly, the cortisol response to methylamphetamine in depressed patients before and after recovery was found to be lower in the depressive phase compared with the recovered phase (Checkley and Crammer, 1977). Attempts to identify diagnostic subtypes of depression using this measure appear to support the distinction between endogenous and non-endogenous forms of depression. When compared with reactive depressives and other non-depressed psychiatric patients, the cortisol response to methylamphetamine was blunted only in endogenous depressives (Checkley, 1979). In a larger replication using dextroamphetamine, the cortisol response to this NA and dopamine releasing agent was also found to be diminished in endogenous depressed patients compared with healthy controls (Sachar *et al.*, 1980, 1985). However, when the cortisol response to dextroamphetamine was assessed at 8 a.m. rather than the 4 p.m. time used in the previous studies (Checkley and Crammer, 1977; Checkley, 1979; Sachar *et al.*, 1980, 1985), no difference was noted between depressed patients and healthy subjects (Feinberg *et al.*, 1981).

The cortisol response to methylamphetamine or dextroamphetamine is not affected by tricyclic antidepressant treatment or ECT (Checkley, 1979; Sachar *et al.*, 1980).

5.4.5 Desipramine

Desipramine is a tricyclic antidepressant; it is a relatively selective NA reuptake inhibitor with significant anticholinergic and antihistaminic effects as well. Single oral doses of desipramine cause a dose-dependent increase in growth homone, cortisol (Laakmann *et al.*, 1977, 1986) and MHPG (Charney *et al.*, 1981a). The growth hormone response to desipramine is blocked by the non-selective α-adrenergic antagonist, phentolamine, and the α_2-adrenergic antagonist, yohimbine, and potentiated by the non-selective β-adrenergic antagonist, propranolol, while the selective α_1-adrenergic antagonist, prazosin, had no effect, suggesting that at least the growth hormone response to desipramine is mediated by stimulation of postsynaptic α_2-adrenergic receptors (Laakmann *et al.*, 1977).

The growth hormone response to desipramine has been reported to be blunted in pre-menopausal female endogenous depressives (Meesters *et al.*, 1985) and male endogenous depressives (Laakmann *et al.*, 1986) compared with healthy subjects. The cortisol response to desipramine has also been reported to be blunted in endogenous depressed patients (Asnis *et al.*, 1986; see also Chapter 7).

5.4.6 Exposure to light

Nocturnal melatonin secretion is mediated by direct stimulation of β-adrenergic receptors by NA released from noradrenergic neurones (Brownstein and Axelrod, 1974). In humans, treatment with the β-adrenergic receptor antagonist, propranolol, blocks night-time melatonin secretion (Hanssen *et al.*, 1977). Environmental light treatment also decreases nocturnal melatonin secretion (Lewy *et al.*, 1980) and this is thought to be due to a decrease in noradrenergic neurotransmission induced by bright light (Brownstein and Axelrod, 1974; Frazer *et al.*, 1986).

The night-time increase in melatonin secretion is blunted in depressed patients compared with healthy subjects (Wetterberg, 1983; Frazer *et al.*, 1986). Treatment with the antidepressant medications desipramine (Cowen *et al.*, 1985b), clorgyline and tranylcypromine (Murphy *et al.*, 1986) elevate plasma melatonin levels, presumably by increasing noradrenergic neurotransmission. However, this is unexpected, since chronic antidepressant treatment decreases β-adrenergic receptor function (Heninger *et al.*, 1990). It is interesting to note that 1 week of desipramine treatment in healthy subjects increases melatonin secretion but after 3 weeks of treatment this response appears to adapt and return to pretreatment levels (Cowen *et al.*, 1985b).

5.4.7 Summary

Neuroendocrine challenge studies of noradrenergic function in depression have suggested that postsynaptic abnormalities may be present in some depressed patients. Table 3 describes the results of neuroendocrine studies of the NA system. While pretreatment abnormalities have been identified, most antidepressant treatments do not consistently modify neuroendocrine measures of noradrenergic function.

Measures of postsynaptic noradrenergic activity suggest that there is a functional blunting of the responsiveness of α_2-adrenergic receptors. The strongest support of this hypothesis has come from investigations demonstrating

Table 3 Neuroendocrine abnormalities of the noradrenergic system in depressed patients and effects of antidepressant treatments.

Receptor subtype/location	Stimulus	Response	Type of abnormality in patients	Effect of ADT	Type of ADT
Postsynaptic α_2-adrenergic	Clonidine	⇑ Growth hormone	Blunted response	None	Desipramine Amitriptyline Mianserin Trazodone MAOI
	Guanfacine	⇑ Growth hormone	None	Not tested	
	Desipramine	⇑ Growth hormone	Blunted response	Not tested	
Postsynaptic α_1-adrenergic	Amphetamine	⇑ Cortisol	Blunted response	None	TCA ECT
Postsynaptic β-adrenergic	Diurnal variation	⇑ Melatonin	Blunted response	Increase response	Desipramine MAOI
	Artificial light	⇓ Melatonin	Blunted	Not tested	
Presynaptic α_2-adrenergic	Desipramine	⇑ MHPG	None	Not tested	
	Yohimbine	⇑ MHPG	None	Not tested	

ADT, antidepressant treatment; MAOI, monoamine oxidase inhibitors; TCA, tricyclic antidepressants; ECT, electroconvulsive therapy; MHPG, 3-methoxy-4-hydroxyphenylethyleneglycol.

a blunted growth hormone response to clonidine. The blunted growth hormone response to desipramine further supports this hypothesis. Moreover, the failure to identify significant patient–control differences in the growth hormone response to the dopamine agonist, apomorphine, suggests that this abnormality may be specific to the noradrenergic system. Likewise, since the growth hormone response to amphetamine is most likely mediated via the stimulation of postsynaptic dopaminergic as well as α_2-adrenergic receptors, it is not surprising to see no patient–control difference using this probe. Still unexplained is the failure to identify differences between depressed patients and healthy subjects using the more selective α_2-adrenergic agonist, guanfacine.

Another postsynaptic abnormality is the blunted cortisol response to amphetamine and desipramine. The cortisol response to noradrenergic agonists is thought to reflect activation of postsynaptic α_1-adrenergic receptors. This blunting of this response is interesting because it is presumably mediated through hypothalamic CRH secretion, although direct effects on the adrenal gland have not been excluded. However, no relationship between the cortisol response to either desipramine or amphetamine has been found to dexamethasone non-suppression.

Assessment of postsynaptic β-adrenergic receptor function has not been as well studied as the other adrenergic receptor subtypes. The primary marker utilized has been the melatonin response to light or the natural night-time melatonin surge. Unfortunately, a melatonin response to β-adrenergic agonists has not been achieved. However, the blunted nocturnal melatonin surge and the fact that depressed patients maintain an enhanced night-time melatonin surge after long-term desipramine treatment, while healthy subjects demonstrate a return to baseline melatonin levels after long-term desipramine treatment, suggests possible differences in β-adrenergic receptor regulation between healthy subjects and depressed patients.

Presynaptic dysregulation of the noradrenergic system has not been identified. The lack of difference in the MHPG, blood pressure and sedative responses to desipramine between healthy subjects and depressed patients suggests relatively normal presynaptic noradrenergic activity using this paradigm. The failure to identify a difference between healthy subjects and depressed patients in the behavioural response to yohimbine further highlights this issue.

Perhaps most important of all has been the lack of a consistent effect of antidepressant treatments on neuroendocrine measures of noradrenergic activity. While some antidepressant treatments affect some of the neuroendocrine measures, there is a glaring lack of discernable pattern across antidepressant treatments.

Behavioural effects of most of the neuroendocrine measures offer some interesting data. Clonidine generally causes sedative type of behavioural effects while yohimbine generally causes anxiety and behavioural activation. Neither drug has striking effects on mood, although yohimbine has caused manic responses in bipolar patients (Price *et al.*, 1984). Amphetamine causes an elevation of mood in healthy subjects and some depressed patients, but this effect may be due to the increase in dopamine release rather than the increased NA release (Wald *et al.*, 1978).

Overall it appears that postsynaptic abnormalities in α_1- and α_2-adrenergic receptor function may exist in some depressed patients but antidepressant treatments do not have consistent effects on neuroendocrine measures of noradrenergic function. Further, treatment with the tyrosine hydroxylase inhibitor, AMPT, did not reverse antidepressant response to imipramine in a small number of patients (Shopsin *et al.*, 1975). These data suggest that the NA system may be involved in depression, but that changes in noradrenergic activity are not a common mechanism of action of antidepressant treatments. It is not possible to exclude the possibility that specific antidepressant medications may, in part or whole, mediate their therapeutic effects by altering noradrenergic activity.

5.5 Assessment of dopaminergic function

Relative to the studies investigating noradrenergic and 5-HT function in affective disorders there has been little study of dopaminergic activity. Some investigators have hypothesized that dysfunction of dopaminergic neurotransmission may be involved in depression, and especially in mania (Jimerson, 1987). This hypothesis is based on the observations that some dopamine agonists, such as L-dopa, amphetamine, methylphenidate and bromocriptine, have been associated with the development of mania, and that dopamine antagonists are efficacious in the treatment of mania. Further, drugs such as bupropion and nomifensine, both of which enhance dopaminergic activity, are effective antidepressants.

However, none of the above drugs are specific dopaminergic agonists and antagonists and most have pronounced effects on the noradrenergic system. Antidepressant trials with more selective dopaminergic agonists such as piribedil, while apparently efficacious in some patients, have, on the whole, been disappointing. Further, cocaine, which has potent effects on the release of dopamine, appears not to be an effective antidepressant in most depressed patients (Post *et al.*, 1974), although this may only apply to a subset of depressed patients, since many dysthymic patients and mildly depressed patients report improvement of depression early in the use of cocaine, with the subsequent development of more dysphoric reactions (personal observations).

Most dopaminergic cell bodies are located in the ventral mesencephalon; these project widely throughout the CNS, giving rise to the nigrostriatal, mesocortical and mesolimbic dopaminergic projections. These projections and others arising from the ventral mesencephalon comprise a diverse and complexly regulated group of projections. Considerable anatomical and functional overlap exists between these projections, as well as a surprising degree of heterogeneity and uniqueness.

The heterogeneity appears related to the diversity of nerve terminal systems, feedback loops, enzyme composition, co-released peptides, and differences in autoreceptor sensitivity within different target brain regions (see Roth et al., 1987, for review).

The dopaminergic cell bodies projecting to the hypothalamus and pituitary arise from a different brain region and are referred to as the tuberoinfundibular (TIDA) and tuberohypophyseal (THDA) neurones. These cell bodies are located primarily in the arcuate nucleus. The THDA neurones project ventrally to the neurointermediate lobe of the pituitary and the TIDA neurones project to the hypothalamus and the hypothalamic–hypophyseal portal system (Moore, 1987). Dopaminergic TIDA projections are involved in the tonic inhibition of prolactin secretion as well as stimulating the release of growth hormone.

Neuroendocrine challenge strategies designed to assess dopaminergic function in depressed patients have used the prolactin and growth hormone responses to direct and indirect dopaminergic agonists as measures of dopaminergic tone. It is worth noting that considerable evidence supports the observations that the TIDA and THDA dopaminergic neurones are regulated differently and may not provide an accurate index of the functional state of the mesolimbic or mesocortical dopaminergic projections (Jimerson, 1987; Moore, 1987).

5.5.1 Apomorphine

Apomorphine is a direct-acting postsynaptic and presynaptic dopamine-2 receptor agonist. Apomorphine leads to an increase in the secretion of growth hormone, ACTH, cortisol and β-endorphin, and a decrease in the secretion of prolactin in humans (Brown et al., 1979; Jezova and Vigas, 1988). Limiting factors in the use of apomorphine have been the occurrence of nausea, which itself could confound results by causing indirect effects on the release of hormones, and the fact that decreasing levels of prolactin, which is already released in small amounts, are difficult to detect.

Neuroendocrine responses to apomorphine have been studied in depression and, for the most part, no difference in the suppression of prolactin or in increased release of growth hormone between healthy subjects and depressed patients have been identified (Willner, 1983; Jimerson, 1987).

ECT has been reported to enhance the growth hormone response to apomorphine in depressed patients and amitriptyline appears to blunt the growth hormone response in both healthy subjects and depressed patients to a similar degree (Balldin *et al.*, 1982; Costain *et al.*, 1982; Cowen *et al.*, 1984).

5.5.2 Amphetamine

The neuroendocrine effects of amphetamine, reviewed in the preceding section on assessment of noradrenergic function, have produced mixed results, with some studies reporting a blunted growth hormone response and others reporting no difference between depressed patients and controls (see Jimerson, 1987; Matussek, 1988, for reviews).

More interesting is the rapid but transient improvement of mood in some depressed patients after acute administration of amphetamine (Fawcet and Siomopoulos, 1971; Joyce, 1985). Although it has been suggested that the improvement of mood following amphetamine in depressed patients predicts subsequent antidepressant response (Fawcet and Siomopoulos, 1971), this has not been fully verified or aggressively followed up.

5.5.3 L-Dopa and bromocriptine

L-Dopa is the immediate precursor for the synthesis of NA and dopamine. L-Dopa has also been used to assess dopaminergic and noradrenergic activity in depression, although, as for amphetamine, it cannot be established with certainty which neurotransmitter is responsible for the neuroendocrine profile. For the most part, the growth hormone and prolactin responses to L-dopa and bromocriptine in depressed patients have been found to be no different than for healthy subjects (see Jimerson, 1987, for review).

5.5.4 Summary

As described above, neuroendocrine abnormalities of the dopamine system have not been established in depression. While mixed dopaminergic–noradrenergic releasing agents, such as amphetamine, methylphenidate and cocaine, appear to cause an elevation of mood and even mania-like states in healthy subjects, and mood elevation in some depressed patients, this does not appear to be related to any neuroendocrine abnormalities in depression.

The lack of neuroendocrine abnormalities of the dopamine system in depression may be because of the distinct nature of the regulation of the TIDA and THDA neurones, but suggests that abnormalities of dopaminergic function may not be involved in most forms of depression. Futher evidence in support of this view is the lack of depressogenic effect of dopaminergic antagonists in either healthy subjects or depressed patients. However, the antidepressant drugs nomifensine and bupropion may in fact be mediating their therapeutic effects through the dopamine system and may indicate that a subgroup of depressed patients may have abnormalities of the dopamine system.

5.6 Assessment of cholinergic function

The cholinergic hypothesis of depression was postulated in the context of data which documented significant anticholinergic properties of most antidepressant drugs and of the mood-altering properties of cholinomimetics and anti-cholinergics in both healthy subjects and affective disorder patients (Janowski and Risch, 1987). This hypothesis stated that excess cholinergic activity was involved in depression and that mania was due to an imbalance between the noradrenergic (increased) and cholinergic (decreased) systems (Janowski et al., 1972).

Even though acetylcholine was the first neurotransmitter identified, research on the behavioural aspects of the CNS cholinergic systems has lagged behind our understanding of the behavioural aspects of the noradrenergic, 5-HT and dopaminergic systems. This appears to have been due primarily to the extensive involvement of the cholinergic mechanisms in the regulation of the parasympathetic nervous system and in the regulation of voluntary movement, which made difficult and tended to obscure research on the behavioural effects of acetycholine (Bartus et al., 1987).

5.6.1 Cholinergic agonists and antagonists

Considerable research has been focused on the behavioural effects of anticholinergic drugs and cholinomimetic drugs and relatively less on the neuroendocrine aspects. Cholinomimetic drugs appear to cause robust behavioural depression in healthy humans (El-Yousef et al., 1973), unlike the modest behavioural effects of dopaminergic, noradrenergic, 5-HT and opiate antagonists. Organophosphate insecticides (Gershon and Shaw, 1961) and physostigmine (Janowski et al., 1973), drugs which greatly enhance CNS cholinergic activity by interfering with the enzyme acetylcholinesterase, lead to behavioural depression in healthy humans and patients with affective disorders. Further, the direct cholinergic agonist, arecoline, exacerbates depressive symptoms (Risch *et al.*, 1982; Nurnberger *et al.*, 1983). Qualitatively, however, the euphoria-producing effects of anticholinergics (Bolin, 1960) do not appear as closely related to mania as are the euphoria-producing effects of the NA and dopamine releasers, cocaine and amphetamine.

Cholinomimetic drugs elevate ACTH, cortisol and β-endorphin secretion in humans (Janowski and Risch, 1987). Physostigmine infusions have been the most studied in depression and lead to increases in ACTH, cortisol and β-endorphin (Risch *et al.*, 1982). Physostigmine reverses the normal suppression of cortisol by dexamethasone in healthy subjects (Carroll *et al.*, 1980; Doerr and Berger, 1983). Further, depressed patients demonstrate an enhanced release of ACTH and β-endorphin (Risch, 1982).

5.6.2 Summary

Robust depressogenic effects of cholinomimetic drugs have been reported. Further, the neuroendocrine effects of cholinomimetic drugs on hypothalamic–pituitary–adrenal (HPA) function in healthy subjects appear to mimic the alterations seen in some depressed patients. However, relatively little has been done to elucidate these phenomena and the enhanced ACTH and β-endorphin release reported in depression has not been further studied to date. Also, the receptor types and subtypes mediating the behavioural and neuroendocrine effects of cholinomimetic drugs remain to be elucidated.

Muscarinic cholinergic receptors may exist in two subtypes, designated as M1 and M2, with each utilizing a different G-protein second messenger system (Avissar and Schreiber, 1989). Selective agonists at each of these receptor subtypes may provide new avenues for further study, and antagonists for these receptor subtypes may be evaluated as potential antidepressants.

5.7 Neuroendocrine aspects of opiate receptor activation in depression

Opioid peptides and various opiate receptor agonists and antagonists have pronounced effects on the release of pituitary and adrenal hormones. After the discovery of endogenously occurring opioid peptides and the characterization of opiate receptors, the uncovering of some of the behavioural effects of the opioid peptides, and the involvement of these substances in 'stress' responses in laboratory animals, a heightened level of interest in the neuroendocrine effects of opioid peptides and other opiates ensued.

5.7.1 Opiate agonists

Some of the first studies of the neuroendocrine effects of opiates in humans were investigations assessing the effects of methadone (Gold *et al.*, 1980) and β-endorphin (Catlin *et al.*, 1980) on plasma cortisol levels, and morphine and methadone on plasma prolactin (Extein *et al.*, 1980). While most (Extein *et al.*, 1980; Judd *et al.*, 1982; Robertson *et al.*, 1984), but not all (Zis *et al.*, 1985a), investigators have found a blunted prolactin response to morphine and methadone in depressed patients compared with healthy controls, the prolactin response to the specific μ-opiate receptor agonist, fentanyl, was not different from controls (Matussek and Hoehe, 1989), and the cortisol response to morphine has been variable, with a subgroup of depressed patients demonstrating an 'escape' of the suppression of cortisol by these opiates (Zis *et al.*, 1985b, 1985c; Banki and Arato, 1987; Zis, 1988). In these studies many of the patients with an 'escape' of suppression of cortisol also had abnormal dexamethasone suppression tests (Zis, 1988).

The neuroendocrine profiles of opiate antagonists have also been investigated in depressed patients and, although robust increases in cortisol have been noted, these are not different from those found in healthy subjects (Zis, 1988, for review).

5.7.2 Summary

A blunted prolactin response to morphine and methadone has been the only consistently identified neuroendocrine abnormality of the opioid system in depressed patients. However, the neuroendocrine effects of opiates may be mediated through catecholaminergic and indoleamine neurotransmitter systems. For example, opiate-induced increases in growth hormone secretion may be mediated via changes in the noradrenergic system (Koenig *et al.*, 1980; Eriksson *et al.*, 1981), and possibly the histaminergic and cholinergic systems (Penalva *et al.*, 1983), and increases in prolactin secretion may be mediated through the dopaminergic (Grandison and Guidotti, 1977; Tolis *et al.*, 1978) and/or serotonergic (Spampinato *et al.*, 1979) systems. This makes interpretation of the blunted prolactin response to opiate agonists difficult, since blunting of the prolactin response to various 5-HT probes is a consistently replicated finding in depressed patients (Heninger *et al.*, 1990). It is interesting that in some studies the euphoric response to fentanyl is blunted in depressed patients compared with healthy controls (Matussek and Hoehe, 1989).

5.8 Investigation of hypothalamic–pituitary–adrenal (HPA) axis function

Abnormalities of the HPA axis have been some of the most studied biological abnormalities in depression. There has been extensive research into the preclinical and clinical aspects of HPA function because of the abnormal cortisol response to stress and to the synthetic steroid dexamethasone seen in many depressed patients (Carroll *et al.*, 1968, 1976, 1981). Cortisol production by the adrenal cortex is stimulated primarily by the hormone ACTH, whose release is in turn stimulated primarily by CRH and vasopressin and inhibited by glucocorticoids. CRH secretion is enhanced by 5-HT, and noradrenergic and cholinergic inputs, and diminished by GABA and glucocorticoids (Holsboer, 1989). Further, CRH feeds back to the locus coeruleus and increases its firing rate.

5.8.1 Dexamethasone

Abnormal levels of basal cortisol in depression were identified almost 30 years ago (Gibbons, 1964). Shortly after this, Carroll reported the lack of normal suppression of cortisol following an oral dose of the synthetic corticosteroid, dexamethasone (Carroll *et al.*, 1968). Although the sensitivity of the dexamethasone suppression test (DST) for diagnosing depression is not adequate and only tentative predictive validity for the DST has been established (Carroll *et al.*, 1981), the lack of normal suppression of plasma cortisol in depressed patients has continued to be replicated. Given the current level of understanding of the regulation of the HPA axis, considerable research is now being focused on attempting to understand the pathophysiology which underlies DST non-suppression in depressed patients.

5.8.2 CRH

Since the identification and synthesis of CRH in the early 1980s (Speiss *et al.*, 1981, Shibahara *et al.*, 1983), CRH has become available as a neuroendocrine probe of HPA activity. The ACTH response to CRH infusion is blunted in depressed patients compared with controls (Holsboer *et al.*, 1984) but cortisol release is exaggerated and the cortisol response to CRH is therefore not different between depressed patients and healthy subjects (Holsboer, 1989). Further, the blunting of the ACTH response is reversed when cortisol biosynthesis is blocked by metyrapone, suggesting that the blunting of the ACTH response is caused in part by feedback inhibition of ACTH release by circulating cortisol (Von Bardeleben *et al.*, 1988). Based on the above, it has been hypothesized that the reasons for hypercortisolism in depression must be related to hypersecretion of CRH (Holsboer, 1989).

Recent investigations add support to this hypothesis, in that depressed patients have been found to have elevated CSF levels of CRH compared with healthy subjects and non-depressed psychiatric patients (Nemeroff *et al.*, 1984; Banki *et al.*, 1987). However, the specificity of these findings is unclear, since both elevated CSF levels of CRH and a blunted ACTH response to CRH are found in underweight anorexia nervosa patients (Taylor and Fishman, 1988).

5.8.3 Summary

Considerable work remains to be done to clarify the nature of the HPA axis abnormality in some depressed patients. The DST has been assessed in patients receiving a number of other challenge tests. However, no correlations between DST non-suppression and blunting of the prolactin response to TRP or fenfluramine or the blunted growth hormone response to clonidine have been identified, although the lack of suppression of cortisol in response to opiate agonists may be a related abnormality.

5.9 Comment

Is there a common pathophysiology of depression, or are there subgroups of depressed patients with discrete abnormalities of certain neurotransmitter systems but not others? Have the monoamine and indoleamine deficiency, or receptor sensitivity, or dysregulation hypotheses of depression been supported? Is there a common mechanism of action of antidepressant treatments or are there many?

In reviewing the neuroendocrine challenge strategies used to assess the above questions it must be stated that, at this time, complete answers remain elusive. A common pathophysiology of depression has not been identified. The data reviewed suggest that there may be multiple pathophysiological abnormalities present in the depressed state. These abnormalities appear to include at least presynaptic 5-HT and/or postsynaptic NA function, but the involvement of other neurotransmitter systems is likely.

A unitary mechanism of antidepressant action has not been identified. The original deficiency hypotheses have not been supported and considerable evidence suggests that it is unlikely that a monoamine or indoleamine deficiency is involved in depression, and simply increasing synaptic concentrations of monoamines or indoleamines does not rapidly reverse depression (see Charney *et al.*, 1981b, for review).

Although there have been discrete abnormalities of 5-HT and NA function identified in some depressed patients, these abnormalities have not had predictive validity for course of illness, diagnostic subtype or treatment response. Therefore, it is not known whether these abnormalities are central to the illness or epiphenomena.

The reasons for this failure to establish predictive validity are unclear. It may be that our predictors of outcome (such as treatment response to NA or 5-HT reuptake inhibitors) or diagnostic clusters (endogenous versus non-endogenous and melancholic versus non-melancholic, bipolar versus unipolar depressions) are inappropriate to the biology of the illness. For example, would an antidepressant medication which enhanced the function of the 5-HT system be more or less likely to work in a patient with an abnormality of the 5-HT system? If an abnormality of the 5-HT system was presynaptic and impaired the release of 5-HT, a 5-HT reuptake inhibitor may be an ineffective treatment. On the other hand, if the abnormality was postsynaptic, a 5-HT reuptake inhibitor might be more effective than other antidepressant treatments. What if the abnormality was an inability to regulate receptor sensitivity? In this case it might be predicted that the 5-HT reuptake inhibitor would be unable to induce the same receptor sensitivity changes which it did in 'normal' laboratory animals, and thus be rendered ineffective.

The above scenarios are just a few of the ways in which biological heterogeneity may underlie functional homogeneity. One could propose many more possible biological abnormalities which would lead to similar functional disturbances of one or more neurotransmitter systems, and thus similar symptoms. Therefore, biological heterogeneity may further limit the interpretations arrived at from neuroendocrine challenge studies.

Most investigators today will quickly point out that they believe that depression is a biologically heterogeneous disorder; in fact a syndrome. It would be highly unlikely, given the great deal of duplication and interplay of CNS neurotransmitter systems, that only one type of abnormality, whether inherited or environmentally caused, was responsible for all forms of depression. In fact we now know that certain types of cerebral infarcts (Robinson and Chait, 1985), hypothyroidism (Sachar, 1973), some of the porphyrias, acquired immune deficiency syndrome (Perry, 1990) and numerous types of drugs can cause very similar or indistinguishable symptoms to those found in depressions of unknown aetiology.

However, even though there may be biological heterogeneity underlying depressive states, it is still possible that functional homogeneity exists. An example of this type of situation is parkinsonism. The symptoms of parkinsonism can be caused by numerous drugs, which lead to an actual or functional deficiency of dopaminergic activity in the nigrostriatal dopaminergic projections as well as naturally occurring forms of the illness. It is the dysfunction of the nigrostriatal system which leads to similar symptoms, regardless of the cause. The question of functional homogeneity in depressive states is important because knowing whether this exists will help us focus our investigations on those systems.

If some degree of functional homogeneity exists in depression, then one would predict that drugs which change the overall level of activity of a given neurotransmitter system might consistently alter mood, even though the neuroendocrine profile may differ between patients. Some clues as to whether this is the case may be found by examining the behavioural effects of drugs which increase or decrease the state of activation of various neurotransmitter systems. In healthy subjects, rapidly increasing the release of dopamine and NA with cocaine or amphetamine (Fawcet and Siomopoulos, 1971), or of 5-HT with 3,4-methylenedioxymethamphetamine (MDMA, Ecstasy), results in an elevation of mood (Price et al., 1989c). The mood response to dopamine and NA releasers more closely resembles mania (Meyendorff et al., 1985), while the mood response to MDMA involves more of a sense of mellow well-being (Price et al., 1989c). Interestingly, amphetamine and cocaine do not consistently improve mood in depressed patients (Fawcet and Siomopoulos, 1971; Post et al., 1974). MDMA has not been studied in depression, and although fenfluramine releases 5-HT it does not have the same behavioural profile as MDMA.

AMPT, which rapidly diminishes brain dopamine and NA content, does not cause depression in non-psychiatric patients (Engelman et al., 1968) but can exacerbate depression in some depressed patients and sometimes reduces manic symptoms (Brodie et al., 1970). Physostigmine, which increases brain acetylcholine, can cause depressive symptoms in healthy subjects and some depressed patients (Janowski and Risch, 1987). PCPA, which decreases brain 5-HT content, does not consistently cause depressive symptoms in non-psychiatric patients (Carpenter, 1970), and rapid dietary TRP depletion does not worsen depressive symptoms in (drug-free) depressed patients (Delgado et al., 1988). The behavioural effects of various treatments which specifically alter NA, dopaminergic, and 5-HT function are presented in Table 4.

Interestingly, PCPA and TRP depletion rapidly and transiently reverse antidepressant response (see Table 1) to a variety of antidepressant drugs (Shopsin et al., 1975, 1976; Delgado et al., 1990a), whereas AMPT may not (Shopsin et al., 1975). This suggests that enhancement of at least the brain 5-HT system may be a necessary, but not sufficient, condition for anti-depressant action with some medications.

When the above are considered in light of the behavioural findings with PCPA, TRP depletion, AMPT, cocaine, amphetamine, MDMA and

Table 4 Behavioural effects of various drugs/procedures in healthy subjects and affective disorder patients.

Drug/procedure	Biological effect	Response in healthy subjects	Response in manic patients	Response in depressed patients	Response in antidepressant-treated depressives
Cocaine/amphetamine	⇑ NA/DA	⇑ Mood	⇑ Mania	⇑ Anxiety/⇑ mood	⇑ Mood (anecdotal)
Fenfluramine	⇑ 5-HT	Nausea/sedation	Not tested	Nausea/sedation	Nausea/sedation
Yohimbine	⇑ NA	⇑ Anxiety	⇑ Anxiety	⇑ Anxiety (manic symptoms in some)	⇑ Anxiety
MDMA	⇑ 5-HT	⇑ Mood	Not tested	Not tested	Not tested
AMPT	⇓ NA/DA	Sedation	⇓ Mania	⇓ Mood	Sedation
PCPA	⇓ 5-HT	Confusion ⇓ Energy	Not tested	No effect	Relapse
TRP depletion	⇓ 5-HT	⇓ Concentration (± ⇓ mood)	Not tested	No effect	Relapse

NA, noradrenaline; 5-HT, serotonin; DA, dopamine; TRP, tryptophan; MDMA, 3,4-methylenedioxymethamphetamine; AMPT, α-methyl-p-tyrosine; PCPA, parachlorophenylalanine.

physostigmine in drug-free depressed patients and healthy subjects, the possibility that 5-HT, NA and possibly acetylcholine are interacting with each other, or influencing some other neurotransmitter system or brain regions which are involved in regulating mood, becomes a very real possibility. Therefore, better understanding of the interrelationships between these systems and how other brain regions and transmitter systems are influenced by these systems becomes essential.

It is clear that our understanding of how brain function is altered in various 'normal' mood states, depression and mania, and by antidepressants, is far from complete. However, there is an unmistakable convergence of data from preclinical and clinical studies utilizing a wide variety of experimental conditions suggesting that at least the brain NA and 5-HT systems are involved in depression and antidepressant action.

5.10 Future directions

The era of the neuroendocrine challenge study may be drawing to an end. However, numerous studies of this type still need to be completed. Several unanswered questions remain; these can and should be addressed through the use of neuroendocrine challenge studies. For example, do patients with abnormal growth hormone responses to clonidine also have blunted prolactin responses to TRP or fenfluramine? What is the significance of these abnormal responses? Do patients with abnormal responses to clonidine or 5-HT agonists represent meaningful subgroups? Also, what is the reason for DST non-suppression?

Considerable interaction exists between CNS neurotransmitter systems. For example, NA denervation prevents tricyclic antidepressants from causing a sensitization of forebrain neurones to 5-HT in laboratory animals (Gravel and de Montigny, 1987). Lesions of the 5-HT system prevent the reduction of β-adrenergic receptor density usually produced by desipramine in rats (A. Janowski et al., 1982). Depletion of both NA and dopamine in rats results in a greater blunting of the growth hormone response to clonidine than depletion of NA alone (Soderpalm et al., 1987). Long-term treatment with the β-adrenergic agonist, clenbuterol, causes an increase in $5-HT_{1A}$ receptors in mouse brain (Frances et al., 1987). The above suggest that future studies should begin systematically to investigate these possible interactions between neurotransmitter systems with neuroendocrine challenge studies.

Brain imaging with positron emission tomography (PET) and single photon emission tomography (SPECT) promise the type of technology which may ultimately answer the questions of pathophysiology and antidepressant action in affective disorders. Pharmacological challenge strategies combined with PET or SPECT may provide a better 'window' into the CNS than neuroendocrine parameters. Better, more specific probes of neurotransmitter receptors need to continue to be developed and probes of second and third messenger function also need to be developed. Studies need to begin to look beyond the monoamine and indoleamine transmitters and to assess co-released transmitters and neuropeptides. Somatostatin, neuropeptide-Y and CRH are peptides which are either co-released with, or highly influenced by, the classical neurotransmitters and deserve close attention.

References

Aghajanian, G.K. (1981) In *Serotonin Neurotransmission and Behavior* (eds Jacobs, B.L. & Gelperin, A.), pp 156–185. Cambridge, MIT Press.

Aghajanian, G.K., Sprouse, J.S. & Rassmussen, K. (1987) In *Psychopharmacology: The Third Generation of Progress* (ed. Meltzer, H.Y.), pp 141–150. New York, Raven Press.

Anderson, I.M. & Cowen, P.J. (1986) *Psychopharmacology* **89**, 131–133.

Anderson, I.M., Cowen, P.J. & Grahame-Smith, D.C. (1990) *Psychopharmacology* **100**, 498–503.

Ansseau, M., Scheyvaerts, M., Doumont, A., Poirrier, R., Legros, J.J. & Franck, G. (1984) *Psychiatry Res.* **12**, 261–272.

Ansseau, M., Von Frenckell, R., Cerfontaine, R. *et al.* (1988) *Br. J. Psychiatry* **153**, 65–71.

Arato, M., Rihmer, Z., Banki, C.M. & Grof, P. (1983) *Prog. Neuropharmacol. Biol. Psychiatry* **7**, 715–718.

Asberg, M., Schalling, D., Traskman-Bendz, L. & Wagner, A. (1987) In *Psychopharmacology: The Third Generation of Progress* (ed. Meltzer, H.Y.), pp 655–668. New York, Raven Press.

Asnis, G.M., Lemus, C.Z. & Halbreich, U. (1986) *Psychopharmacol. Bull.* **22**, 571–578.

Asnis, G.M., Eisenberg, J., van Praag, H.M., Lemus, C.Z., Friedman, H. & Miller, A. (1988) *Biol. Psychiatry* **24**, 117–120.

Avissar, S. & Schreiber, G. (1989) *Biol. Psychiatry* **26**, 113–130.

Balldin, J., Granerus, A.K., Lindstedt, G., Modigh, K. & Walinder, J. (1982) *Psychopharmacology* **76**, 371–376.

Banki, C.M. & Arato, M. (1987) *Psychoneuroendocrinology* **12**, 3–11.

Banki, C.M., Bissette, G., Arato, M., O'Connor, L., Nemeroff, M.S. & Nemeroff, C.B. (1987) *Am. J. Psychiatry* **144**, 7.

Bartus, R.T., Dean, R.L. & Flicker, C. (1987) In *Psychopharmacology: The Third Generation of Progress* (ed. Meltzer, H.Y.), pp 219–232. New York, Raven Press.

Bianchi, G., Caccia, S., Vedova, F.D. & Garattini, S. (1988) *Eur. J. Pharmacol* **151**, 365–371.

Blier, P., de Montigny, C. & Azzaro, A.J. (1986) *J. Pharmacol. Exp. Ther.* **237**, 987–994.

Blier, P., de Montigny, C. & Chaput, Y. (1990) *J. Clin. Psychiatry* **51** (Suppl.), 14–20.
Bolin, R.R. (1960) *J. Nerv. Ment. Dis.* **131**, 256–259.
Boyer, P., Schaub, C. & Pichot, P. (1982) *Neuroendocrinol. Lett.* **4**, 178.
Brambilla, F., Catalano, M., Lucca, A. & Smeraldi, E. (1988) *Eur. J. Clin. Pharmacol.* **35**, 601–605.
Briley, M., Raisman, R., Sechter, D., Zarifian, E. & Langer, S.Z. (1980) *Neuropharmacology* **19**, 1209–1210.
Brodie, H.K.H., Murphy, D.L., Goodwin, F.K. & Bunney, W.E. (1970) *Clin. Pharmacol. Ther.* **12**, 218–224.
Brown, G.M., Freind, W.C. & Chambers, J.W. (1979) In *Clinical Neuroendocrinology. A Pathophysiological Approach* (eds Tolis, G., Labrie, F., Martin, J.B. & Naftolin, F.), pp 47–81. New York, Raven Press.
Brownstein, M. & Axelrod, J. (1974) *Science* **184**, 163–165.
Bunney, W.E. Jr. & Davis, J.M. (1965) *Arch. Gen. Psychiatry* **13**, 483–494.
Carlsson, A. & Lindqvist, M. (1978) *J. Neural Transm.* **43**, 73–91.
Carpenter, W.T. (1970) *Ann. Int. Med.* **73**, 607–629.
Carroll, B.J., Martin, F.I. & Davies, B.M. (1968) *Br. Med. J.* **3**, 285–287.
Carroll, B.J., Curtis, G.C. & Mendels, J. (1976) *Arch. Gen. Psychiatry* **33**, 1039–1044.
Carroll, B.J., Greden, J.F., Haskett, R. *et al.* (1980) *Acta Psychiatr. Scand.* **61** (Suppl. 280), 183–199.
Carroll, B.J., Feinberg, M., Greden, J.F. *et al.* (1981) *Arch. Gen. Psychiatry* **38**, 15–22.
Catlin, D.H., Poland, R.E., Gorelick, D.A. *et al.* (1980) *J. Clin. Endocrinol. Metab.* **50**, 1021–1025.
Chan-Palay, V. & Asan, E. (1989) *J. Comp. Neurol.* **287**, 357–372.
Charig, E.M., Anderson, I.M., Robinson, J.M. *et al.* (1986) *Hum. Psychopharmacol.* **1**, 93–97.
Charney, D.S. & Redmond, D.E. (1983) *Neuropharmacology* **22**, 1531–1536.
Charney, D.S., Heninger, G.R., Sternberg, D.E. & Roth, R.H. (1981a) *Psychiatry Res.* **5**, 217–229.
Charney. D.S., Menekes, D.B. & Heninger, G.R. (1981b) *Arch. Gen. Psychiatry* **38**, 1160–1180.
Charney, D.S., Heninger, G.R., Sternberg, D.E. *et al.* (1981c) *Arch. Gen. Psychiatry* **38**, 1334–1340.
Charney, D.S., Heninger, G.R., Renhard, J.F., Sternberg, D.E. & Hafstead, K.M. (1982a) *Psychopharmacology* **77**, 217–222.
Charney, D.S., Heninger, G.R., Sternberg, D.E., Hafstead, K.M., Giddings, S. & Landis, H. (1982b) *Arch. Gen. Psychiatry* **39**, 290–294.
Charney, D.S., Heninger, G.R. & Sternberg, D.E. (1982c) *Psychiatry Res.* **7**, 135–138.
Charney, D.S., Heninger, G.R. & Sternberg, D.E. (1982d) *Life Sci.* **30**, 2033–2041.
Charney, D.S., Heninger, G.R. & Sternberg, D.E. (1984a) *Arch. Gen. Psychiatry* **41**, 359–365.
Charney, D.S., Heninger, G.R. & Sternberg, D.E. (1984b) *Br. J. Psychiatry* **144**, 407–416.
Charney, D.S., Woods, S.W., Goodman, W.K. & Heninger, G.R. (1987) *Psychopharmacology* **92**, 14–24.
Charney, D.S., Southwick, S.M., Delgado, P.L. & Krystal, J.H. (1990) In *Pharmacotherapy of Depression* (ed. Amsterdam, J.D.), pp 13–34. Basel, Marcel Dekker.
Checkley, S.A. (1979) *Psychol. Med.* **9**, 107–115.
Checkley, S.A. & Crammer, J.L. (1977) *Br. J. Psychiatry* **131**, 582–586.
Checkley, S.A., Slade, A.P. & Shur, E. (1981) *Br. J. Psychiatry* **138**, 51–55.

Checkley, S.A., Glass, J.B., Thompson, C., Corn, T. & Robinson, P. (1984) *Psychol. Med.* **14**, 773–777.

Chouinard, G. (1985) *J. Clin. Psychiatry* **46**, 32–37.

Clemens, J.A., Bennett, D.R. & Fuller, R.W. (1980) *Horm. Metab. Res.* **12**, 35–38.

Coccaro, E.F., Siever, L.J., Klar, H.M. *et al.* (1989) *Arch. Gen. Psychiatry* **46**, 587–599.

Coppen, A. (1967) *Br. J. Psychiatry* **113**, 1237–1264.

Costain, D.W., Cowen, P.J., Gelder, M.G. & Grahame-Smith, D.G. (1982) *Lancet* **ii**, 400–404.

Cowen, P.J. (1988) *Am. J. Psychiatry* **145**, 740–741.

Cowen, P.J. & Anderson, I.M. (1986) In *Advances in the Biology of Depression* (eds Deakin, J.F.W. & Freeman, H.), pp 71–89. London, Royal College of Psychiatrists.

Cowen, P.J. & Charig, E.M. (1987) *Arch. Gen. Psychiatry* **44**, 958–966.

Cowen, P.J., Braddock, L.E. & Gosden, B. (1984) *Psychopharmacology* **83**, 378–379.

Cowen, P.J., Gadhvi, H., Godsen, B. & Koloakowska, T. (1985a) *Psychopharmacology* **86**, 164–169.

Cowen, P.J., Green, A.R., Grahame-Smith, D.G. & Braddock, L.E. (1985b) *Br. J. Psychiatry* **19**, 799–805.

Cowen, P.J., McCance, S.L., Cohen, P.R. *et al.* (1989) *Psychopharmacology* **99**, 230–232.

Cowen, P.J., Anderson, I.M. & Grahame-Smith, D.G. (1990) *J. Clin. Psychopharmacology* **10**(Suppl. 3), 21S–25S.

Culley, W.J., Saunders, R.N., Mertz, E.T. & Jolly, D.H. (1963) *Proc. Soc. Exp. Biol. Med.* **113**, 645–648.

Curzon, G. (1979) *J. Neural Transm.* **15**(Suppl.), 93–105.

Curzon, G. (1981) In *Serotonin: Current Aspects of Neurochemistry and Function* (eds Haber, B. & Gabay, S.) pp 207–219. New York, Plenum Press.

Dahlstrom, A. & Fuxe, K. (1964) *Acta Physiol. Scand.* **62**(Suppl. 232), 1–55.

Deakin, J.F.W., Pennell, I., Upadhyaya, A.J. & Lofthouse, R. (1990) *Psychopharmacology* **101**, 85–92.

Delgado, P.L., Price, L.H., Charney, D.S., Aghajanian, G.K., Landis, H. & Heninger, G.R. (1988) *American Psychiatric Association 141st Annual Meeting*, Montreal, New Research Abstract 164.

Delgado, P.L., Charney, D.S., Price, L.H., Landis, H. & Heninger, G.R. (1989) *Life Sci.* **45**, 2323–2332.

Delgado, P.L., Charney, D.S., Price, L.H., Aghajanian, G.K., Landis, H. & Heninger, G.R. (1990a) *Arch. Gen. Psychiatry* **47**, 411–418.

Delgado, P.L., Fischette, C., Seibyl, J.P. *et al.* (1990b) *American Psychiatric Association 143rd Annual Meeting*, New York, New Research Abstract 184.

de Montigny, C. & Blier, P. (1984) *Adv. Biochem. Psychopharmacol.* **39**, 223–240.

Doerr, P. & Berger, M. (1983) *Biol. Psychiatry* **18**, 261–268.

Dolan, R.J. & Calloway, S.P. (1986) *Am. J. Psychiatry* **143**, 772–774.

Elphick, M., Yang, J. & Cowen, P.J. (1990) *Arch. Gen. Psychiatry* **47**, 135–140.

El-Yousef, M.K., Janowski, D.S., Davis, J.M. & Rosenblatt, J.E. (1973) *Br. J. Addict.* **68**, 321–325.

Engelman, K., Horwitz, D., Jequier, E. & Sjoerdsma, A. (1968) *J. Clin. Inv.* **47**, 577–594.

Eriksson, E., Eden, S. & Modigh, K. (1981) *Neuroendocrinology* **33**, 91–96.

Eriksson, E., Balldin, J., Lindstedt, G. & Modigh, K. (1988) *Psychiatry Res.* **26**, 59–67.

Extein, L., Pottash, A.L.C., Gold, M.S., Sweeney, D.R., Martin, D.M. & Goodwin, F.K. (1980) *Am. J. Psychiatry* **137**, 845–846.

Fawcet, J. & Siomopoulos, V. (1971) *Arch. Gen. Psychiatry* **25**, 244–247.

Feinberg, M., Greden, J.F. & Carroll, B.J. (1981) *Psychoneuroendocrinology* **6**, 355–357.

Fernstrom, J.D. (1977) *Metabolism* **26**, 207–223.

Fernstrom, J.D. & Hirsch, M.J. (1975) *Life Sci.* **17**, 455–464.

Fernstrom, J.D., Larin, F. & Wurtman, R.J. (1973) *Life Sci.* **13**, 517–524.

Frances, H., Bulach, C., Simon, P., Fillion, M. & Fillion, G. (1987) *J. Neural Transm.* **67**, 215–224.

Frazer, A., Brown, R., Kocsis, J. *et al.* (1986) *J. Neural Transm.* **21** (Suppl.), 269–290.

Frohman, L.A. & Jansson, J.-O. (1986) *Endocr. Rev.* **7**, 223–253.

Furchgott, R.F. (1972) In *Catecholeamines* (eds Blaschko, H. & Muscholl, E.) pp 283–385, Springer-Verlag, Berlin.

Fuxe, K., Butcher, L.L. & Engel, J. (1971) *J. Pharm. Pharmacol.* **23**, 420–424.

Fuxe, K., Ogren, S., Benfenati, F. & Agnati, L. (1984) *Adv. Biochem. Psychopharmacol.* **39**, 271–284.

Gal, E.M. & Dreses, P.A. (1962) *Proc. Soc. Exp. Biol. Med.* **110**, 368–371.

Gershon, S. & Shaw, F.H. (1961) *Lancet* **i**, 1371–1374.

Gibbons, J.L. (1964) *Arch. Gen. Psychiatry* **10**, 572.

Gibbons, J.L., Barr, G.A., Bridger, W.H. & Leibowitz, S.F. (1979) *Brain Res.* **169**, 139–153.

Gold, P.W., Extein, I., Pickar, D., Rebar, R., Ross, R. & Goodwin, F.K. (1980) *Am. J. Psychiatry* **137**, 862–863.

Goldberg, M.R., Jackson, R.V., Krakau, J., Island, D.P. & Robertson, D. (1986) *Life Sci.* **39**, 395–398.

Golden, R.N., Hsiao, J.K., Lane, E., Hicks, R., Rogers, S. & Potter, W.Z. (1989) *J. Clin. Endocrinol. Metab.* **68**, 632–637.

Golden, R.N., Hsiao, J.K., Lane, E. *et al.* (1990) *Psychiatry Res.* **31**, 39–47.

Gonzalez-Heydrich, J. & Peroutka, S.J. (1990) *J. Clin. Psychiatry* **51** (Suppl.), 5–12.

Grandison, L. & Guidotti, A. (1977) *Nature* **270**, 357–359.

Gravel, P. & de Montigny, C. (1987) *Synapse* **1**, 233–239.

Halbreich, U., Sachar, E.J., Asnis, G.M. *et al.* (1982) *Arch. Gen. Psychiatry* **39**, 189–192.

Hanssen, T., Heyden, T., Sundberg, I. & Wetterberg, L. (1977) *Lancet* **ii**, 309–310.

Harper, A.E., Benevenga, N.J. & Wohlhueter, R.M. (1970) *Physiol. Rev.* **50**, 428–548.

Heninger, G.R. & Charney, D.S. (1987) In *Psychopharmacology: The Third Generation of Progress* (ed. Meltzer, H.Y.), pp 535–544. New York, Raven Press.

Heninger, G.R., Charney, D.S. & Sternberg, D.E. (1984) *Arch. Gen. Psychiatry* **41**, 398–402.

Heninger, G.R., Charney, D.S. & Price, L.H. (1988) *Arch. Gen. Psychiatry* **45**, 165–175.

Heninger, G.R., Charney, D.S., Price, L.H., Delgado, P.L., Woods, S. & Goodman, W. (1989) In *Psychophamacology Series 7: Clinical Pharmacology in Psychiatry* (eds Dahl, S.G. & Gram, L.F.), pp 95–104. Berlin, Springer-Verlag.

Heninger, G.R., Charney, D.S. & Delgado, P.L. (1990) In *Review of Psychiatry*, vol. 9 (eds Tasman, A., Goldfinger, S.M. & Kaufman, C.A.), pp 33–58. Washington DC, American Psychiatric Press.

Holsboer, F. (1989) *Eur. Arch. Psychiatr. Neurol. Sci.* **238**, 302–322.

Holsboer, F., von Bardeleben, U., Gerken, A., Stella, G.K. & Muller, O.A. (1984) *N. Engl. J. Med.* **311**, 1127.

Idzikowski, C., Cowen, P.J., Nutt, D. & Mills, F.J. (1987) *Psychopharmacology* **93**, 416–420.

Janowski, A., Okada, F., Manier, H., Applegate, C.D., Sulser, F. & Steranka, L.R. (1982) *Science* **218**, 900–901.

Janowski, D.S. & Risch, S.C. (1987) In *Psychopharmacology: The Third Generation of Progress* (ed. Meltzer, H.Y.), pp 527–533. New York, Raven Press.

Janowski, D.S., El-Yousef, M.K., Davis, J.M. & Sekerke, H.J. (1972) *Lancet* **ii**, 632–635.

Janowski, D.S., El-Yousef, M.K., Davis, J.M. & Sekerke, H.J. (1973) *Arch. Gen. Psychiatry* **28**, 542–547.

Jezova, D. & Vigas, M. (1988) *Psychoneuroendocrinology* **13**, 479–485.

Jimerson, D.C. (1987) In *Psychopharmacology: The Third Generation of Progress* (ed. Meltzer, H.Y.), pp 505–511. New York, Raven Press.

Joyce, P.R. (1985) *Biol. Psychiatry* **20**, 598–604.

Judd, L.L., Risch, S.C., Parker, D.C., Janowski, D.S., Segal, D.S. & Huey, L.Y. (1982) *Arch. Gen. Psychiatry* **39**, 1413–1416.

Kahn, R.S., Wetzler, S., Asnis, G.M., Kling, M.A., Suckrow, R.F. & van Praag, H.M. (1990) *Psychopharmacology* **100**, 339–344.

Katona, C.L.E., Theodorou, A.E., Davies, S.L. *et al.* (1986) In *The Biology of Depression* (ed. Deakin, J.F.W.), pp 121–136. London, Gaskell.

Koenig, J., Mayfield, M.A., Coppings, R.J., McCann, S.M. & Krulich, L. (1980) *Brain Res.* **197**, 453–468.

Kuhar, M.J., Roth, R.H. & Aghajanian, G.K. (1971) *Brain Res.* **35**, 167–176.

Laakmann, G., Schumacher, G., Benkert, O. & v. Werder, K. (1977) *J. Clin. Endocrinol. Metab.* **44**, 1010–1013.

Laakmann, G., Zygan, K., Schoen, H.W. *et al.* (1986) *Psychoneuroendocrinology* **11**, 447–461.

Lal, S., Tolis, G., Martin, J.B., Brown, G.M. & Guyda, H. (1975) *J. Clin. Endocrinol. Metab.* **41**, 827–832.

Langer, G., Heinze, G., Reim, B. & Matussek, N. (1975) *Neurosci. Lett.* **1**, 185–189.

Langer, G., Heinze, G., Reim, B. & Matussek, N. (1976) *Arch. Gen. Psychiatry* **33**, 1471–1475.

Leckman, J.F., Redmond, D.E. & Heninger, G.R. (1981) *Life Sci.* **26**, 2179–2185.

Lesch, K.P., Rupprecht, R., Poten, B. *et al.* (1989) *Biol. Psychiatry* **26**, 203–205.

Lesch, K.P., Mayer, S., Disselkamp-Tietze, J., Hoh, A., Schoelnhammer, G. & Schulte, H.M. (1990a) *Life Sci.* **46**, 1271–1277.

Lesch, K.P., Disselkamp-Tietze, J. & Schmidtke, A. (1990b) *J. Neural Transm.* **80**, 157–161.

Lewy, A.J., Wehr, T.A., Goodwin, F.K., Newsome, D.A. & Markey, S.P. (1980) *Science* **210**, 1267–1269.

Lytle, L.D., Messing, R.B., Fisher, L. & Phebus, L. (1975) *Science* **190**, 692–694.

McCance, S.L., Cohen, P.R. & Cowen, P.J. (1989) *Psychopharmacology* **99**, 276–281.

McCance, S.L., Cowen, P.J., Waller, H. & Grahame-Smith, D.G. (1987) *J. Psychopharmacol.* **2**, 90–94.

McIndoe, J.H. & Turkington, R.W. (1973) *J. Clin. Invest.* **52**, 1972–1978.

Mann, J.J., Stanley, M., McBride, P.A. & McEwen, B.S. (1986) *Arch. Gen. Psychiatry* **43**, 954–959.

Mason, J., Sachar, E.J., Fishman, J., Hamburg, D. & Handlon, J. (1965) *Arch. Gen. Psychiatry* **13**, 1.

Matussek, N. (1988) *Curr. Top. Neuroendocrinol.* **8**, 145–182.

Matussek, N. & Hoehe, M. (1989) *Neuropsychobiology* **21**, 1–8.

Matussek, N., Ackenheil, M., Hippius, H. *et al.* (1980) *Psychiatry Res.* **2**, 25–36.

Meesters, P., Kerkhofs, M., Charles, G., Decoster, C., Vanderelst, M. & Mendlewicz, J. (1985) *Eur. Arch. Psychiatry Neurol. Sci.* **235**, 140–142.

Meltzer, H.Y. & Lowy, M.T. (1987). In *Psychopharmacology: The Third Generation of Progress* (ed. Meltzer, H.Y.), pp 513–526. New York, Raven Press.

Meltzer, H.Y., Flemming, R. & Robertson, A. (1983) *Arch. Gen. Psychiatry* **40**, 1099–1102.

Meltzer, H.Y., Umberkoman-Wiita, B., Robertson, A., Tricou, B.J., Lowy, M. & Perline, R. (1984) *Arch. Gen. Psychiatry* **41**, 366–374.

Messing, R.B., Fisher, L.A., Phebus, L. & Lytle, L.D. (1976) *Life Sci.* **18**, 707–714.

Meyendorff, E., Lerer, B., Moore, N.C., Bow, J. & Gershon, S. (1985) *Psychiatry Res.* **16**, 303–308.

Mitchell, P. & Smythe, G. (1990) *J. Affective Disord.* **19**, 43–51.

Moir, A.T.B. & Eccleston, D. (1968) *J. Neurochem.* **15**, 1093–1108.

Moja, E.A., Mendelson, W.B., Stoff, D.M., Gillin, J.C. & Wyatt, R.J. (1979) *Life Sci.* **24**, 1467–1470.

Moja, E.A., Cipollo, P., Castoldi, D. & Tofanetti, O. (1989) *Life Sci.* **44**, 971–976.

Molliver, M.E. (1987) *J. Clin. Psychopharmacol.* **7**, 3S–23S.

Moore, K.E. (1987) *Biol. Reprod.* **36**, 47–58.

Mueller, E.A., Murphy, D.L. & Sunderland, T. (1985) *J. Clin. Endocrinol. Metab.* **61**, 1179–1184.

Muhlbauer, H.D. (1984) *Pharmacopsychiatry* **17**, 191–193.

Muhlbauer, H.D. & Muller-Oerlinghausen, B. (1985) *J. Neural Transm.* **61**, 81–94.

Murphy, D.L., Cambell, I. & Costa, J.L. (1978) In *Psychopharmacology: A Generation of Progress* (eds Lipton, M.A., DiMascio, A. & Killam, K.F.), pp 1235–1247. New York, Raven Press.

Murphy, D.L., Tamarkin, L., Sunderland, T., Garrick, N.A. & Cohen, R.M. (1986) *Psychiatry Res.* **17**, 119–127.

Murphy, D.L., Mueller, E.A., Hill, J.L., Tolliver, T.J. & Jacobsen, F.M. (1989) *Psychopharmacology* **98**, 275–282.

Nemeroff, C., Widerlov, E., Bissette, G. *et al.* (1984) *Science* **226**, 1342–1344.

Ng, L.K.Y., Chase, T.N., Colburn, R.W. & Kopin, I.J. (1972) *Brain Res.* **45**, 499–505.

Nurnberger, J.I. Jr., Gershon, E.S., Jimerson, D.C. *et al.* (1982) *Psychoneuroendocrinology* **7**, 163–176.

Nurnberger, J.I., Jimerson, D.C., Simmons-Alling, S. *et al.* (1983) *Psychiatry Res.* **9**, 191–200.

Nurnberger, J.I., Berrettini, W., Simmons-Alling, S., Lawrence, D. & Brittain, H. (1989) *Psychiatry Res.* **31**, 57–67.

Parent, A., Descarries, L. & Beaudet, A. (1981) *Neuroscience* **6**, 115–138.

Penalva, A., Villaneueva, L., Casanueva, F., Cavagnini, F., Gomez-Pan, A. & Muller, E.E. (1983) *Psychopharmacology* **80**, 120–124.

Peroutka, S.J. (1988) *Trends Neurosci.* **11**, 496–500.

Perry, S.W. (1990) *Am. J. Psychiatry* **147**, 696–710.

Post, R.M., Kopin, J. & Goodwin, F.K. (1974) *Am. J. Psychiatry* **131**, 511–517.

Price, L.H., Charney, D.S. & Heninger, G.R. (1984) *Am. J. Psychiatry* **141**, 1267–1268.

Price, L.H., Charney, D.S. & Heninger, G.R. (1985) *Life Sci.* **37**, 809–818.

Price, L.H., Charney, D.S. & Heninger, G.R. (1986) *Psychopharmacology* **89**, 38–44.

Price, L.H., Charney, D.S., Delgado, P.L. & Heninger, G.R. (1989a) *Arch. Gen. Psychiatry* **46**, 13–19.

Price, L.H., Charney, D.S., Delgado, P.L. & Heninger, G.R. (1989b) *Arch. Gen. Psychiatry* **46**, 625–631.

Price, L.H., Charney, D.S., Delgado, P.L. *et al.* (1990) *J. Clin. Psychiatry* **51** (Suppl.), 44–50.

Quattrone, A., Tedeschi, G., Aguglia, U., Scopascasa, F. & Direnzo, G.F. (1983) *Br.*

J. Clin. Pharmacol. **16**, 471–475.

Redmond, D.E. (1987) In *Psychopharmacology: The Third Generation of Progress* (ed. Meltzer, H.Y.), pp 967–975. New York, Raven Press.

Risch, S.C. (1982) *Biol. Psychiatry* **17**, 1071–1079.

Risch, S.C., Janowski, D.S., Judd, L.J. *et al.* (1982) *Peptides* **3**, 319–322.

Robertson, A.G., Jackman, H. & Meltzer, H.Y. (1984) *Psychiatry Res.* **11**, 353–364.

Robinson, D.S., Rickels, K., Feighner, J. *et al.* (1990) *J. Clin. Psychopharmacol.* **10**(Suppl.), 67S–76S.

Robinson, R.G. & Chait, R.M. (1985) *Crit. Rev. Clin. Neurobiol.* **1**, 285–318.

Rose, W.C., Haines, W.J. & Warner, D.T. (1954) *J. Biol. Chem.* **206**, 421–430.

Roth, R.H., Wolf, M.E. & Deutch, A.Y. (1987) In *Psychopharmacology: The Third Generation of Progress* (ed. Meltzer, H.Y.), pp 81–94. New York, Raven Press.

Sachar, E.J. (1973) In *Biological Psychiatry* (ed. Mendels, J.), pp 175–197. New York, Wiley.

Sachar, E.J., Finkelstein, J. & Hellman, L. (1971) *Arch. Gen. Psychiatry* **25**, 263.

Sachar, E.J., Asnis, G., Nathan, R.S., Halbreich, U., Tabrizi, M.A. & Halpern, F.S. (1980) *Arch. Gen. Psychiatry* **37**, 755–757.

Sachar, E.J., Puig-Antich, J., Ryan, N.D. *et al.* (1985) *Acta Psychiatr. Scand.* **71**, 1–8.

Schildkraut, J.J. (1965) *Am. J. Psychiatry* **122**, 509–522.

Schittecatte, M., Charles, G., Machowski, R. & Wilmotte, J. (1989) *Br. J. Psychiatry* **154**, 858–863.

Seyle, H. (1936) *Br. J. Exp. Path.* **17**, 234.

Shapira, B., Reiss, A., Kaiser, N., Kindler, S. & Lerer, B. (1989) *J. Affective Disord.* **16**, 1–4.

Shapira, B., Lerer, B., Litchenberg, P., Kindler, S. & Calev, A. (1990) *American Psychiatric Association 143rd Annual Meeting*, New York, New Research Abstract 413.

Shibahara, S., Morimoto, Y., Furutani, Y. *et al.* (1983) *EMBO J.* **2**, 775–779.

Shopsin, B., Gershon, S., Goldstein, M., Friedman, E. & Wilk, S. (1975) *Psychopharmacol. Commun.* **1**, 239–249.

Shopsin, B., Friedman, E. & Gershon, S. (1976) *Arch. Gen. Psychiatry* **33**, 811–891.

Siever, L.J. & Davis, K.L. (1985) *Am. J. Psychiatry* **142**, 1017–1031.

Siever, L.J., Uhde, T.W., Silberman, E.K. *et al.* (1982a) *Psychiatry Res.* **6**, 171–183.

Siever, L.J., Uhde, T.W., Insel, T.R., Roy, B.F. & Murphy, D.L. (1982b) *Psychiatry Res.* **7**, 139.

Siever, L.J., Murphy, D.L., Slater, S., de la Vega, E. & Lipper, S. (1984) *Life Sci.* **34**, 1029–1039.

Smith, S.E., Pihl, R.O., Young, S.W. & Ervin, F.R. (1987) *Psychopharmacology* **91**, 451–457.

Soderpalm, B., Andersson, L., Carlsson, M., Modigh, K. & Eriksson, E. (1987) *J. Neural Transm.* **69**, 105–114.

Spampinato, S., Locatelli, V., Cocchi, D. *et al.* (1979) *Endocrinology* **105**, 163–170.

Speiss, J., Rivier, J., Rivier, C. & Vale, W. (1981) *Proc. Natl Acad. Sci. USA* **78**, 6517–6521.

Stanley, M. & Mann, J.J. (1983) *Lancet* **i**, 214–216.

Stanley, M., Virgilio, J. & Gershon, S. (1982) *Science* **216**, 1337–1339.

Tagliamonte, A., Biggio, G., Vargiu, L. & Gessa, G.L. (1973) *Life Sci.* **12**, 277–287.

Taylor, A.L. & Fishman, L.M. (1988) *N. Engl. J. Med.* **319**, 213–222.

Tolis, G., Dent, R. & Gupta, H. (1978) *J. Clin. Endocrinol. Metab.* **47**, 200–203.

Van de Kar, L.D., Karteszi, M., Bethea, C.L. & Ganong, W.F. (1985) *Neuroendocrinology* **41**, 380–384.

Vergnes, M. & Kempf, E. (1981) *Psychopharmacol. Aggr. Soc. Behav.* **14**, 19–23.

von Bardeleben, U., Stalla, G.K., Muller, O.A. & Holsboer, F. (1988) *Biol. Psychiatry* **24**, 782–786.

Wald, D., Ebstein, R.P. & Belmaker, R.H. (1978) *Psychopharmacology* **57**, 83–87.

Walters, J.K., Davis, M. & Sheard, M.H. (1979) *Psychopharmacology* **62**, 103–109.

Weizman, A., Mark, M., Gil-Ad, I., Tyano, S. & Laron, Z. (1988) *Clin. Neuropharmacol.* **11**, 250–256.

Wetterberg, L. (1983) *Psychoneuroendocrinology* **8**, 75–80.

Willner, P. (1983) *Brain Res. Rev.* **6**, 237–246.

Winokur, A., Lindberg, N.D., Lucki, I., Phillips, J. & Amsterdam, J.D. (1986) *Psychopharmacology* **88**, 213–219.

Woodward, D.J., Moises, H.C., Waterhouse, B.D., Hoffer, B.J. & Freedman, R. (1979) *Fed. Proc.* **38**, 2109–2116.

Wurtman, R. (1970) In *Hypophysiotropic Hormones of the Hypothalamus* (ed. Meites, J.), pp 184–194. Baltimore, Williams & Wilkins.

Young, S.N., Smith, S.E., Pihl, R.O. & Ervin, F.R. (1985) *Psychopharmacology* **87**, 173–177.

Young, S.N., Ervin, F.R., Pihl, R.O. & Finn, P. (1989) *Psychopharmacology* **98**, 508–511.

Young, V.R., Hussein, M.A., Murray, E. & Scrimshaw, N.S. (1969) *Am. J. Clin. Nutr.* **22**, 1563–1567.

Young, V.R., Hussein, M.A., Murray, E. & Scrimshaw, N.S. (1971) *J. Nutr.* **101**, 45–60.

Zis, A.P. (1988) *Psychoneuroendocrinology* **13**, 419–430.

Zis, A.P., Haskett, R.F., Albala, A.A., Carroll, B.J. & Lohr, N.E. (1985a) *Biol. Psychiatry* **20**, 287–292.

Zis, A.P., Haskett, R.F., Albala, A.A., Carroll, B.J. & Lohr, N.E. (1985b) *Psychiatry Res.* **15**, 91–95.

Zis, A.P., Haskett, R.F., Albala, A.A., Carroll, B.J. & Lohr, N.E. (1985c) *Arch. Gen. Psychiatry* **42**, 383–386.

CHAPTER 6

POST-MORTEM STUDIES OF NEUROTRANSMITTER BIOCHEMISTRY IN DEPRESSION AND SUICIDE

S.C. Cheetham[1], C.L.E. Katona[2] and R.W. Horton[3]

[1] Boots Pharmaceuticals Research Department, R3, Nottingham NG2 3AA.

[2] Department of Psychiatry, University College and Middlesex School of Medicine, London W1N 8AA.

[3] Department of Pharmacology and Clinical Pharmacology, St George's Hospital Medical School, London W17 0RE.

Table of Contents

BIOLOGICAL ASPECTS OF AFFECTIVE DISORDERS
ISBN 0-12-356510-3

S.C. Cheetham, C.L.E. Katona and R.W. Horton

6.1 Background

The neurochemical disturbances that underlie depressive illness remain elusive. Investigations of an association between depression and central neurotransmitter abnormalities dominate research in this area. However, attempts to identify such abnormalities in depressed patients are limited by ethical and practical considerations to relatively indirect approaches, such as measurement of neurotransmitters and their metabolite concentrations in body fluids, neuroendocrine responses to specific pharmacological challenges and the study of peripheral receptor systems with properties similar to neuronal receptors. All these approaches have disadvantages and problems of interpretation. Clearly it is advantageous to adopt a more direct approach and study brain tissue from depressed patients. At present most neurochemical analysis of human brain involves tissue obtained post-mortem, as the availability of biopsy material is limited. Neurochemical examination of post-mortem brain tissue has proved valuable in the investigation of brain disorders that are neurodegenerative in nature, such as Alzheimer's disease and Huntington's disease. Disorders not involving gross neuropathology have also been studied. Whilst there are numerous studies involving subjects with schizophrenia, the affective disorders have received less attention.

Several factors may influence the findings of post-mortem brain studies and their interpretation. These range from the obvious issue of post-mortem stability to the characteristics of individual subjects, such as age, gender, manner of death, and to techniques under the control of the investigator, such as dissection and storage (reviewed by Perry and Perry, 1983). Although the number of factors that need to be considered is rather daunting, none are insurmountable. Normal and pathological groups should be matched, as far as is possible, with regard to age, gender, post-mortem delay, storage time and manner of death. In addition, neurochemical data should be analysed in relation to as many of the above variables as possible.

Two strategies have been used to study depression using post-mortem tissue. The most widely used approach is the study of tissue from suicide victims. The rationale is based on the well-documented relationship between suicide and depression (reviewed by Barraclough and Hughes, 1987). Studies of suicide victims do however pose additional problems with regard to interpretation, as the majority of studies have not attempted psychiatric definition or classification. Although depression is the most frequent psychiatric correlate of suicide, suicide victims are a diagnostically heterogeneous group in which a wide range of psychiatric illnesses other than depression, such as schizophrenia, personality disorder, alcoholism or drug abuse, may be present. Furthermore, suicide may be associated with traumatic life events in the absence of psychiatric illness. Studies of undefined suicide victims will therefore almost certainly be heterogeneous in relation to psychiatric illness. Although studies of such subjects may identify biological abnormalities related to suicide, extrapolation of findings to depression is unwarranted. However, some studies have been more selective in their choice of suicide subjects and have excluded certain psychiatric diagnoses, such as schizophrenia and alcoholism. Our own approach has been to restrict studies to those suicides for whom there was documentary medical evidence of depression, in the absence of symptoms of other psychiatric and neurological disorders. Under these circumstances we feel it is more justified to relate our findings to depression.

An additional problem is that few studies have distinguished between drug-free and drug-treated, particularly antidepressant-treated, subjects. It is crucial to make this distinction in attempting to distinguish biological differences that underlie the illness from those associated with drug treatment.

An alternative strategy is the study of post-mortem brain tissue from patients with a well-documented history of depressive illness, for whom psychiatric assessment was performed prior to their death by natural causes. The difficulty of identifying suitable patients has limited this approach to studies involving relatively few subjects. The subjects are mostly elderly, often die after prolonged periods of physical illness and are rarely drug-free at the time of death.

Research into the biological basis of depressive illness and the mechanism of action of antidepressant drugs and electroconvulsive shock therapy (ECT) has been dominated for the last 20 years by the 'monoaminergic hypotheses' involving the neurotransmitters serotonin (5-hydroxytryptamine, 5-HT) and noradrenaline (NA). As a consequence, post-mortem studies relating to depression and suicide have concentrated on these two monoamines, with few studies involving other neurotransmitters. The aim of this chapter is to provide a comprehensive review and critical assessment of these studies. Although the main emphasis will lie with the monoamines, other neurotransmitters, such as γ-aminobutyric acid (GABA) and acetylcholine, will be discussed.

6.2 Monoamines and monoamine metabolite concentrations

6.2.1 5-Hydroxytryptamine

Low concentrations of 5-hydroxyindoleacetic acid (5-HIAA), the major metabolite of 5-HT metabolism, have been reported in the cerebrospinal fluid

(CSF) of depressed patients (Ågren, 1980; Åsberg *et al.*, 1984), but not consistently replicated (reviewed by Gjerris, 1988). Only a proportion of depressed patients appear to have low CSF 5-HIAA concentrations, particularly those who had recently attempted suicide by violent methods (Åsberg *et al.*, 1976; Brown and Goodwin, 1986). This correlation between low CSF 5-HIAA concentration and violent suicidal behaviour provides support for a decrease in central 5-HT turnover in some depressed patients.

Several groups have measured 5-HT and/or 5-HIAA concentrations in post-mortem brain tissue from suicides. Demographic and clinical details of the subjects included in these studies are summarized in Table 1 and the results of post-mortem analysis are given in Table 2.

The earliest studies were limited to the brain stem (hindbrain) from suicides. In these studies Shaw *et al.* (1967) and Pare *et al.* (1969) reported lower concentrations of 5-HT in suicides compared with controls. In contrast, Bourne *et al.* (1968) found no difference in brain stem 5-HT concentration between suicides and controls, but observed a significantly lower concentration of 5-HIAA, a finding Pare *et al.* (1969) did not reproduce. Subsequent studies investigated discrete regions from the brain stem. Lloyd *et al.* (1974) found lower concentrations of 5-HT throughout the raphe nuclei of suicides when compared with controls, reaching statistical significance in the raphe nuclei dorsalis and centralis inferior, but found no differences in 5-HIAA concentrations. In contrast, Beskow *et al.* (1976) and Cochran *et al.* (1976) reported no differences in 5-HT concentration. Beskow *et al.* (1976) did however find significantly lower concentrations of 5-HIAA in mesencephalon, pons and medulla oblongata but attributed these to differences in post-mortem delay between suicides and controls. A more recent study reported no differences in 5-HT or 5-HIAA in brain stem areas between suicides and controls (Korpi *et al.*, 1986).

The majority of studies in suicides have found no significant differences in 5-HT and/or 5-HIAA concentrations in frontal cortex (Cochran *et al.*, 1976; Crow *et al.*, 1984; Korpi *et al.*, 1986; Arato *et al.*, 1987; Cheetham *et al.*, 1989). Beskow *et al.* (1976) attributed the lower concentration of 5-HIAA between suicides and controls to differences in post-mortem delay.

Alterations in 5-HT and 5-HIAA in other regions of the brain have also been reported, but not consistently replicated (see Table 2).

Thus the most consistent, but by no means universally replicated finding, is a significantly lower concentration of 5-HT or 5-HIAA in the brain stem of suicides (Shaw *et al.*, 1967; Bourne *et al.*, 1968; Pare *et al.*, 1969; Lloyd *et al.*, 1974; Beskow *et al.*, 1976).

A number of factors have been proposed to explain the inconsistencies between studies. Post-mortem delay, age, gender, seasonal and diurnal variations may all influence 5-HT and/or 5-HIAA concentrations (Carlsson

Post-mortem studies of neurotransmitter biochemistry in depression and suicide

Reference	No. controls/ suicides	No. depressed	Mean age (years)	Post-mortem delay (range) (h)	Cause of death	Drug treatment
Shaw et al. (1967)	17/11	8 (3 probable)	54 (C) 49 (S)	24–96	Overdose (6) Other (5)	Not known
Bourne et al. (1968)	28/23	16	60 (C) 49 (S)	24–96	Overdose (13) Other (10)	No information
Pare et al. (1969)	15/26	23 (15 endogenous; 8 reactive/ neurotic)	63 (C) 49 (S)	No information	Carbon monoxide poisoning (26)	Imipramine or amitriptyline (5)
Lloyd et al. (1974)	14/7	No information	28–93 (C) 24–51 (S) (range)	6–33	Overdose (3) Other (4)	Drug treated (3)
Moses and Robins (1975)	19/25	14 depressed (11 alcoholics)	56 (C) 47 (S)	4–33	Overdose (3) Other (22)	No information
Beskow et al. (1976)	62/23	11 (1 endogenous)	60 (C) 47 (S)	45 (C) 94 (S) (means)	Overdose (10) Other (13)	No information
Cochran et al. (1976)	12/19	10 depressed (9 alcoholics)	54 (C) 48 (S)	5–33	Overdose (1) Other (18)	Tricyclic antidepressants (2)
Crow et al. (1984)	19/10	7	56 (C) 50 (S)	No information	Overdose (5)	No information
Owen et al. (1986)	19/19	3 (6 possible)	54 (C) 45 (S)	44 (C) 48 (S) means	No information	Antidepressant (7)
Korpi et al. (1986)	29/14	No information	44 (C) 37 (S)	3–31	Overdose (3) Other (11)	Tricyclic antidepressants (6) Flurazepam (1)
Arato et al. (1987)	13/14	No information	No information	4–6	Overdose (0) Other (14)	Antidepressant (2)
Cheetham et al. (1989)	19/19	19	40 (C) 39 (S)	16–72	Overdose (5) Other (14)	Antidepressant (3) Antidepressant and benzodiazepine (2) Benzodiazepine (1)

C, controls; S, suicides; others include carbon monoxide poisoning, hanging, jumping, self-inflicted wounding, drowning, suffocation, burns, explosion, electrocution and gunshot wounds. Number of subjects is given in parentheses.

195

Table 2 Differences in 5-HT and 5-HIAA concentrations in post-mortem brain tissue from suicides and controls.

Reference	No. regions studied	Brain stem		Frontal cortex		Other regions	
		5-HT	5-HIAA	5-HT	5-HIAA	5-HT	5-HIAA
Shaw et al. (1967)	1	↓19%					
Bourne et al. (1968)	1	↑	↓28%				
Pare et al. (1969)	1	↓11%	↑				
Lloyd et al. (1974)	14	↓29%ᵃ	↑			↑	↑
Beskow et al. (1976)	9	↑	↓26%ᵇ		↓43%	↑	↓18%ᶜ
Cochran et al. (1976)	33	↑		↑		↑	
Crow et al. (1984)	1				↑		
Owen et al. (1986)	2					→↑97%↓50%ᵉ	→↑27%ᵈ
Korpi et al. (1986)	14	↑	↑	↑	↑		→↓41%ᶠ
Arato et al. (1987)	1			↑	↑		
Cheetham et al. (1989)	6			↑	↑	↑	→↑25%ᵍ

ᵃ 30% lower in raphe nuclei dorsalis and 28% lower in raphe central inferior, four other regions of raphe no significant difference.
ᵇ 23% lower in mesencephalon, 30% lower in pons and 26% lower in medulla oblongata.
ᶜ 18% lower in thalamus and 17% lower in putamen.
ᵈ Hippocampus.
ᵉ 108% higher in globus pallidus, 86% higher in putamen, 50% lower in hypothalamus.
ᶠ Nucleus accumbens.
ᵍ Amygdala (antidepressant-free suicides only).
→, No significant difference; ↓, lower, ↑, higher than controls; →↓↑, different regions.

et al., 1980; Bucht *et al.*, 1981; McIntyre and Stanley, 1984), although reports of post-mortem stability of brain 5-HT and 5-HIAA are contradictory (McIntyre and Stanley, 1984). Few studies have taken all these factors into account. Analytical methods and dissection techniques may also be important. Early studies used fluorometric detection techniques which are less accurate and sensitive than the more recently used high performance liquid chromatography with electrochemical detection. Furthermore, early studies assayed relatively large areas of the brain whilst more recently anatomically distinct regions have been studied. 5-HT and 5-HIAA concentrations exhibit wide regional variation not only between different brain regions but also within the same region (Cochran *et al.*, 1976; McIntyre and Stanley, 1984).

Interhemispheric differences in neurotransmitter concentrations have been found in post-mortem human brain and this may contribute to the conflicting findings (Oke *et al.*, 1978; Glick *et al.*, 1982). Two studies have measured 5-HT and 5-HIAA concentrations in tissue from left and right hemispheres from suicides and controls. No significant asymmetry in 5-HT or 5-HIAA concentrations was found in frontal cortex (Arato *et al.*, 1987; Cheetham *et al.*, 1989). Interhemispheric differences were however observed in 5-HT concentrations in hippocampus and amygdala and 5-HIAA concentrations in temporal cortex of controls, with higher concentrations of 5-HT and lower concentrations of 5-HIAA in the right than the left hemisphere. No such hemispheric differences were observed in suicides (Cheetham *et al.*, 1989).

The inconsistencies may be related to the lack of sufficient psychiatric definition of the suicide groups and failure to distinguish between drug-free and drug-treated subjects. Although several studies have attempted retrospective diagnosis, only one study has compared drug-free and antidepressant-treated depressed suicides (Cheetham *et al.*, 1989).

Mode of death may also be important, as low CSF 5-HIAA concentration appears to be most marked in those depressed patients exhibiting violent suicidal behaviour (Åsberg *et al.*, 1976). Thus low concentrations of 5-HT and/or 5-HIAA may be confined to, or at least more apparent in, suicides who die violently. Only two studies have investigated 5-HT and 5-HIAA concentrations in brain tissue from suicides in relation to violence of death. Neither study found evidence of lower 5-HT or 5-HIAA concentrations for suicides who died violently when compared with those who died non-violently or to controls (Korpi *et al.*, 1986; Cheetham *et al.*, 1989).

Similar studies in depressed patients dying of natural causes are few. Demographic and clinical details of the subjects included in these studies are summarized in Table 3 and results are given in Table 4. The concentration of 5-HIAA did not differ in frontal or occipital cortex or hippocampus between depressed patients and controls (Crow *et al.*, 1984; Ferrier *et al.*, 1986; McKeith *et al.*, 1987). The lack of difference in 5-HIAA concentration in frontal cortex

Table 3 Monoaminergic studies: demographic and clinical details of elderly depressed patients and controls.

Reference	No. controls/ depressed subjects	Psychiatric history	Mean age (years)	Post-mortem delay (range) (h)	Cause of death	Treatment
Riederer et al. (1980)	16/10	Endogenous unipolar type depression. Hospitalized 2–8 years	67 (C) 69 (D)	3–15	Bronchopneumonia (4) Cardiac failure (6)	Long term treatment tri- or tetracyclics. Final dose 2–5 days prior to death
Perry et al. (1983)	14/11	Intermittent unipolar depression	78 (C) 79 (D)	19 (C) 21 (C) (means)	No information	Dothiepin (3) Imipramine (1) No antidepressants (4) Not known (3)
Crow et al. (1984)[c]	22/9	Unipolar (4) Bipolar (1) Reactive (3) Schizoaffective (1)	79 (C) 76 (D)	4–69	No information	Tricyclics (7) Uncertain (1) None (1)
Ferrier et al. (1986)[d] McKeith et al. (1987)[e]	6/9[a]/7[b]	Major affective disorder[a] (9). Dysthymia[b] (7). Hospitalized (majority)	76 (C) 75 (D[a]) 81 (D[b])	28 (C) 28 (D[a]) 30 (D[b]) (mean)	No information	Antidepressants 6 > 1/12, 5 < 1/12, 3 none, 2 uncertain. ECT in past 6 > 1/12 Neuroleptics (7)

[c-e] Studies including same major affective disorder group.
[d,e] Studies including same controls and depressed subjects.
C, controls; D, depressed subjects. Number of subjects is given in parentheses.

198

Table 4 Differences in monoamines and/or their metabolite concentrations between elderly depressed patients and controls.

Reference	Regions studied	5-HIAA	NA	MHPG	HVA
Riederer et al. (1980)	Basal ganglia (3)		↑	→↓64%[a]	
	Diencephalon (3)			→↓57%[b]	
	Brain stem (3)		→↓72%[c]	→↓46%[d]	
	Limbic structures (5)		↑	→↓34%[e]	
Crow et al. (1984)[f]	Frontal cortex	↑		↑	↑
	Occipital cortex	↑		↑	↑
	Hippocampus	↑		↑	→↓51%
Ferrier et al. (1986)[g]	Frontal cortex	↑			
McKeith et al. (1987)[h]	Frontal cortex				

[a] Globus pallidus.
[b] 63% lower in hypothalamus and 50% lower in mammillary bodies.
[c] Red nucleus.
[d] 41% lower in substantia nigra and 50% lower in raphe and reticular formation.
[e] Nucleus accumbens.
[f-h] Studies including same major affective disorder group.
[d,e] Studies including same controls and depressed subjects.
→, No significant difference; ↓, lower than controls; →↓, different regions.

is in agreement with previously discussed suicide studies. Frontal cortical 5-HIAA concentration for those depressed patients who were not receiving drug treatment for at least 1 month prior to death was significantly lower than for those patients receiving drugs up to their deaths (Ferrier *et al.*, 1986). However, the number of subjects in the drug-free and drug-treated groups was too small (4 in each group) to allow firm conclusions to be drawn.

6.2.2 Noradrenaline and dopamine

The catecholamines NA and dopamine (DA) and their respective major central metabolites, 3-methoxy-4-hydroxyphenylethylene glycol (MHPG) and homovanillic acid (HVA), have received less attention than 5-HT and 5-HIAA. Demographic and clinical details of the subjects studied and results are summarized in Tables 3–5. Noradrenaline concentrations were first measured in the hindbrain of depressed and non-depressed suicides and controls by Bourne *et al.* (1968) who found no significant differences. Pare *et al.* (1968) who found no significant differences. Pare *et al.* (1969) subsequently reported no differences in the concentration of NA in hypothalamus of suicides and controls, a finding replicated by Beskow *et al.* (1976). Moses and Robins, (1975) studied 30 distinct areas of the brain, and found significantly higher NA concentrations in two out of eight areas of the hypothalamus and in hippocampal gyrus of depressed suicides than controls. However, they suggested that sampling error could account for these differences, owing to the small amount of tissue sampled (often less than 10 mg for hypothalamic areas). No significant differences in MHPG, DA or HVA concentrations have been reported between suicides and controls (Pare *et al.*, 1969; Moses and Robins, 1975; Beskow *et al.*, 1976; Crow *et al.*, 1984).

Table 5 Differences in catecholamines and their metabolite concentration in post-mortem brain tissue from suicides and controls.

Reference	Number of regions	NA	MHPG	DA	HVA
Bourne *et al.* (1968)	1	→			
Pare *et al.* (1969)	2	→		→	
Moses and Robins (1975)	30	→↑105%[a]		→	
Beskow *et al.* (1976)	4	→		→	→
Crow *et al.* (1984)	1			→	→

[a] 120% higher in hippocampal gyrus, 95% higher in anterior medial ventral hypothalamus and 99% higher in anterior lateral ventral hypothalamus.
→, No significant difference; ↑, higher than controls; →↑, different regions.

Two studies have determined NA and/or MHPG concentrations in brain from depressed patients and controls. Riederer *et al.* (1980) reported lower concentrations of MHPG in six out of 14 brain areas from depressed patients than controls, whereas significantly lower NA concentrations were found only in the red nucleus. Crow *et al.* (1984) found no differences in MHPG concentration between depressed patients and controls in frontal or occipital cortex or hippocampus. However, none of these regions were included in the study of Riederer *et al.* (1980).

Thus studies of catecholamines and their metabolites have not revealed consistent abnormalities in suicides and depressed patients.

6.3 Monoamine biosynthetic and degradative enzymes

Monoamine biosynthetic and degradative enzymes have received little attention in post-mortem brain studies relating to suicide and depression. The three studies carried out to date relate to suicide victims. Grote *et al.* (1974) examined monoamine oxidase (MAO) A and B, catechol-*O*-methyltransferase, tyrosine hydroxylase and dopamine-β-hydroxylase activity in suicides categorized as suffering from affective disorder (depression) or alcoholism and controls. No significant differences were found between controls and suicides in the 28 brain regions studied, with the sole exception of higher tyrosine hydroxylase activity in substantia nigra of the depressed suicides than alcoholic suicides and controls. In contrast, Gottfries *et al.* (1975) reported significantly lower MAO-A and MAO-B activity in several brain regions from alcoholic suicides when compared with controls, but found no differences between non-alcoholic suicides and controls. No significant differences in MAO-A and MAO-B activity with respect to both maximum velocity (V_{max}) and substrate affinity (K_m) were found in frontal cortex of a group of suicide victims, the majority of whom died by violent means, when compared with control subjects matched for age, sex and post-mortem delay (Mann and Stanley, 1984).

Although it is unwise to draw any firm conclusions at this stage due to the small number of studies, there is no evidence of an abnormality in MAO (A or B) activity in non-alcoholic suicides.

6.4 Monoamine neurotransmitter receptor binding and uptake sites

Neurotransmitter receptor binding and uptake sites appear to be stable measures of neurotransmitter biochemistry after death. Under simulated autopsy conditions, the stability of several classes of receptor binding site in rat brain has been demonstrated for up to 96 h after death (Whitehouse *et al.*, 1984). Furthermore, an impressive number of studies in man have reported that no relationship exists between measures of several classes of receptor binding site and post-mortem interval (Bennett *et al.*, 1979; Cash *et al.*, 1984; Cross *et al.*, 1984; Marcusson *et al.*, 1984a, 1984b; Cheetham *et al.*, 1988a; De Paermentier *et al.*, 1990; Lawrence *et al.*, 1990b).

There have been relatively few receptor binding and uptake site studies in depressed patients; the majority relate to suicide deaths. Demographic and clinical details of the subjects studied are summarized in Tables 3 and 6 and results are given in Tables 7 and 8.

6.4.1 5-HT uptake sites

Evidence for an association between depressive illness and an abnormality in 5-HT uptake arises from studies of blood platelets, which actively accumulate 5-HT by a carrier-mediated mechanism similar to neuronal 5-HT uptake (Stahl and Meltzer, 1978). A lower number of platelet 5-HT uptake sites has been widely reported for drug-free depressed patients compared with controls. Platelet [3H]imipramine binding, which is associated with the 5-HT uptake system, has also been extensively studied. The number of platelet [3H]imipramine binding sites has been reported to be significantly lower in drug-free depressed patients than controls. However, this finding remains contentious as a significant number of studies have not found differences (see Chapter 4).

Studies of 5-HT uptake sites in brain tissue from suicides and depressed patients have in the main used [3H]imipramine as the radioligand. These have yielded inconsistent results. Decreased (Stanley *et al.*, 1982), increased (Meyerson *et al.*, 1982) and unaltered (Crow *et al.*, 1984, Arora and Meltzer, 1989a) [3H]imipramine binding has been reported in frontal cortex of suicides compared with controls. Crow *et al.* (1984) reported significantly lower [3H]imipramine binding in a small subgroup of suicides with a history of depression. However, a subsequent study by Crow and co-workers found no differences in [3H]imipramine binding in frontal or occipital cortex or hippocampus from a group of suicides compared with controls, or when the comparison was repeated in a smaller subgroup who were definitely or probably suffering from depression (Owen *et al.*, 1986), and thus did not replicate their earlier findings. A recent detailed autoradiographic study by Gross-Isseroff *et al.* (1989) quantitated [3H]imipramine binding in 42 regions from suicides and controls. Binding was found to be lower in suicides in postcentral gyrus, insular cortex and claustrum, higher in most areas of the hippocampal formation and unaltered in prefrontal cortex.

Subject selection is likely to be a major contributing factor to these discrepancies. Crow *et al.* (1984) and Owen *et al.* (1986) included subjects with definite and probable depression, schizophrenia, personality disorder and those for whom no diagnosis could be made, although they did report results for the subgroup of depressed and probably depressed suicides. Gross-Isseroff *et al.* (1989) excluded subjects with a known history of schizophrenia, alcoholism and drug abuse, whilst the remaining studies gave no information on the psychiatric history of the suicides (Meyerson *et al.*, 1982; Stanley *et al.*, 1982; Arora and Meltzer, 1989a). Two studies made specific reference to mode of suicide: Arora and Meltzer (1989a) compared suicides who died by violent and non-violent methods; these groups did not differ from each other or from controls. Stanley *et al.* (1982) restricted their comparison to violent suicides and controls.

Drug treatment prior to death, in particular with antidepressant drugs, may also be a critical factor. Stanley *et al.* (1982) and Crow *et al.* (1984) provided no information on drug treatment, whilst Owen *et al.* (1986) included several antidepressant-treated suicides. Two studies were virtually restricted to drug-free subjects (Meyerson *et al.*, 1982; Arora and Meltzer, 1989a), whereas Gross-Isseroff *et al.* (1989) studied only suicides who were drug-free at the time of death.

A further confounding factor is the recent reports of hemispheric asymmetry in [^{3}H]imipramine binding in post-mortem human frontal cortex. The number of [^{3}H]imipramine binding sites was double in the right than left hemispheres of controls (Arato *et al.*, 1987; Demeter *et al.*, 1988; 1989). This asymmetry was reversed in suicides (Arato *et al.*, 1987), and in homicide victims with a history of psychiatric illness, including depression, schizophrenia and alcoholism (Demeter *et al.*, 1988; 1989).

Choice of radioligand may also be an important factor. [^{3}H]Imipramine labels multiple sites in human brain, only one of which is thought to be related to the 5-HT uptake site (Cash *et al.*, 1985; Bäckström *et al.*, 1989). When desmethylimipramine or amitriptyline is used to define non-specific binding, both 5-HT uptake and 'other' sites are quantitated, the proportion of non-5-HT uptake sites being dependent on the radioligand concentration and brain region. These two compounds have been used to define non-specific [^{3}H]imipramine binding in most studies of suicides. Therefore conflicting results may relate to the proportion of non-5-HT uptake sites labelled, especially as some studies were carried out at only one or two radioligand concentrations (Meyerson *et al.*, 1982; Crow *et al.*, 1984; Owen *et al.*, 1986).

Recently the more selective 5-HT uptake inhibitor, paroxetine has been developed as a radioligand for the 5-HT uptake site (Habert *et al.*, 1985; Mellerup and Plenge, 1986). Although this radioligand labels a small proportion of non-5-HT uptake sites, 5-HT and citalopram displace [^{3}H]par-oxetine binding from a single class of protease-sensitive binding sites related

Table 6 Monoaminergic studies: demographic and clinical details of suicides and controls.

Reference	No. controls/ suicides	No. depressed	Mean age (years)	Post-mortem delay (mean) (h)	Cause of death	Treatment
Meyerson et al. (1982)	10/8	No information	No information	<48	Violent (8)	None detected but no information on prior treatment
Stanley et al. (1982)	9/9	No information	35 (C) 34 (C)	20 (C) 22 (S)	Violent (9)	No information
Stanley and Mann (1983)	11/11	No information	33 (C) 35 (S)	21 (C) 18 (S)	Violent (9)	No information
Crow et al. (1984)	19/10	7	56 (C) 50 (S)	No information	Violent (4) Non-violent (6)	No information
Mann et al. (1986)	21/21	No information	32 (C) 36 (S)	16 (C) 20 (S)	Violent (17) Non-violent (4)	No information
Owen et al. (1986)	19/19	3 (6 possible)	54 (C) 45 (S)	44 (C) 48 (S)	No information	Antidepressants (7)
Arato et al. (1987)	13/14	No information	No information	4–6 (range)	Violent (14)	Antidepressants (2)
Meana and Garcia-Sevilla (1987)	10/5	5	46 (C) 46 (S)	22 (C) 26 (S)	Violent (5)	Amitriptyline (12) Drug free 2–3 weeks (3)
Biegon and Israeli (1988)	14/14	No information	43 (C) 44 (S)	<48	No information	Drug free at time of death
Cheetham et al. (1988a) Cheetham et al. (1990)	19/19	19	41 (C) 39 (S)	41 (C) 39 (S)	Violent (8) Non-violent (11)	Antidepressant (3) Antidepressant and Benzodiazepine (2) Benzodiazepine (1)
Gross-Isseroff et al. (1988)	12/12	No information	No information	No information	Violent (8) Non-violent (2) Unknown (2)	No barbiturates, analgesics, phenothiazines or salicylates

Study					
Arora and Meltzer (1989a)	28/28	No information	44 (C) / 46 (S)	13 (C) / 15 (S)	Violent (16) / Non-violent (12)	Antidepressant (1)
Arora and Meltzer (1989b)	37/32	No information	45 (C) / 48 (S)	14 (C) / 15 (S)	Violent (21) / Non-violent (11)	No information
Gross-Isseroff et al. (1989)	12/12	No information	45 (C) / 47 (S)	21 (C) / 18 (S)	Violent (8) / Non-violent (2) / Unknown (2)	Drug free at time of death
De Paermentier et al. (1990)	20/21	21	43 (C) / 42 (S)	40 (C) / 35 (S)	Violent (10) / Non-violent (11)	Antidepressant free at time of death
Lawrence et al. (1990b)	20/22	22	43 (C) / 42 (S)	40 (C) / 35 (S)	Violent (12) / Non-violent (10)	Antidepressant free at time of death

C, controls; S, suicides. Violent deaths include hanging, jumping, gunshot wounds and self-inflicted wounding; non-violent deaths include overdoses, carbon monoxide poisoning, suffocation and drowning. Number of subjects is given in parentheses.

Table 7 Differences in monoamine neurotransmitter receptor binding sites in post-mortem brain tissue from suicides and controls.

Reference	No. regions studied	5-HT uptake	5-HT$_1$	5-HT$_2$	NA uptake	β	α$_2$
Meyerson et al. (1982)	1	↑35%				↑	
Stanley et al. (1982)	1	↓44%					
Stanley and Mann (1983)	1			↑44%			
Crow et al. (1984)	1	→(↓19%)	↑	→↑		→↑	
Mann et al. (1986)	1		↑	↑28%		↑73%	
Owen et al. (1986)	3	→↑	↑	↑			
Arato et al. (1987)	2	→↓^{R}48%↑^{L}154%					
Meana and Garcia-Sevilla (1987)	1						↑72%
Biegon and Israeli (1988)	7			→↓23%		→↑↑48%	
Cheetham et al. (1988a)	5	→↓					
Gross-Isseroff et al. (1988)	9				↑		
Arora and Meltzer (1989a)	1	↑					
Arora and Meltzer (1989b)	1			↑35%			
Gross-Isseroff et al. (1989)	42	→↓49%↑75%					
Cheetham et al. (1990)	5		→↓20%				
De Paermentier et al. (1990)	9					→↓16%	
Lawrence et al. (1990b)	10	→↑					

R and L, right and left hemispheres.

→, No significant difference; ↓, lower; ↑, higher than controls; →↓↑, different brain regions.

Table 8 Differences in monoamine receptor binding and uptake sites between depressed patients and controls.

Reference	Regions studied	5-HT uptake	5-HT$_1$	5-HT$_2$	β	α_1	α_2
Perry et al. (1983)	Hippocampus	↓47%[a]					
	Occipital cortex	↓33%[a]					
Crow et al. (1984)[c]	Hippocampus				↓42%	↓50%	↑
	Occipital cortex				↑	↑	↑
Ferrier et al. (1986)[d]	Frontal cortex	→[b]					
McKeith et al. (1987)[e]	Frontal cortex		↑	↑			

[a] [^{3}H]imipramine binding.
[b] [^{3}H]paroxetine binding.
[c–e] Studies including same major affective disorder group.
[d,e] Studies including same controls and depressed subjects.
→, No significant difference; ↓, lower than controls.

to 5-HT uptake (Bäckström *et al.*, 1989). In human frontal cortex the number of [^{3}H]paroxetine binding sites is much lower than the number of [^{3}H]imipramine sites, when the latter is defined with desmethylimipramine or amitriptyline but similar when defined with 5-HT (Arora and Meltzer, 1989a).

Using this radioligand Lawrence *et al.* (1990a, 1990b) have studied brain tissue from suicides and controls. No asymmetry of [^{3}H]paroxetine binding sites was found in frontal cortex, putamen or substantia nigra of controls and suicides (Lawrence *et al.*, 1990a), which is in contrast to the findings using [^{3}H]imipramine (Arato *et al.*, 1987; Demeter *et al.*, 1988; 1989). Furthermore, no differences in the number or affinity were found between suicides and controls in cortex (frontal, temporal and occipital), hippocampus, caudate, thalamus, putamen, amygdala and substantia nigra (Lawrence *et al.*, 1990b). However, unlike previous studies, suicides were limited to those for whom a firm retrospective diagnosis of depression could be established. Therefore findings are more likely to relate specifically to depression. In addition, only suicides who had not recently been prescribed antidepressant drugs were included, thus minimizing the possible confounding effects of treatment.

To date only one study has quantitated [^{3}H]imipramine binding in brain tissue from depressed patients (Perry *et al.*, 1983). They reported lower binding in hippocampus and occipital cortex. A further study of subjects with a pre-mortem diagnosis of major affective disorder found no differences in frontal cortical [^{3}H]paroxetine binding, albeit at a single ligand concentration (Ferrier *et al.*, 1986), which is in agreement with the findings in depressed suicides (Lawrence *et al.*, 1990b).

Thus post-mortem studies do not provide convincing evidence of an abnormality in 5-HT uptake sites in depression and/or suicide.

6.4.2 5-HT receptor binding sites

Animal studies indicate that the therapeutic mechanism of action of antidepressant drugs and ECT may involve 5-HT receptor mechanisms. Hence, abnormal 5-HT receptor functioning may be involved in the aetiology of depression. In rat frontal cortex the number of 5-HT$_2$ receptor binding sites has been reported to be decreased following chronic administration of most antidepressant drugs and increased following repeated electroconvulsive shocks (ECS). In contrast, rat brain 5-HT$_1$ receptor binding sites have generally been reported to be unaltered following repeated administration of antidepressant drugs and ECS (reviewed by Sugrue, 1983).

No significant differences in 5-HT$_1$ binding have been reported in frontal and occipital cortex between suicides and controls (Crow *et al.*, 1984; Mann *et al.*, 1986; Owen *et al.*, 1986). No differences in 5-HT$_1$ or 5-HT$_{1A}$ binding sites were found in frontal or temporal cortex between a group of depressed suicides who were antidepressant free at the time of death and controls (Cheetham *et al.*, 1990). Furthermore, $5\text{-}HT_1$ binding was found to be unaltered in frontal cortex of depressed patients when compared with controls (McKeith *et al.*, 1987). Thus it would appear that depression and/or suicide are not associated with abnormalities in $5\text{-}HT_1$ binding sites within these cortical regions.

A significantly lower number of $5\text{-}HT_1$ binding sites was found in hippocampus of antidepressant-free depressed suicides than controls. Furthermore, the number of $5\text{-}HT_1$ binding sites was significantly higher and the binding affinity lower in hippocampus of a small group of antidepressant-treated suicides compared with antidepressant-free suicides (Cheetham *et al.*, 1990). In contrast, Owen *et al.* (1986) reported no difference in $5\text{-}HT_1$ binding (at a single ligand concentration) in hippocampus between suicides and controls. However, these studies are not comparable, as Cheetham *et al.* (1990) studied depressed suicides separated into antidepressant-free and antidepressant-treated groups whilst Owen *et al.* (1986) studied suicides with a range of psychiatric diagnoses and made no distinction between antidepressant-free and treated subjects.

$5\text{-}HT_2$ binding sites have been most extensively studied but have yielded conflicting results. Several studies have reported a higher number of $5\text{-}HT_2$ binding sites in frontal cortex of suicides compared with controls (Stanley and Mann, 1983; Mann *et al.*, 1986; Arora and Meltzer, 1989b). In contrast, Crow *et al.* (1984) and Owen *et al.* (1986) found no differences in $5\text{-}HT_2$ binding in frontal cortex and, in the latter study, frontal and occipital cortex between suicides and control. Cheetham *et al.* (1988a) also reported no differences in the number of $5\text{-}HT_2$ binding sites in frontal, temporal and occipital cortex of antidepressant-free depressed suicides and controls, but did find a significantly lower number of sites in hippocampus.

Mode of death appears to be an important factor in explaining these discrepant results. Stanley and Mann (1983) and Mann *et al.* (1986) limited their studies to suicides who died violently. Arora and Meltzer (1989b) reported a significantly higher number of $5\text{-}HT_2$ sites in frontal cortex of violent suicides compared with controls, but found no differences between non-violent suicides and controls. Furthermore, Cheetham *et al.* (1988a) reported a tendency towards an increased number of sites in frontal cortex of depressed suicides who died violently when compared with those who died non-violently. Associations between reduced concentrations of CSF 5-HIAA, violent suicide attempts, aggression and impulsive behaviour have been established. Reduced CSF 5-HIAA is thought to reflect reduced 5-HT turnover in the brain. An increased number of $5\text{-}HT_2$ binding sites in frontal cortex of those suicide victims who died violently may thus be an adaptive response to decreased 5-HT turnover and may be related more to an effect of aggression / impulsivity rather than depression (reviewed by Van Praag *et al.*, 1986).

Information on drug treatment prior to death was presented in only two studies (Owen *et al.*, 1986; Cheetham *et al.*, 1988a). Cheetham *et al.* (1988a) studied separate groups of antidepressant-free and antidepressant-treated suicides. Although the number of antidepressant-treated suicides studied was too small to allow firm conclusions to be drawn, affinity constants were higher in antidepressant-treated depressed suicides than controls, whereas no significant differences in the number of sites were observed. Thus, in contrast to animal studies, there was no evidence of a reduction in the number of frontal cortical 5-HT$_2$ binding sites.

Only one study has quantitated 5-HT$_2$ receptor binding in brain tissue from depressed patients. McKeith *et al.* (1987) reported no significant difference in 5-HT$_2$ binding in frontal cortex of subjects with a history of major affective disorder.

Thus, studies of depressed suicides and depressed patients provide no evidence of a consistent abnormality in cortical 5-HT$_2$ sites in depressive illness. However, studies of suicides who died violently suggest that increased frontal cortical 5-HT$_2$ binding sites may be associated with aggressive/impulsive behaviour, a finding which would appear to be independent of psychiatric diagnosis. An abnormality in serotonergic mechanisms within the hippocampus may be involved in depressive illness and / or suicide, since both 5-HT$_1$ and 5-HT$_2$ binding sites have been reported to be lower in hippocampus of the same group of antidepressant-free depressed suicides (Cheetham *et al.*, 1988a, 1990).

6.4.3 NA uptake sites

In contrast to the number of studies of 5-HT uptake sites in depression and suicide, only one study has measured NA uptake sites. High affinity binding of [^{3}H]desmethylimipramine, a marker for noradrenergic uptake sites, did not differ in prefrontal and frontoparietal cortex and hippocampus between suicides (most of whom died by violent methods) and controls (Gross-Isseroff *et al.*, 1988).

6.4.4 Adrenoceptors

Adrenoceptors have received little attention, even though down-regulation of β-adrenoceptors is the most consistent effect of antidepressants in animals (reviewed by Sugrue, 1983). Mann *et al.* (1986) reported β-adrenoceptor binding in frontal cortex of suicides to be 73% higher than controls.

Subsequently, Biegon and Israeli (1988) reported a greater number of β-adrenoceptors in frontal cortex of drug-free suicide victims than controls; a finding which was largely restricted to the β_1-subtype. In contrast, Meyerson *et al.* (1982) and Crow *et al.* (1984) found no differences in frontal cortical β-adrenoceptor binding between suicides and controls. Furthermore, De Paermentier *et al.* (1990) reported no significant differences in the number of total β- and β_1-adrenoceptors in frontal cortex of antidepressant-free depressed suicides when compared with controls, but a significantly lower number of total β- and β_1-adrenoceptors was found in those suicides who died by violent methods.

Subject selection is likely to be crucial in explaining the apparent discrepancies between studies. De Paermentier *et al.* (1990) restricted their study to suicides for whom there was documentary evidence of depression. Crow *et al.* (1984) also reported results for a small subgroup of depressed suicides, with findings in agreement with those of De Paermentier *et al.* (1990). In contrast, Mann *et al.* (1986) and Biegon and Israeli (1988) studied suicides for whom no psychiatric history was presented. It is likely that Mann *et al.* (1986) and Biegon and Israeli (1988) included suicides with a range of psychiatric illnesses.

The majority of studies have used [^{3}H]dihydroalprenolol (DHA) as the radioligand defined with propranolol. This strategy presents a problem in that some 5-HT receptors may be labelled in addition to β-adrenoceptors. The study of De Paermentier *et al.* (1990) used [^{3}H]CGP 12177, a radioligand which is selective for β-adrenoceptors with higher affinity and lower non-specific binding than [^{3}H]DHA.

No differences in frontal cortical β-adrenoceptor binding were reported for subjects with an ante-mortem DSM-III diagnosis of major depressive disorder who died by natural causes, when compared with controls (Ferrier *et al.*, 1986).

The majority of studies have concentrated on the frontal cortex. De Paermentier *et al.* (1990) also measured β-adrenoceptors in other brain areas. Lower numbers of total β-adrenoceptors were found in Brodmann area 38 and of β_1-adrenoceptors in Brodmann area 21/22 (both areas of temporal cortex) in antidepressant-free depressed suicides compared with controls. No differences were found in occipital cortex, hippocampus, putamen, thalamus and caudate.

Lower α_1-adrenoceptor binding has been reported in hippocampus of depressed patients compared with controls, but was unaltered in occipital cortex (Crow *et al.*, 1984). No differences in α_2-adrenoceptor binding were found in hippocampus and occipital cortex of this same group of depressed patients compared with controls (Crow *et al.*, 1984). However, the number of α_2-adrenoceptors was found to be markedly higher (by 72%) in frontal cortex of a small group of depressed suicides compared with controls (Meana and Garcia-Sevilla, 1987).

6.5 Other neurotransmitters

6.5.1 γ-Aminobutyric acid

Several lines of evidence suggest the involvement of the inhibitory neurotransmitter GABA in depression and antidepressant drug action. The concentration of GABA in CSF and plasma has been proposed to reflect brain GABA concentration (Böhlen et al., 1979; Petty et al., 1987). Significantly lower concentrations of GABA have been reported in CSF and plasma of drug-free depressed patients compared with other psychiatric or neurological disorders, hospitalized medical patients and healthy controls (Gold et al., 1980; Petty and Schlesser, 1981; Kasa et al., 1982; Gerner et al., 1984; Petty and Sherman, 1984; Coffman and Petty, 1986). Furthermore, the GABA mimetics, progabide and fengabine, have been shown to have antidepressant effects in clinical trials (Morselli et al., 1986; Musch, 1986).

GABA exerts its neurotransmitter action via two classes of receptor: bicuculline-sensitive $GABA_A$ receptors, which are linked to benzodiazepine (BZ) binding sites and chloride ion channels (Olsen, 1981), and bicuculline-insensitive $GABA_B$ receptors (Bowery et al., 1983). Alterations in both classes of brain GABA receptors and BZ binding sites have been reported following repeated antidepressant administration to rodents, although the findings are not consistent (Pilc and Lloyd, 1984; Suranyi-Cadotte et al., 1984; Lloyd et al., 1985; Suzdak and Gianutsos, 1985; Gray and Green, 1987; Gray et al., 1987; Kimber et al., 1987; Cross and Horton, 1988).

A limited number of studies have attempted to investigate the role of GABA in depression using post-mortem brain tissue from suicides and depressed patients. Demographic and clinical details of the subjects studied and results are summarized in Tables 9 and 10.

GABA concentration in post-mortem brain (frontal cortex, amygdala, hypothalamus, caudate nucleus and nucleus accumbens) has been reported not to differ between suicides and controls (Korpi et al., 1988). This finding is in contrast to reports of lower CSF and plasma GABA concentration for depressed patients than healthy controls. Brain GABA concentration is known to increase with increasing post-mortem delay in animals. The extent to which this occurs in man is not known but suggests the necessity for rigorous matching with regard to post-mortem delay.

Table 9 GABAergic studies: demographic and clinical details of elderly depressed patients or suicides and controls.

Reference	No. controls/patient group	No. depressed	Mean age (years)	Post-mortem delay (mean) (h)	Cause of death	Treatment
Perry et al. (1977a)	16/8	8	77 (C) 73 (D)	31 (C) 30 (D)	Natural causes	Antidepressant therapy (majority)
Crow et al. (1984)	22/9	9	79 (C) 76 (D)	22 (C) 28 (D)	No information	Tricyclics (7) Uncertain (1) None (1)
Manchon et al. (1987)	5/7	No information	45 (C) 50 (S)	27 (C) 18 (S)	Hanging (6) Jumping (1)	No tricyclic antidepressants or benzodiazepines
Korpi et al. (1988)	25/13	No history of psychosis	45 (C) 36 (S)	14 (C) 16 (S)	Hanging (2), O/D (3) jumping (4), GSW (1), CO poisoning (1), burns (1), self-inflicted wounding (1)	No information
Cross et al. (1988)[a]	20/20	20	39 (C)[d] 39 (S)	39 (C)[d] 34 (S)	Hanging (7), O/D (5), CO poisoning (5), drowning (1), self-inflicted wounding (2)	Antidepressant (3) Antidepressant and neuroleptic or benzodiazepine (2) Benzodiazepine (1)
Cheetham et al. (1988b)[b]	21/21	21	41 (C) 40 (S)	40 (C) 30 (S)	Hanging (7), O/D (6), CO poisoning (5), self-inflicted wounding (2), drowning (1)	Antidepressant (3) Antidepressant and neuroleptic or benzodiazepine (3) Benzodiazepine (2)
Stocks et al. (1990)[c]	19/19	19	41 (C) 40 (S)	40 (C) 32 (S)	Hanging (6), O/D (6), CO poisoning (4), self-inflicted wounding (2), drowning (1)	Antidepressant (3) Antidepressant and benzodiazepine (2) Benzodiazepine (2)

[a-c] Essentially same suicides and controls in all three studies.
[d] Information for 16 controls and 16 suicides only.
C, controls; D, elderly depressed patients; S, suicides; O/D, overdose; GSW, gunshot wounds; CO, carbon monoxide. Number of subjects is given in parentheses.

Table 10 Differences in GABA concentration, GAD activity and GABA related receptor binding sites in depression and suicide.

Reference	No. regions studied	GABA	GAD	$GABA_A$	$GABA_B$	BZ
Perry et al. (1977a)[a]	8		→↓46%[b]			
Crow et al. (1984)[a]	3			↑		↑
Manchon et al. (1987)	1					↑↑
Korpi et al. (1988)	5	↑				
Cross et al. (1988)[e]	3				↑	
Cheetham et al. (1988b)[f]	2		→↑	↑		→↑18%[c]
Stocks et al. (1990)[g]	2					→↑22%[d]

[a] Elderly depressed patients all other studies of suicides.
[b] 41% lower in frontal cortex, 51% lower in occipital cortex, 48% lower in caudate nucleus, 45% lower in substantia nigra.
[c] 18% higher in frontal cortex (all suicides). 16% higher for drug-free suicides and 21% higher for drug-treated suicides.
[d] 22% higher in amygdala of drug-free than drug-treated suicides.
[e-g] All three studies of essentially same suicides and controls.
→, No significant difference; ↓, lower; ↑, higher than controls; →↑, different regions.

The activity of glutamic acid decarboxylase (GAD), the rate limiting enzyme in GABA synthesis, has been reported to be significantly lower in frontal and occipital cortex, caudate and substantia nigra from depressed patients dying of natural causes compared with controls (Perry et al., 1977a). In contrast, Cheetham et al. (1988b) reported no differences in GAD activity in frontal or temporal cortex between depressed suicides, whether antidepressant-free or antidepressant-treated, and controls. GAD activity is markedly reduced by terminal illness, particularly when associated with hypoxia, and with increasing post-mortem delay (Perry et al., 1977a; Spokes, 1979; Agid et al., 1984). Perry et al. (1977a) included patients dying after prolonged periods of illness but argued that the magnitude of the reductions they observed could not entirely be attributed to this factor and was therefore a reflection of depressive illness. The study of Cheetham et al. (1988b) was not complicated by the effects of protracted illness. Furthermore, suicides and controls were well matched for post-mortem delay. Thus, the results of Cheetham et al. (1988b) do not support the view of Perry et al. (1977a) of reduced cortical GAD activity in depression. An unexpected finding was that death by carbon monoxide poisoning was associated with a marked reduction in cortical GAD activity (Cheetham et al., 1988b).

No differences in $GABA_A$ or $GABA_B$ receptor binding sites have been reported between depressed patients or depressed suicides and controls (Crow et al., 1984; Cheetham et al., 1988b; Cross et al., 1988). Results for BZ binding sites are however less consistent. Crow et al. (1984) reported no significant difference in [^{3}H]diazepam binding (albeit at a single ligand concentration) in frontal cortex and hippocampus of depressed patients compared with controls. In agreement, no differences in the number of hippocampal BZ binding sites have been reported between depressed suicides and controls (Stocks et al., 1990) and a small group of psychiatrically undefined suicides and controls (Manchon et al., 1987), although the proportion of BZ type 1 sites was greater in the suicides of the latter study. In contrast to the finding of Crow et al. (1984) a significantly higher number of BZ binding sites was found in frontal cortex of depressed suicides compared with controls, but with no difference in temporal cortex (Cheetham et al., 1988b). This increase was found in drug-free and drug-treated depressed suicides, suggesting that this effect is not wholly drug related. Findings in temporal cortex also support this view.

Thus, to date, post-mortem studies provide no consistent evidence of an abnormality in GABA neurotransmission in depression and/or suicide.

6.5.2 Acetylcholine

Although there is evidence to suggest that depression is associated with increased central cholinergic activity, few studies have examined cholinergic markers in post-mortem brain. Meyerson *et al.* (1982) reported a 47% higher number of frontal cortical muscarinic receptors in a small group of violent suicides, in whose brains antidepressant drugs could not be detected, compared with controls. However, two subsequent studies have not replicated this finding. Stanley (1984) found no difference in frontal cortical muscarinic binding between 22 suicides, or a subgroup who died by violent methods, and matched controls. Kaufmann *et al.* (1984) reported muscarinic binding to be unaltered in frontal cortex and pons of suicides compared with controls, although there was a trend towards a lower number of binding sites in the hypothalamus of suicides.

One study has reported cholinergic markers in a small group of depressed subjects. Muscarinic binding was unaltered in parietal cortex but was moderately reduced in caudate nucleus of depressed subjects compared with controls (Perry *et al.*, 1977b). There was also a trend towards lower choline acetyl transferase in parietal cortex and caudate nucleus (Perry *et al.*, 1977b).

6.5.3 Corticotrophin releasing factor

The increased activity of the hypothalamic–pituitary–adrenal axis in depression is thought to be due, in part, to a hypersecretion of corticotrophin releasing factor (CRF) from the hypothalamus. CRF, as well as functioning as a hormone, also acts as a central neurotransmitter, and CRF concentration is elevated in the CSF of drug-free depressed patients (Nemeroff *et al.*, 1984; Arato *et al.*, 1986; Banki *et al.*, 1987). Although cortical CSF concentration did not differ between depressed suicides and controls (Charlton *et al.*, 1988), the number of CRF receptors has been reported to be 23% lower in frontal cortex of 26 suicides compared with controls (Nemeroff *et al.*, 1988). These authors interpret this finding as an adaptive receptor down-regulation in response to chronic hypersecretion of CRF.

6.6 Future studies

Studies of post-mortem brain tissue from suicide victims provide the most direct and feasible approach to the understanding of the aetiology of suicidal behaviour and depression. In this chapter we have attempted to review and critically assess the relevant studies carried out to date. In doing so we have highlighted a lack of consistency in the results obtained for all neurotransmitter parameters discussed. A number of factors are responsible. However, it is clear that subject selection is likely to be the single most important factor. Although depression is the most frequent psychiatric correlate of suicide (frequency approximately 45%), suicide is associated with a range of psychiatric diagnoses. Thus, extrapolation of results from a general population of suicide victims to depression, an approach which has frequently been adopted, is unwarranted. A choice between the two broad aims of an understanding of the aetiology of suicidal/aggressive behaviour and that of depression must be made in future studies. This decision will clearly affect subject selection. Retrospective psychiatric diagnosis using operationally defined criteria is essential to the selection of those suicide victims with a history of depression. The study of depressed suicide victims is the approach we have adopted as we feel that under these circumstances findings are more likely to be related to depression. However, it must also be borne in mind that depressed patients who commit suicide may not be representative of depressed patients in general and may form a distinct subgroup within the depressed population. Thus, biological abnormalities associated with depressed suicide victims can not necessarily be generalized to depression as a whole.

Although subject selection is crucial several other factors must not be neglected. These include age, gender, post-mortem delay, storage time, mode of death and medication. Rigorous matching of normal and pathological groups would appear to be the most appropriate solution for the majority of these. However, this is not possible for medication. In order to distinguish between changes resulting from the underlying illness and those resulting from drug treatment, both drug-free and drug-treated subjects must be studied separately. Repeated administration of antidepressant drugs to rodents has been shown to alter several classes of neurotransmitter receptor binding sites. Thus, this is of particular relevance to suicide victims with a history of depression, who are more than likely to have been prescribed antidepressant drugs prior to death. We have attempted to study both antidepressant drug-free and antidepressant-treated depressed suicide victims. In doing so we have encountered several problems worthy of note. Collection of a group of depressed suicide victims receiving a single antidepressant was hampered by the fact that a significant proportion of depressed patients receive combination treatment, for example antidepressant and benzodiazepine. Information on duration of treatment and compliance was difficult to obtain retrospectively. Furthermore, antidepressant-treated suicides were more likely to have used drug overdosage than any other mode of death. What effect, if any, this has on neurotransmitter parameters is unknown.

However, if the practical difficulties associated with the management of post-mortem studies relating to suicide and depression can be overcome, then these studies are likely to make an important contribution to the neurochemistry of these disorders in the future.

Acknowledgements

We would like to thank Miss S.M. Hyde for typing this chapter, and Professor W.R. Buckett for constructive criticism and useful comments.

References

Agid, Y., Ploska, A., Monfort, J.C. & Javoy-Agid, F. (1984) *Lancet* **i**, 280.

Ågren, H. (1980) *Psychiatry Res.* **3**, 225–236.

Arato, M., Banki, C.M., Nemeroff, C.B. & Bissette, G. (1986) *Ann. N.Y. Acad. Sci.* **487**, 263–270.

Arato, M., Tekes, K., Tothfalusi, L. *et al.* (1987) *Psychiatry Res.* **21**, 355–356.

Arora, R.C. & Meltzer, H.Y. (1989a) *Psychiatry Res.* **30**, 125–135.

Arora, R.C. & Meltzer, H.Y. (1989b) *Am. J. Psychiatry* **146**, 730–736.

Åsberg, M., Träskman, L. & Thoren, P. (1976) *Arch. Gen. Psychiatry* **33**, 1193–1197.

Åsberg, M., Bertilsson, L., Martensson, B., Scalia-Tomba, G.-P., Thoren, P. & Träskman-Bendz, L. (1984) *Acta Psychiatr. Scand.* **69**, 201–219.

Bäckström, I., Bergström, M. & Marcusson, J. (1989) *Brain Res.* **486**, 261–268.

Banki, C.M., Bissette, G., Arato, M., O'Connor, L. & Nemeroff, C. (1987) *Am. J. Psychiatry* **144**, 873–877.

Barraclough, B. & Hughes, J. (1987) In *Suicide. Clinical and Epidemiological Studies*, pp 8–36. London, Croom Helm.

Bennett, J.P., Enna, S.J., Bylund, D.B., Gillin, C.J., Wyatt, R.J. & Snyder, S.H. (1979) *Arch. Gen. Psychiatry* **36**, 927–934.

Beskow, J., Gottfries, C.G., Roos, B.E. & Winbald, B. (1976) *Acta Psychiatr. Scand.* **53**, 7–20.

Biegon, A. & Israeli, M. (1988) *Brain Res.* **442**, 199–203.

Böhlen, P., Huot, S. & Palfreyman, M.G. (1979) *Brain Res.* **167**, 297–305.

Bourne, H.R., Bunney, W.E., Colburn, R.W. *et al.* (1968) *Lancet* **ii**, 805–808.

Bowery, N.G., Hill, D.R. & Hudson, A.L. (1983) *Br. J. Pharmacol.* **78**, 191–206.

Brown, G.L. & Goodwin, F.K. (1986) *Ann. N.Y. Acad. Sci.* **487**, 175–188.

Bucht, G., Adolfsson, R., Gottfries, C.G., Roos, B.-E. & Winbald, B. (1981) *J. Neural Transm.* **51**, 185–203.

Carlsson, A., Svennerholm, L. & Winbald, B. (1980) *Acta Psychiatr. Scand.* **61** (Suppl. 280), 75–85.

Cash, R., Ruberg, M., Raisman, R. & Agid, Y. (1984) *Brain Res.* **322**, 269–275.

Cash, R., Raisman, R., Ploska, A. & Agid, Y. (1985) *Eur. J. Pharmacol.* **117**, 71–80.

Charlton, B.G., Cheetham, S.C., Horton, R.W., Katona, C.L.E., Crompton, M.R. & Ferrier, I.N. (1988) *J. Psychopharmacol.* **2**, 13–18.

Cheetham, S.C., Crompton, M.R., Katona, C.L.E. & Horton, R.W. (1988a) *Brain Res.* **443**, 272–280.

Cheetham, S.C., Crompton, M.R., Katona, C.L.E., Parker, S.J. & Horton, R.W. (1988b) *Brain Res.* **460**, 114–123.

Cheetham, S.C., Crompton, M.R., Czudek, C., Horton, R.W., Katona, C.L.E. & Reynolds, G.P. (1989) *Brain Res.* **502**, 332–340.

Cheetham, S.C., Crompton, M.R., Katona, C.L.E. & Horton, R.W. (1990) *Psychopharmacol.* **102**, 544–548.

Cochran, E., Robins, E. & Grote, S. (1976) *Biol. Psychiatry* **11**, 283–294.

Coffman, J.A. & Petty, F. (1986) In *GABA and Mood Disorders: Experimental and Clinical Research* (eds Bartholini, G., Lloyd, K.G. & Morselli, P.L.), pp 179–185. New York, Raven Press.

Cross, A.J., Crow, T.J., Ferrier, I.N., Johnson, J.A., Bloom, S.R. & Corsellis, J.A.N. (1984) *J. Neurochem.* **43**, 1574–1581.

Cross, J.A. & Horton, R.W. (1988) *Br. J. Pharmacol.* **9**, 331–336.

Cross, J.A., Cheetham, S.C., Crompton, M.R., Katona, C.L.E. & Horton, R.W. (1988) *Psychiatry Res.* **26**, 119–129.

Crow, T.J., Cross, A.J., Cooper, S.J. *et al.* (1984) *Neuropharmacol.* **23**, 1561–1569.

Demeter, E., Tekes, K., Majorossy, K., Arato, M. & Somogyi, E. (1988) *Acta Psychiatr. Scand.* **77**, 746–747.

Demeter, E., Tekes, K., Majorossy, K. *et al.* (1989) *Life Sci.* **44**, 1403–1410.

De Paermentier, F., Cheetham, S.C., Crompton, M.R., Katona, C.L.E. & Horton, R.W. (1990) *Brain Res.* **525**, 71–77.

Ferrier, I.N., McKeith, I.G., Cross, A.J., Perry, E.K., Candy, J.M. & Perry, R.H. (1986) *Ann. N.Y. Acad. Sci.* **487**, 128–142.

Gerner, R.H., Fairbanks, L., Anderson, G.M. *et al.* (1984) *Am. J. Psychiatry* **141**, 1533–1540.

Gjerris, A. (1988) *Acta Psychiatr. Scand.* **78** (Suppl. 346), 1–35.

Glick, S.D., Ross, D.A. & Hough, L.B. (1982) *Brain Res.* **234**, 53–63.

Gold, B.I., Bowers, M.B., Roth, R.H. & Sweeney, D.W. (1980) *Am. J. Psychiatry*, **137**, 362–364.

Gottfries, C.G., Oreland, L., Wiberg, A. & Winbald, B. (1975) *J. Neurochem.* **25**, 667–673.

Gray, J.A. & Green, A.R. (1987) *Br. J. Pharmacol.* **92**, 357–362.

Gray, J.A., Goodwin, G.M., Heal, D.J. & Green, A.R. (1987) *Br. J. Pharmacol.* **92**, 863–870.

Gross-Isseroff, R., Israeli, M. & Biegon, A. (1988) *Brain Res.* **456**, 120–126.

Gross-Isseroff, R., Israeli, M. & Biegon, A. (1989) *Arch. Gen. Psychiatry* **46**, 237–241.

Grote, S.S., Moses, S.G., Robins, E., Hudgens, R.W. & Croninger, A.B. (1974) *J. Neurochem.* **23**, 791–802.

Habert, E., Graham, D., Tahraoui, L., Claustre, Y. & Langer, S.Z. (1985) *Eur. J. Pharmacol.* **118**, 107–114.

Kasa, K., Otsuki, S., Yamamoto, M., Sato, M., Kuroda, H. & Ogawa, N. (1982) *Biol. Psychiatry* **17**, 877–883.

Kaufmann, C.A., Gillin, J.C., Hill, B. *et al.* (1984) *Psychiatry Res.* **12**, 47–55.

Kimber, J.R., Cross, J.A. & Horton, R.W. (1987) *Biochem. Pharmacol.* **36**, 4173–4175.

Korpi, E.R., Kleinman, J.E., Goodman, S.I. *et al.* (1986) *Arch. Gen. Psychiatry* **43**, 594–600.

Korpi, E.R., Kleinman, J.E. & Wyatt, R.J. (1988) *Biol. Psychiatry* **23**, 109–114.

Lawrence, K.M., De Paermentier, F., Cheetham, S.C., Crompton, M.R., Katona, C.L.E. & Horton, R.W. (1990a) *Biol. Psychiatry* **28**, 544–546.

Lawrence, K.M., De Paermentier, F., Cheetham, S.C., Crompton, M.R., Katona, C.L.E. & Horton, R.W. (1990b) *Brain Res.* **526**, 17–22.
Lloyd, K.G., Farley, I.J., Deck, J.H.N. & Hornykiewicz, O. (1974) *Adv. Biochem. Psychopharmacol.* **11**, 387–397.
Lloyd, K.G., Thuret, F. & Pilc, A. (1985) *J. Pharmacol. Exp. Ther.* **235**, 191–199.
McIntyre, I.M. & Stanley, M. (1984) *J. Neurochem.* **42**, 1588–1592.
McKeith, I.G., Marshall, E.F., Ferrier, I.N. *et al.* (1987) *J. Affective Disord.* **13**, 67–74.
Manchon, M., Kopp, N., Rouzioux, J.J., Lecestre, D., Deluermoz, S. & Miachon, S. (1987) *Life Sci.* **41**, 2623–2630.
Mann, J.J. & Stanley, M. (1984) *Acta Psychiatr. Scand.* **69**, 135–139.
Mann, J.J., Stanley, M., McBride, P.A. & McEwen, B.S. (1986) *Arch. Gen. Psychiatry* **43**, 954–959.
Marcusson, J.O., Morgan, D.G., Winbald, B. & Finch, C.E. (1984a) *Brain Res.* **311**, 51–56.
Marcusson, J., Oreland, L. & Winbald, B. (1984b) *J. Neurochem.* **43**, 1699–1705.
Meana, J.J. & Garcia-Sevilla, J.A. (1987) *J. Neural Transm.* **70**, 377–381.
Mellerup, E.T. & Plenge, P. (1986) *Psychopharmacol.* **89**, 436–439.
Meyerson, L.R., Wennogle, L.P., Abel, M.S. *et al.* (1982) *Pharmacol. Biochem. Behav.* **17**, 159–163.
Morselli, P.L., Fournier, V., Macher, J.P., Orofiamma, B., Bottin, P. & Huber, P. (1986) In *GABA and Mood Disorders: Experimental and Clinical Research* (eds Bartholini, G., Lloyd, K.G. & Morselli, P.L.), pp 119–126. New York, Raven Press.
Moses, S.G. & Robins, E. (1975) *Psychopharmacol. Commun.* **1**, 327–337.
Musch, B. (1986) In *GABA and Mood Disorders: Experimental and Clinical Research* (eds Bartholini, G., Lloyd, K.G. & Morselli, P.L.), pp 171–177. New York, Raven Press.
Nemeroff, C.B., Widerlov, E., Bissette, G. *et al.* (1984) *Science* **226**, 1342–1344.
Nemeroff, C.B., Owens, M.J., Bissette, G., Andorn, A.C. & Stanley, M. (1988) *Arch. Gen. Psychiatry* **45**, 577–579.
Oke, A., Keller, R., Mefford, I. & Adams, R.N. (1978) *Science* **200**, 1411–1413.
Olsen, R.W. (1981) *J. Neurochem.* **37**, 1–13.
Owen, F., Chambers, D.R., Cooper, S.J. *et al.* (1986) *Brain Res.* **362**, 185–188.
Pare, C.M.B., Yeung, D.P.H., Price, K. & Stacey, R.S. (1969) *Lancet* **ii**, 133–135.
Perry, E.K. & Perry, R.H. (1983) *Life Sci.* **33**, 1733–1743.
Perry, E.K., Gibson, P.H., Blessed, G., Perry, R.H. & Tomlinson, B.E. (1977a) *J. Neurol. Sci.* **34**, 247–265.
Perry, E.K., Perry, R.H., Blessed, G. & Tomlinson, B.E. (1977b) *Lancet* **i**, 189.
Perry, E.K., Marshall, E.F., Blessed, G., Tomlinson, B.E. & Perry, R.H. (1983) *Br. J. Psychiatry* **142**, 188–192.
Petty, F. & Schlesser, M.A. (1981) *J. Affective Disord.* **3**, 339–343.
Petty, F. & Sherman, A.D. (1984) *J. Affective Disord.* **6**, 131–138.
Petty, F., Kramer, G. & Feldman, M. (1987) *Biol. Psychiatry* **22**, 725–732.
Pilc, A. & Lloyd, K.G. (1984) *Life Sci.* **35**, 2149–2154.
Riederer, P., Birkmayer, W., Seemann, D. & Wuketich, S. (1980) *Acta Psychiatr. Scand.* **61** (Suppl. 280), 251–257.
Shaw, D.M., Camps, F.E. & Eccleston, E.G. (1967) *Br. J. Psychiatry* **113**, 1407–1411.
Spokes, E.G.S. (1979) *Brain* **102**, 333–346.
Stahl, S.M. & Meltzer, H.Y. (1978) *J. Pharmacol. Exp. Ther.* **205**, 118–132.
Stanley, M. (1984) *Am. J. Psychiatry* **141**, 1432–1436.
Stanley, M. & Mann, J.J. (1983) *Lancet* **i**, 214–216.
Stanley, M., Virgilio, J. & Gershon, S. (1982) *Science* **216**, 1337–1339.

Stocks, G.M., Cheetham, S.C., Crompton, M.R., Katona, C.L.E. & Horton, R.W. (1990) *J. Affective Disord.* **18**, 11–15.

Sugrue, M.F. (1983) *Pharmacol. Ther.* **21**, 1–33.

Suranyi-Cadotte, B.E., Dam, T.V. & Quirion, R. (1984) *Eur. J. Pharmacol.* **106**, 673–675.

Suzdak, P.D. & Gianutsos, G. (1985) *Neuropharmacol.* **24**, 217–222.

Van Praag, H.M., Plutchik, R. & Conte, H. (1986) *Ann. N.Y. Acad. Sci.* **487**, 150–167.

Whitehouse, P.J., Lynch, D. & Kuhar, M.J. (1984) *J. Neurochem.* **43**, 553–559.

CHAPTER 7

BIOLOGICAL RHYTHMS IN THE PATHOPHYSIOLOGY AND TREATMENT OF AFFECTIVE DISORDERS

Janis L. Anderson[1,2] and Anna Wirz-Justice[2]

[1]Laboratory for Circadian and Sleep Disorders Medicine, Brigham and Women's Hospital and Harvard Medical School, 221 Longwood Avenue, Boston, Massachusetts 02115, USA

[2]Chronobiology Laboratory, Psychiatrische Universitätsklinik, Wilhelm Klein Strasse 27, CH-4025 Basel, Switzerland

Table of Contents

J.L. Anderson and A. Wirz-Justice

7.1 Introduction

The body is like a clock: if one wheel be amiss, all the rest are disordered, the whole fabric suffers. (Burton, 1638)

In the endogenous depressive, we see a shift in the 24-hour rhythm, a phase shift, ...the night becomes day... Anyone knowing the material would look for the CNS origin in the midbrain, where the entire vegetative nervous system is controlled by a central clock whose rhythmicity regulates and balances the biological system. (Georgi, 1947)

The remarkable periodicities of mood and its disorders have intrigued scientists for centuries (cf. Menninger-Lerchenthal, 1960; Wehr, 1989; Wehr and Rosenthal, 1989). Key clinical observations have included the classic daily rhythmic symptoms of melancholia: diurnal variation of mood, early morning awakening, and disturbances of sleep timing and architecture; as well as regular patterns of recurrence of depressive and manic episodes (see Checkley, 1989; Wehr, 1990a). In addition, appealing analogies have been drawn between the syndrome of depression and certain behaviour patterns of animals, such as hibernation (Giedke, 1986) (however, for discussion of the limitation of these analogies, see Mrosovsky, 1988; Zucker, 1988).

The contemporary resurgence of interest in biological rhythms and affective disorders has come at a propitious time. Clinical researchers have benefitted from and contributed to significant recent discoveries in basic circadian neuroscience. New hypotheses that have been proposed concerning depression and biological rhythms have incorporated three important developments in *chronobiology* (the study of time-related processes in living systems) which are reviewed in greater detail below. First, the principal circadian pacemaker in mammals has been located in the suprachiasmatic nuclei (SCN) of the anterior hypothalamus. Light has been identified as the most powerful *external* synchronizer of this pacemaker, and additional evidence has suggested that melatonin, a hormone of the pineal gland, may be one of the principal *internal* synchronizers of circadian rhythms. Both light and melatonin (Arendt, 1989) have become important tools in basic and clinical research.

Second, the characteristics of circadian and seasonal rhythms have been rigorously formalized. The products of these analyses have guided the formulation of hypotheses, crafting of specific treatment parameters and interpretation of resulting data. They have allowed circadian hypotheses of affective disorders to be more explicit and more testable. Interestingly, these models, which were greatly influenced by experiments on unicellular organisms and insects, have been found to apply across a wide range of species including *Homo sapiens* (Pittendrigh and Bruce, 1957; Pittendrigh, 1979; Czeisler *et al.*,

224

1989; Wever, 1989). Physiological investigations based on the formal analyses have provided feedback to chronobiology researchers, helping to recast key issues and to raise further questions (Rusak, 1989; Remé *et al.*, 1990, 1991).

Finally, as discussed below, pharmacological agents used in the treatment of depression have been prominent among the substances found to affect biological rhythmicity.

On the basis of this body of research, both therapeutic manipulations of sleep rhythms and specific light therapy regimens have been developed. These interventions have been shown to induce dramatic, although sometimes transient, improvements in the symptoms of some depressed patients and patients with certain types of insomnia or premenstrual dysphoria. Efforts are underway to expand on these initial discoveries and develop their clinical utility. In addition, this area of research has provided an important conceptual framework for beginning to construct biological hypotheses about affective disorders which integrate molecular and neuronal events into the larger physiological systems that ultimately must be involved in the expression of clinical symptoms.

After reviewing major discoveries and principles of chronobiology, this chapter summarizes recent tests of circadian hypotheses in human subjects and considers the developing models of sleep and affective disorders that are based on a chronobiological approach, their experimental predictions and clinial implications.

It will be seen that circadian medicine is a growing field which has served to remind modern science of the daily impact on human biology of the cycles of our geophysical environment, and has demonstrated that this interface is vulnerable to dysregulation. Evidence suggests that mood and sleep disorders at times arise directly from such dysregulation. This has opened exciting new avenues of inquiry into physiological processes that may be involved in the whole spectrum of affective disorders.

7.2 Circadian timing system

The frequencies of rhythms observed in nature reflect every division of time, from milliseconds to years. Likewise, these oscillations occur at all levels of organization, from chemical reactions to gene products, single cells, networks and tissues, organs, whole organisms and populations (Pittendrigh, 1960, 1974; Cummings, 1975; Moore-Ede *et al.*, 1982; Rapp, 1987). The most prominent rhythms are those which oscillate with a frequency corresponding to that of a major environmental periodicity: daily, lunar or seasonal. This has led to speculation that in the course of evolution, external periodicity has been internalized in the form of a 'biological clock' (Pittendrigh and Bruce, 1957; Pittendrigh, 1979). In this view, internal timing systems serve to coordinate the temporal sequence of metabolic and physiological events, synchronizing interdependent functions, segregating incompatible ones, and allowing organisms to anticipate, prepare for, and use to advantage the major changes that predictably recur in their external environment (Pittendrigh, 1979; Moore-Ede, 1986; Wehr *et al.*, 1988; Rusak, 1989). Thus, organisms can adapt to 'niches in time' (Aschoff, 1981c).

7.2.1 Circadian rhythms

Circadian rhythms are perhaps the most extensively studied of all biological oscillations. They are genetically determined rhythms of nearly 24 h (*circa diem* = about a day: Halberg, 1959) that are found in all eukaryotic organisms (Pittendrigh, 1960; Aschoff, 1981b; Minors and Waterhouse, 1981). Circadian rhythms persist in the absence of external time cues (or *zeitgebers*), even in spacecraft orbiting the Earth (e.g. Sulzman *et al.*, 1984); therefore, the source of circadian rhythmicity is an *internal* oscillator (de Mairan, 1729; Bünning, 1935; Aschoff, 1979). Light is the dominant external zeitgeber and in many species probably the only agent that *entrains* (synchronizes) the circadian system to a 24-h day.

The SCN appears to be the primary endogenous pacemaker for mammalian circadian rhythms[1] (Rusak and Zucker, 1979; Moore, 1983; Turek, 1985; Pickard *et al.*, 1987). As schematically illustrated in Figure 1, information about the environmental light–dark cycle is directly transmitted from the retina to the SCN, via the retinohypothalamic tract.

As also suggested in Figure 1, light sensitivity in human beings demonstrates circadian rhythmicity (Knörchen *et al.*, 1976; Bassi and Powers, 1986), and the retina may contain a secondary oscillator that actively gates light input (Terman and Terman, 1985; Remé *et al.*, 1991). The circadian pacemaker may also receive feedback from the rest–activity cycle. At certain circadian phases, activity in animals has been reported to re-entrain the circadian system after phase shifts (Mrosovsky and Salmon, 1987). The acceleration in phase shifting after the administration of a benzodiazepine, triazolam, has been shown to be mediated by locomotor activity (Turek, 1989; Van Reeth and Turek, 1989).

[1] Whether mammals actually possess more than one endogenous circadian oscillator is the subject of ongoing debate (e.g. Wever, 1975; Moore-Ede and Czeisler, 1984; Illnerová *et al.*, 1985; Czeisler *et al.*, 1986a; Rosenwasser and Adler, 1986; Honma *et al.*, 1987a, 1989; Remé *et al.*, 1991).

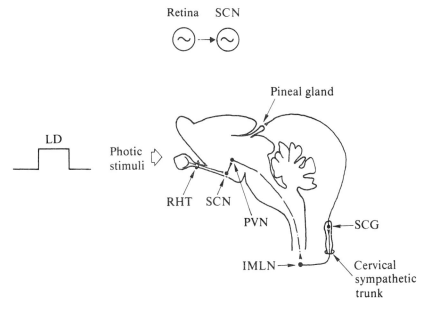

Figure 1 Retinal afferent cells convey information about the environmental light–dark cycle (LD) to the superchiasmatic nuclei (SCN) of the hypothalamus via direct bilateral retinohypothalamic tracts (RHT). Among several efferent pathways from the SCN is a link to the pineal gland, by way of synapses in the paraventricular nucleus (PVN), the intermediolateral cell column of the spinal cord (IMLN) and the superior cervical ganglion (SCG).

The SCN has efferent projections to several brain regions (Meijer and Rietveld, 1989). Among these is a multisynaptic pathway, illustrated in Figure 1, that connects the SCN to the pineal gland (Klein *et al.*, 1983), which is the primary site of synthesis of the methoxyindole hormone, melatonin (a small amount of melatonin is also produced in the retina). In all species studied, whether they are usually day-active (diurnal), night-active (nocturnal), or active at dawn and dusk (crepuscular), melatonin is secreted only at night.

The extremely stable rhythm of pineal melatonin synthesis is regulated by input from the SCN (Tamarkin *et al.*, 1985; Illnerová, 1988) and is also subject to direct suppression by bright light (Lewy *et al.*, 1980; Bojkowski *et al.*, 1987; Illnerová, 1988) (see below). In many species the nocturnal duration of melatonin secretion is directly related to the duration of summer or winter darkness. Thus melatonin has been described as an 'internal zeitgeber' (Armstrong, 1989), transducing the light–dark signal from the SCN to internal tissues of the organism.

Pineal melatonin may also play a role in its own regulation (Redman *et al.*, 1983; Illnerová, 1988), and a relatively high density of melatonin receptors has been found in the human SCN (Reppert *et al.*, 1988). Melatonin has been reported to have limited phase-shifting effects on the circadian pacemaker (Armstrong, 1989; Sack *et al.*, 1990), and preliminary data from melatonin administration in blind subjects support such a possibility (R.L. Sack *et al.*, 1988, 1990; Sarrafzadeh *et al.*, 1990). However, other experiments have failed to demonstrate a melatonin effect on the circadian pacemaker (Wever, 1989; Folkard *et al.*, 1990).

In human beings, unlike some other species, light intensities typically encountered indoors (< 500 lx) have not been observed to suppress melatonin synthesis dramatically. However, in 1980, Lewy *et al.* (also chronicled in Eastman, 1991) discovered that human melatonin secretion could be suppressed by sunshine[2] as well as by artificial light of intensities around 2500 lx or more. This key finding influenced the revival of light exposure treatments for affective disorders (Kripke *et al.*, 1983a, 1983b) and reopened the investigation of light as a zeitgeber in human beings (Czeisler *et al.*, 1981b, 1986a; Wever *et al.*, 1983; Czeisler and Allan, 1987; Dijk *et al.*, 1987; Honma *et al.*, 1987a, 1987b; Lewy *et al.*, 1987; Wever, 1989) by prompting investigators to use brighter light in studies of human subjects. It also figured prominently in the revival of interest in annually-recurring affective disorders (see historical reviews in Wehr, 1989; Wehr and Rosenthal, 1989).

Evidence now suggests that nocturnal species tend to be more sensitive to light than are diurnal creatures, and also that the timing and intensity of previous light exposures can alter the sensitivity of an individual organism (Illnerová, 1988). In recent human studies, certain individuals have shown suppression of melatonin by 200–500 lx (Bojkowski *et al.*, 1987; McIntyre *et al.*, 1989). While there are individual differences in the absolute sensitivity of human beings to the suppression of melatonin by light, an intensity–response relationship remains, with greater suppression by higher light intensities (McIntyre *et al.*, 1989).

Experiments using bright light to manipulate circadian rhythms in human beings have raised new questions. As further discussed below, the relationship between the melatonin rhythm and other circadian rhythms is the subject of ongoing research. At the present time the precise relationship between light effects on melatonin secretion and effects on other circadian rhythms remains to be specified.

In the past decade, awareness of the importance of bright light exposure has grown, particularly as its clinical application in the treatment of autumn/winter seasonal depression and other disorders has spread. Efforts

---

[2] Light intensity outdoors at noon on a sunny day can reach as much as 100 000 lx.

have been made to document carefully actual light exposure in human subjects. Average daily exposure to bright light in a Southern California sample was only 90 min in young adults (Okudaira *et al.*, 1983) and 60 min in elderly subjects (Campbell *et al.*, 1988), with women receiving less light than men. Even when a young adult subject was enabled to spend summer hours in Hawaii as she liked, her actual amounts of light exposure were surprisingly modest (Kripke and Gregg, 1990). Thus, the findings of Kripke and associates suggest that chronically low levels of light exposure may be common enough to play a significant aetiological role in some sleep and mood disturbances. At polar latitudes, specific sleep and affective disorders, discussed in greater detail below, have been known to stem from the extremely long winter nights (Bohlen, 1979; Lingjärde *et al.*, 1985).

7.2.2 Seasonal rhythms

Physiological and behavioural processes which cycle on a yearly basis, even under constant conditions (without external seasonal cues), are called *circannual*. Light is also the principal zeitgeber for these rhythms. Day length (photoperiod) is the most precise and reliable aspect of the yearly environmental cycle (for review, see Gwinner, 1981).

'Photoperiodism' refers to significant changes in an organism's physiology or behaviour that depend upon the amount of its light and dark exposure per 24-h cycle (Pittendrigh, 1988). Seasonal behaviours, such as migration, reproduction and hibernation, can be evoked by simulated photoperiods (Gwinner, 1981). If melatonin is administered at times that are equivalent to those of its secretion under a particular light–dark schedule, the seasonal physiological and behavioural changes typical of that light–dark schedule can be induced. While in some species (such as Siberian hamster, sheep and monkey) it has been established that the photoperiodic information is transduced by the duration of the nightly episode of melatonin secretion (Tamarkin *et al.*, 1985), the range of species for whom melatonin duration plays a role in mediating seasonal rhythms remains to be completely documented (Arendt and Broadway, 1987). In some cases, such as the rat and the Syrian hamster, melatonin onset has been reported to begin much after dusk. Although the timing of this rise was considered crucial as a cue for seasonal rhythms (Tamarkin *et al.*, 1985), newer experiments show that it is the duration of secretion that is important (Maywood *et al.*, 1990).

Definitive data from human subjects regarding the degree of seasonal changes in melatonin duration have not been collected. It appears that factors such as latitude and life-style may affect the degree to which people exhibit seasonal changes in the duration of their episodes of melatonin secretion (Beck-Friis *et al.*, 1984; Illnerová *et al.*, 1985; Bojkowski and Arendt, 1988;

Illnerová, 1988). Some data suggest that seasonal melatonin rhythms in human beings may be similar to those described above for the rat and the Syrian hamster (Arendt *et al.*, 1989).

Melatonin may not be the only transducer of seasonal cycles. The relative timing of cortisol and prolactin rhythms have also been proposed as mediators of certain seasonal changes in vertebrate behaviour and physiology (Meier *et al.*, 1971; Cincotta *et al.*, 1989; Meier and Cincotta, 1990), although this hypothesis has been challenged (Borer *et al.*, 1990).

In recent times people have become increasingly shielded from the geophysical environment, and data suggest that the amplitude of a number of seasonal rhythms has decreased from the last century to this (Aschoff, 1981a; Roenneberg and Aschoff, 1990a, 1990b). However, many seasonal rhythms are still observed in human populations. A large number of the neurobiological systems studied with respect to affective disorders demonstrate marked seasonal variation, including: central nervous system (CNS) neurotransmitters, neuroendocrine systems, sleep, temperature regulation and metabolism (for extensive review, see Lacoste and Wirz-Justice, 1989). Human subjects have maintained seasonality even when studied in an environment free from time cues (Wirz-Justice *et al.*, 1984).

Population statistics document that rates of depression, suicide and mania each continue to vary with time of year (Aschoff, 1981a; also see reviews in Carney *et al.*, 1989; Thompson, 1989; Wehr and Rosenthal, 1989). Circannual patterns have been of particular interest to investigators studying seasonal affective disorders (SAD), such as depressions that recur in some patients each autumn/winter (see below).

7.2.3 Formal properties

The output of the hypothalamic circadian pacemaker has not been measured directly in human subjects. Instead, variables known to be tightly regulated by the pacemaker, such as core body temperature, have been used to assess pacemaker functioning (Aschoff and Wever, 1962). These studies have confirmed that the human circadian timing system demonstrates the same basic properties as those previously observed in other organisms.

Current understanding of circadian principles and physiology has been well reviewed by several authors (see e.g. Wever, 1979, 1989; Czeisler *et al.*, 1987; Illnerová, 1988). Two properties are of concern here. First, under constant conditions (without external time cues) the period of an observed rhythm reflects the *intrinsic frequency* of the endogenous pacemaker. As shown in Figure 2, the circadian system in most human beings has a slightly longer than 24-h intrinsic frequency; thus, human subjects without time cues live on a nearly 25-h day. Outside of the laboratory, one common reflection of this internal periodicity may be the natural tendency of people to sleep later when

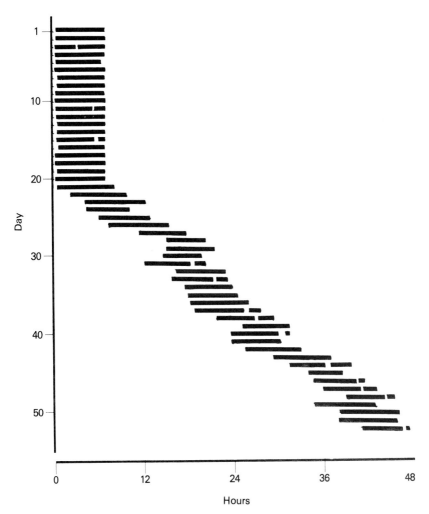

Figure 2 The timing of the sleep–wake cycle of a healthy young man who was initially synchronized to a 24-h cycle length (sleep allowed in dark from midnight to 7 a.m.) for 3 weeks, and who thereafter selected his own schedule with time cues eliminated from his environment. The ordinate presents time (hours) with reference to the habitual bedtime at home (time 0), as recorded in a diary during the preceding week. The abscissa presents successive days. Dark bars indicate time spent asleep in bed during the entrained and then the free-running segments of the experiment. The free-running period was about 25.3 h (Redrawn from data of Czeisler *et al.*, 1981a).

social conditions permit, such as on holidays and weekends (Borbély, 1984) (see Figure 3), or during student life at Oxford (Wirz-Justice and Pringle, 1987).

Second, the endogenous oscillations are influenced by environmental and by internal stimuli, thus giving the rhythms *entrainability* (Pittendrigh, 1979). The amount of shift in a rhythm after external perturbation (such as by a pulse of light) depends on the time in the circadian cycle at which the perturbation occurred. Systematic application of a stimulus at different circadian phases allows one to document this relationship, which can be summarized in a plot (Hastings and Sweeney, 1958) such as in Figure 4, that has come to be known as a phase response curve (PRC). The PRCs to light that have been obtained to date have similar characteristics across species (Pittendrigh, 1979; Czeisler *et al.*, 1989). Figure 4 illustrates the finding that light pulses are normally only effective in shifting circadian rhythms if they are presented between dusk and dawn. Light pulses given around dusk induce *phase delays* (shifts of the circadian cycle to a later time), while light pulses given around dawn induce *phase advances* (shifts of the circadian cycle to an earlier time) (Hastings and Sweeney, 1958; Pittendrigh, 1979; Czeisler *et al.*, 1986a, 1989; Illnerová *et al.*, 1989)[3]. The closer in time a light pulse is to the centre of the dark phase, the greater the magnitude of the phase shift that it will produce.

Recent experiments suggest that, throughout the phylogenetic tree, light also modifies the amplitude of oscillation in endogenous circadian pacemakers (Winfree, 1980; Czeisler *et al.*, 1987, 1989; Jewett *et al.*, 1991). It has been shown that light stimuli of specific intensity and timing can drive circadian pacemakers into virtual arrhythmicity (known theoretically as the point of 'singularity'; Winfree, 1980, 1987).

The shape and amplitude of a PRC is dependent on:

1. The circadian period of the underlying oscillator and the amplitude of its oscillation.
2. The sensitivity of the oscillator to the zeitgeber.
3. The strength of the zeitgeber.

Under natural conditions it is these characteristics which determine the exact phase relationships of rhythms to their entraining zeitgebers

---

[3] A study of the rest–activity cycle in free-running humans did not demonstrate phase delay shifts following bright light (Honma *et al.*, 1987a), but the validity of rest–activity as a circadian marker in humans has been questioned (Czeisler *et al.*, 1989). However a human PRC to a single bright light pulse has recently been obtained with both delays and advances (using the core temperature rhythm as a marker) (Minors *et al.*, unpublished data). More recent studies using a constant routine protocol to assess circadian phase changes following bright light exposure have also failed to find phase delays after evening exposures (Campbell and Dawson, 1990; Clodore *et al.*, 1990). The reason for the apparent discrepancy between these studies and those of Czeisler *et al.* (1989) are currently unknown.

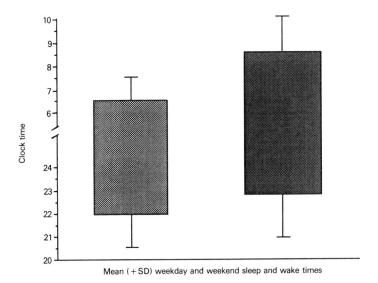

Figure 3 Tendency of people to sleep later when social conditions permit is reflected in the responses of 1000 residents of Switzerland, ages 15–74 years, who reported average sleep lengths of 7–8 h on weeknights (left) and 8–9 h on weekend nights (right). Those describing regular sleep habits, which was more frequently the case in older subjects, reported somewhat later mean times of going to bed on weekend nights and also later mean times of arising on weekend mornings, thus representing a phase delay as well as overall lengthening of sleep (Redrawn from data of Borbély, 1984).

(Pittendrigh, 1979; Aschoff, 1981b; Pittendrigh, 1981), and to one another (Wever, 1989). In human beings these parameters therefore play a major role in determining influential rhythms such as the timing of the sleep–wake cycle, daily times of maximal alertness and efficiency, cycles of mood, and also the peak (acrophase) and nadir of secretion of many hormones, including melatonin, cortisol, thyroid stimulating hormone and prolactin.

These principles have been used as a basis for hypotheses that implicate internal and external phase relationships in symptom formation of certain sleep and affective disorders. As discussed below in greater detail, circadian dysfunctions can be hypothesized to involve abnormalities of the period, phase or amplitude of the endogenous circadian pacemaker, relative insensitivity of the pacemaker to entraining stimuli, or decreased strength of zeitgeber inputs.

Any agent or situation that disrupts our intricately synchronizedphysiological cycles can have pervasive effects on health and behaviour. Phenomena such as jet lag reflect the acute and reversible effects of dramatic shifts in the timing pattern of environmental demands relative to internal circadian processes. The consequences of repeated, frequent disruptions can be extremely

233

HAMSTER PHASE RESPONSE CURVES

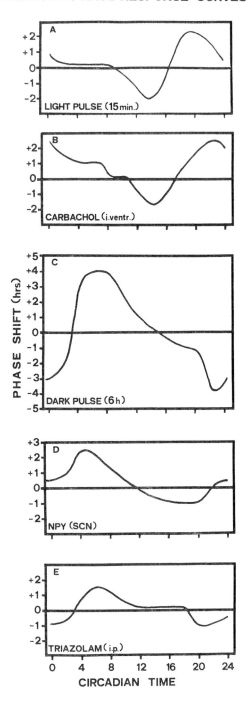

pernicious. As discussed below, a growing research literature on shiftwork documents the toll that is taken on physical and mental health, and in some circumstances the immediate danger of accidents that is created, when people are required to be alert and efficient at the circadian hours of physiological unpreparedness, the time when they are most susceptible to fatigue and error (Dinges *et al.*, 1989). Behavioural and environmental situations such as depression, confinement, or extremes of environmental temperature that result in persistent withdrawal from adequate light may also mediate dysfunctional circadian changes.

Measurement of the human PRC to light has provided information about the mechanism by which the non-24-h intrinsic period of the endogenous circadian oscillator is normally synchronized to the external 24-h light–dark cycle (Pittendrigh, 1979; Czeisler *et al.*, 1989). This PRC also provides a basis for evaluating the impact of specific light–dark (and to some extent sleep–wake) schedules on the circadian timing system.

Under normal circumstances, phase shifts need only result in a < 1-h advance per day in order to synchronize human circadian rhythms to the 24-h light–dark cycle. Human time-cue isolation studies have suggested that such adjustments can be accomplished by cycles of ordinary room light and darkness (Czeisler *et al.*, 1981b). Moreover, Aschoff and Wever (1981) have shown that certain individuals in time-isolation experiments maintain entrainment of their core body temperature rhythm to indoor light–dark cycles even though their sleep–wake cycle begins to free run.

Figure 4 Phase response curves (PRCs) summarize the shifts in circadian phase produced in hamsters by perturbations applied at different times in the circadian cycle. (**A**) In a standard plot of the PRC, the phase position of the perturbing stimulus (in this case a 15-min pulse of 100 lx light) is plotted on the ordinate, and the shift in circadian rhythms produced by the light pulse is plotted on the abscissa. Circadian time (CT) is a standardized measure, calculated by dividing the animal's free running period by 24 (CT 12 designates the beginning of the active phase for nocturnal rodents). Phase delays usually occur after a pulse in the early subjective night, between (CT 10–15 h), phase advances occur after a light pulse in the late subjective night (CT 16–24 h). During the subjective day, light has little or no effect, hence this area of the PRC is often referred to as the 'dead zone'. (**B**) The PRC to intraventricular application of carbachol mimics the PRC to a light pulse (Zatz and Herkenham, 1981; Earnest and Turek, 1985; Mistlberger and Rusak, 1986). (**C**) The PRC to a long dark pulse (Boulos and Rusak, 1982; Ellis *et al.*, 1982) shows a different timing of phase advances and delays than does the PRC to light. (**D**) The PRC to neuropeptide-Y (NPY) infused into the SCN (Albers and Ferris, 1984) shows similarities to the PRC produced by applications of a dark pulse. (**E**) The PRC to triazolam given i.p. (Rietveld and Wirz-Justice, 1986) also resembles the PRC to a dark pulse.

235

Recent studies indicate that to produce sizeable phase shifts of the human circadian pacemaker, *bright* light exposures, precisely timed, of relatively long duration, and perhaps in repeated pulses, may be required (Czeisler *et al.*, 1986a, 1989; Wever, 1989). Based on time-cue isolation experiments, where the light exposure history of human subjects could be quantified over a considerable time, Wever has concluded, '...light in the commonly used intensity range of artificial illumination has only marginal influence on human circadian rhythms...' (Wever, 1989, p. 173). Periods of exposure to dimmer light can modulate responses to bright light pulses. In the carefully controlled constant routine studies of Czeisler *et al.*, the timing and duration of room light exposures influenced the outcome of circadian-phase resetting protocols, just as did the timing of dark exposures (Czeisler *et al.*, 1989). In addition, bright light pulses administered in a daily series did not produce simple additive effects (see also, Strogatz, 1990). Results suggested that the ultimate phase-shifting effect of a series of bright light pulses in human subjects is dependent in part on the amplitude of oscillation of the circadian pacemaker (Czeisler *et al.*, 1989), as had previously been shown for other organisms.

During the 1980s, much of the clinical work on phototherapy for affective and related disorders focused on phase-shifting properties of light. However, any regimen of light exposure has other circadian effects as well (Wever, 1989). As reviewed below, more recent observations have enriched the analysis of light therapy with propositions concerning the role of endogenous circadian amplitude and also the role of variations in retinal sensitivity.

7.3 Sleep and depression

Sleep–wake behaviour is also a rhythmic daily cycle. Much of its function remains a mystery. During the past half-century, a great deal has been learned about the sleep process and questions have emerged regarding the relationship of the sleep–wake cycle to other circadian rhythms. This work has been of interest to students of affective disorders, since sleep disturbances are common in affectively disordered patients (e.g. see reviews by Reynolds, 1987; Reynolds and Kupfer, 1987; Wehr, 1988). Ironically, one of the most common sleep complaints in affective disorders is insomnia, yet sleep deprivation can be therapeutic, as discussed below.

Several different conceptual approaches have been taken in order to understand sleep and its relationship to affective disorders. Rapid eye movement (REM) sleep, first investigated in the 1950s (Aserinsky and

Kleitman, 1955) has been of interest to students of affective disorder for several reasons. Abnormalities of REM sleep are also among the features that have been described in many depressed patients (see reviews by Wehr and Wirz-Justice, 1982; Reynolds, 1987; Reynolds and Kupfer, 1987; Wehr, 1988), deprivation of REM sleep has been used as an antidepressant treatment (Vogel *et al.*, 1980), and, finally, REM has been suspected of playing a role in the relapse seen after sleep deprivation treatments (e.g. Riemann *et al.*, 1990; see also review by Wu and Bunney, 1990). One heuristic model has been proposed which relates the REM abnormalities frequently described in depressed patients to the functioning of brain stem noradrenergic and cholinergic neuronal systems that control the occurence of REM episodes (McCarley, 1982).

Other investigators have looked more specifically at possible circadian aspects of REM abnormalities. The propensity for REM sleep is known to have a circadian rhythm (e.g. Zulley, 1990). Under usual conditions, the greatest propensity for REM sleep in human subjects occurs later in the sleep episode, during early morning hours (Weitzman *et al.*, 1974; Hume and Mills, 1977; see also Avery, 1987). During the same hours, the endogenous circadian rhythm of core body temperature typically reaches its *minimum* (Czeisler *et al.*, 1980a, 1980b; Zulley *et al.*, 1981; see also hypothesis of Beersma *et al.*, 1984; and reviews by Avery, 1987; Wehr, 1989). The inevitability of their co-occurence has been disputed on the basis of data from entrained subjects (Lund *et al.*, 1984), and the physiological consequences of their interaction remains to be demonstrated. In fact, the relationship between REM propensity and the circadian temperature rhythm is only one aspect of the poorly understood, but clearly complex, temporal relationship between body temperature and the various components of sleep (e.g. Zulley *et al.*, 1981; Gillberg and Åkerstedt, 1982; Schulz and Lund, 1985; van den Hoofdakker and Beersma, 1985; Sewitch *et al.*, 1990; and see reviews of Avery, 1987; Beersma *et al.*, 1987; Wever, 1989; Wehr, 1989).

The proposed close temporal relationship between the rhythms of core body temperature and REM propensity is of particular interest, since, by contrast, the propensity to go to sleep is itself not as tightly regulated. In the classic studies of human circadian rhythms, including studies of temporal isolation carried out by Aschoff and Wever (Aschoff and Wever, 1962; Wever, 1975, 1989; Aschoff, 1979, 1981b), and later extended by Mills (Mills *et al.*, 1974) and Czeisler and Weitzman (Czeisler *et al.*, 1980a), the sleep–wake cycle often desynchronized from the circadian rhythm of body temperature (Aschoff *et al.*, 1967). Thus, healthy, euthymic subjects behaviourally exhibited very long or very short days, changing the length of time they remained awake and then slept, even while many of their circadian variables, including core temperature and REM propensity, continued to display near-24-h

237

rhythms, a process known as 'internal desynchronization' (Wever, 1989) (see Figure 5a).

Wever has modelled this phenomenon using two circadian oscillators. One drives the sleep–wake cycle; the other drives the rhythm of core body temperature and rhythms that maintain similar periods to that of core temperature even after desynchronization, such as melatonin, and REM sleep (Wever, 1975). As discussed below, this model and the desynchronization phenomena from which it was taken have influenced many circadian hypotheses of affective disorders.

The timing of REM sleep, non-REM sleep, and waking, and their relationship to the circadian timing system have also been modelled using

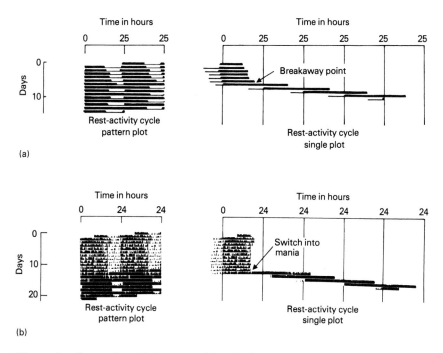

Figure 5 Comparison of the rest-activity rhythm: (**a**) in a control subject isolated from time cues (drawn on the 25-h timescale of a free running rhythm); with (**b**) a manic-depressive patient entrained to 24 h. A characteristic of many subjects in temporal isolation is the phenomenon of 'internal desynchronisation' between the sleep–wake and temperature cycles. This can develop into circabidian days (c. 50 h), as shown here. The pattern is strikingly similar to the spontaneous sleep deprivation exhibited by many depressed patients who then switch into mania (Wehr and Wirz-Justice, 1982; Wehr *et al.*, 1982), and can develop recurring 48-h cycles of sleepless nights, such as shown in the actogram. (Data from T.A. Wehr, with permission.)

one circadian oscillator (Daan *et al.*, 1988). This parsimonious model has been applied to the analysis of sleep disorders seen in patients with depression in the form of a two-process model of sleep regulation.

7.3.1 Two-process model of sleep regulation

In the two-process model of sleep regulation (Borbély, 1982; Daan *et al.*, 1988), although two oscillatory processes are incorporated, only one is a circadian pacemaker (process C) (Figure 6). This self-sustaining oscillator modulates the thresholds for sleep onset and termination. Sleep is represented by a relaxation oscillator, whose intensity increases with wake time and declines during sleep (process S). The interaction of these two processes is proposed to determine the timing and structure of sleep.

When applied to the sleep of patients with affective disorders, the model has suggested an impairment of process S in depression, rather than of the circadian pacemaker (Borbély and Wirz-Justice, 1982; Borbély, 1987). It has been hypothesized that process S accumulates too slowly in depressed patients. Resulting neurophysiological signals can therefore convey a false impression that sleep need is lower than it actually is, in some cases leading to frequent sleep interruptions or to early awakening. Since low amounts of process S are hypothesized to be associated with depression, sleep deprivation and the

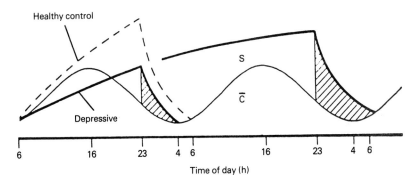

Figure 6   The two-process model of sleep regulation applied to the sleep of patients with affective disorders (Borbély and Wirz-Justice, 1982; Borbély, 1987). Two oscillatory processes are schematically represented with reference to the time of day (hours) over 48 h. Process C is a circadian pacemaker (a self-sustaining oscillator) that modulates the thresholds for sleep onset and termination. Process S is a relaxation oscillator whose intensity increases with wake time and declines during sleep (hatched areas). The interaction of these two processes determine the timing and structure of sleep. An impairment of process S in this model produces a sleep pattern with several features that are frequently found in the sleep of depressed patients.

resulting build-up of process S might be associated with normal or even euphoric mood. A further hypothesis based on traditional EEG scoring categories is that the weakened process S interacts reciprocally with REM propensity, hence accounting for both decreased REM latency and decreased amounts of stages 3 and 4 sleep seen in depressed patients. This has been empirically challenged (Schulz and Lund, 1985; van den Hoofdakker and Beersma, 1985). In addition, careful examination of EEG sleep stages, in some cases with concurrent core temperature measurements, have raised important questions about the nature and extent of circadian involvement in the REM abnormalities found in some depressed patients (Schulz and Lund, 1985; van den Hoofdakker and Beersma, 1985; Avery, 1987; von Zerssen, 1987; Buysse et al., 1990).

A second empirical measure that has been proposed for the assessment of process S is the power density in the delta band (0.25–4.00 Hz) of the EEG. Experimental tests of the Borbély and Wirz-Justice hypothesis using this parameter have yielded inconsistent results (see reviews in Wehr, 1988; Mendelson, 1989), and impaired sleep intensity in depression has not been found in all studies (Daan et al., 1984; Beersma et al., 1987). Efforts are underway to clarify this issue.

While debate continues regarding the most useful ways to conceptualize the interrelationships among circadian rhythms such as core body temperature and various aspects of sleep, one conclusion is clear. In considering the effects of stimuli such as light, dark, and drugs on circadian rhythmicity, care must be taken (and experiments appropriately planned) to differentiate effects on the circadian process from those on the sleep dependent process, and to evaluate the degree of their interaction.

The evidence presently available for the locus of the phase shifting effects of bright light indicates that they result from a direct action on the endogenous circadian pacemaker via the retina, and not from an action on sleep (Czeisler et al., 1981b, 1986a; Wever et al., 1983; Beersma et al., 1987; Czeisler and Allan, 1987; Dijk et al., 1987; Honma et al., 1987a, 1987b; Lewy et al., 1987).[4] The same appears to be true of the urinary melatonin rhythm (Wever, 1989).

Recent data on the temporal regulation of hormone secretion suggest that in the case of certain hormones, such as cortisol, the pulses of hormone released vary in amplitude in conjunction with the activity of the endogenous circadian oscillator, whereas they vary in frequency in association with events of the sleep–wake cycle (E. van Cauter et al., 1990, personal communication; also see Born et al., 1986).

---

[4] In some protocols sleep can have an indirect effect by modifying the light–dark cycle, if the subject has at least some light exposure, since when the subject's eyes are closed, his or her light exposure is thereby reduced (Carpenter and Grossberg, 1984).

When attempting to understand the behavioural and physiological effects of modifications in the timing of sleep itself, it can be particularly difficult to separate sleep-dependent from other circadian aspects of the manipulations. However, experimental and clinical evidence suggest that such an analysis may yield important insights. Modifications in the timing of sleep have been shown to have powerful clinical effects on affective disorders.

7.3.2 Changing the timing of sleep

In view of the prominence of insomnias in the symptom picture of depressions, it may appear paradoxical that after deprivation of sleep, a rapid (although usually transient) improvement is often seen in symptoms of major depression, including in sleep symptoms (Schulte, 1959; Pflug and Tölle, 1971; Kuhs and Tölle, 1986; van den Hoofdakker et al., 1990). This phenomenon has recently been reviewed by Wu and Bunney (1990), who found that 59% of patients among 1700 in the research literature of the past 21 years demonstrated a marked decrease in depressive symptoms following a night of total sleep deprivation. The percentage was higher among those with a more endogenous depression, regardless of unipolar versus bipolar diagnosis, and particularly marked among those with classic diurnal mood variation (Haug, 1990 (personal communication); Reinink et al., 1990a, 1990b). Among unmedicated patients, 83% of sleep deprivation responders went on to relapse after the first night of sleep.

Data also suggest that it is the timing, rather than the amount of sleep deprivation that is crucial. Whereas partial sleep deprivation in the first half of the night has little effect, partial sleep deprivation in the second half of the night has been found to produce improvements in mood which are equivalent to those produced by total sleep deprivation (Schilgen and Tölle, 1980; Götze and Tölle, 1981; Sack et al., 1988). Models that attempt to account for the antidepressant effects of sleep deprivation were also reviewed by Wu and Bunney (1990). One hypothesis is that wakefulness in the second half of the night is more important for antidepressant action than is reducing the number of hours slept. This is further supported by the finding that remissions in depression can be induced by abruptly phase advancing the sleep episode by several hours (Wehr et al., 1979; Elsenga and van den Hoofdakker, 1985; Sack et al., 1985; Souêtre et al., 1987). These observations have led to suggestions that there may be a critical circadian interval during which wakefulness can allow a patient to switch out of depression (Wehr and Wirz-Justice, 1981). Since depression often returns when the individual next goes to sleep, some investigators suspect that there is an aspect of sleep which can have depressogenic effects in susceptible individuals (Wehr and Wirz-Justice, 1981, 1982; Borbély and Wirz-Justice, 1982; see also reviews in Wehr,

1988; Wehr and Rosenthal, 1989; Wu and Bunney, 1990). In addition, it appears that sleep deprivation may be a precipitant of manic episodes. This has led to suggestions that some aspect of prolonged wakefulness may be euphorogenic (Wehr *et al.*, 1987; Wu and Bunney, 1990).

The clinical course and rest–activity cycle of a bipolar patient who undertook serial sleep deprivations and also phase advance of her sleep–wake cycle is documented in Figure 7.

The mechanisms underlying such profound and immediate clinical changes are currently unknown. One important line of ongoing research concerns the thermoregulatory impact of sleep deprivation (Wehr *et al.*, 1989b). In addition, the optimal parameters for clinical use of alterations in sleep timing need to be defined (Southmayd *et al.*, 1985; Wiegand *et al.*, 1987; Giedke, 1988; Southmayd and David, 1989, 1990). For instance, the length of time awake appears to affect the antidepressant response. Two hours of wakefulness in the second half of the night has been reported to have a mild therapeutic effect, whereas 4 h were fully effective (Giedke, 1988). Repetition of sleep deprivation (or partial deprivation) on successive nights may enhance its effectiveness (Holsboer-Trachsler *et al.*, 1988; Sack *et al.*, 1988). Finally,

Figure 7 Comparison of the clinical state and the circadian rest–activity cycle in a manic-depressive woman (bipolar II, 57 years old) for 125 consecutive days. This long-term study illustrates the close relationship of mood state to manipulations of sleep. Left: daily behavioural ratings of depth of depression or mania that were made by experienced nursing staff on a standardized scale. Right: Data from a wrist activity monitor that was worn continuously (with data collected in 15-min bins) plotted as an actogram. The *x* axis is a time scale of 24 h (7 a.m.–7 a.m.). The rhythms of successive days are plotted beneath one another. The entire display is double-plotted to the right to facilitate perception of the overall pattern across time. Thus, two broad, dark vertical bands result from high activity during the daytime; two light vertical bands result from low levels of activity during sleep. Daytime activity levels are higher (darker) during mania compared with depression. The succession of clinical states is summarized on the far right. The following manipulations of sleep were studied: (1) while the patient was depressed, total sleep deprivation (appearing in the actogram as continuation of activity throughout the former sleep phase) was carried out on each of 5 nights during consecutive weeks, in each case followed by partial or complete improvement of depressive symptoms that lasted only 1 day; (2) a phase shift (described in Wehr *et al.*, 1979) in which the sleep–wake cycle was advanced by 6 hours so that sleep occurred from 5 p.m. to 1 a.m; within a day of the phase advance, depression ratings started to decrease, and by the third day the patient was in remission; after a slightly hypomanic phase that was characterized by increased activity and lasted for 2 weeks, the patient relapsed again into depression; (3) a second phase advance was implemented (sleep time from 11 a.m. to 7 p.m.), with a similar remission; (4) an attempt was made at prophylactic phase advance before the relapse, but was unsuccessful. (Data from Wehr *et al.* (1979), T.A. Wehr with permission.)

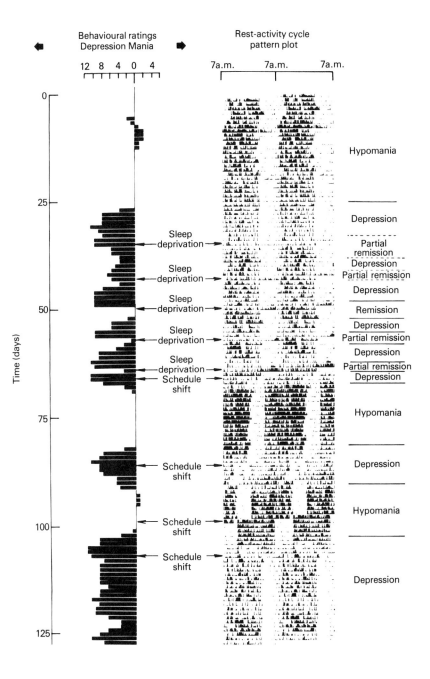

the combination of sleep deprivation or partial sleep deprivation with antidepressant pharmacotherapy has appeared in some patients to produce greater benefits than either treatment alone (Wirz-Justice *et al.*, 1979; Baxter *et al.*, 1986; Holsboer-Trachsler *et al.*, 1988).

No other treatment acts with such alacrity and efficacy on severe depression; therefore, sleep deprivation has also become an important theoretical focus of research (Wehr *et al.*, 1988). The advantage of this particular focus is that the depressive state, therapeutic response, and relapse all occur within a short span of time, making it practical to monitor closely neuroendocrinological parameters and sleep-related physiology. Furthermore, the basic manipulation is non-pharmacological, so a major source of physiological artifacts can be eliminated. This latter is also true of phototherapy manipulations.

A small literature has developed regarding the effects of artificial bright light exposure in healthy controls on sleep (Saletu *et al.*, 1986; Dijk *et al.*, 1987, 1989; Badia *et al.*, 1990; Benoit and Foret, 1990; Tzischinsky and Lavie, 1990) as well as on night-time core body temperature (Engelmann *et al.*, 1985; Badia *et al.*, 1990; Tzischinsky and Lavie, 1990). Careful naturalistic observations have suggested that daily changes in outdoor light exposure can have immediate effects on sleep (Kripke and Gregg, 1990). This is consistent with the finding that light therapy affects sleep duration and EEG architecture in hypersomnic patients with autumn/winter seasonal depression (Anderson *et al.*, 1990a). Following bright light treatment in these patients, sleep efficiency was improved and delta sleep increased, while density of REM was decreased. The effects of bright light exposure on sleep in other types of affective disorder have also begun to be studied (Dietzel *et al.*, 1986).[5]

7.4 Circadian models of affective disorders

Over the past few decades, clinical studies have been conducted to specify the types of circadian abnormalities manifested by patients with affective disorders. The results of basic chronobiological experiments have then been used to formulate hypotheses regarding possible circadian disturbances that could underlie the observed abnormalities. As discussed above, the articulation

[5] Although light therapy reduces daytime sleepiness in hypersomnic patients with autumn/winter seasonal depression, similar bright light treatment has not been found to benefit narcoleptics (Hajek *et al.*, 1987). However, studies of circadian physiology have led to the development of chronobiological treatments, including light therapy, for certain circadian-related disorders of sleep, described in greater detail below, such as delayed sleep phase syndrome, sleep disorders occuring at polar latitudes, and sleep disorders associated with blindness.

of formal properties of the circadian system has provided a basis for classifying possible rhythm disturbances.

For instance, the sleep–wake phase shift described by Georgi in depressed patients (1947) is a form of phase abnormality. Aschoff (1983) has succinctly summarized possible circadian disturbances that could underlie phase abnormalities in affective disorders; these are as follows: (1) partially or completely free-running rhythms; (2) shift of phase with clinical state; (3) stable phase advance or phase delay; and (4) instability of phase. These disturbances could arise from one or more modifications of the circadian system, shortened or lengthened period of the underlying pacemaker, reduced amplitude of pacemaker oscillation, increased or decreased sensitivity to light, and disturbed coupling between oscillators, or between oscillators and the light–dark cycle. The last has been discussed as a problem of appropriate entrainment (von Zerssen, 1987).

Although investigators have long been aware that the phases of certain events tends to be systematically abnormal in many depressed patients (such as with early morning awakening), more precise documentation of phase abnormalities has been difficult to obtain. This has complicated efforts to identify possible underlying circadian disturbances. It is known from the time–isolation studies discussed above that the core temperature minimum of healthy subjects under entrained conditions occurs near the end of sleep. As subjects live without time cues, this phase relationship is able to undergo a change: the sleep–wake cycle lengthens, and the time when core temperature is lowest advances towards the beginning of sleep. The temporal dissociation between these two rhythmic processes in healthy, euthymic subjects formed the basis for some circadian hypotheses of affective illnesses.

Temporal dissociation between rhythms can occur to varying degrees (e.g. Wever, 1989). Extreme temporal dissociation, such as occurs in internal desynchronization after circadian rhythms free run, has been used as a model for some circadian abnormalities in affective disorders. Halberg's internal desynchronization hypothesis concerned the switch process in rapidly-cycling bipolar illness (Halberg, 1968). These switches can occur with great temporal regularity. Halberg's hypothesis involved a proposed interaction between two circadian oscillators that had different periods, with one of them running unentrained. The interaction as these oscillating processes moved in and out of synchrony was hypothesized to account for the temporal pattern of mood shifts in rapidly-cycling bipolar illness. However, in subsequent studies few depressed patients have appeared to show free-running circadian rhythms (Kripke et al., 1978; Pflug et al., 1983; Pollak et al., 1989a, 1989b).

Disorders in which free-running rhythms have been implicated in the pathophysiology have been sleep rather than psychiatric disorders. For instance, free-running rhythms have produced phase or period abnormalities in blind subjects (Lund, 1974), who have only social and behavioural but not photic zeitgebers (these disorders are further discussed below). In the case of depressive disorders, a slightly different proposal, known as the phase advance hypothesis, has received more extensive research attention.

7.4.1 Phase advance hypothesis

Phase advance hypotheses address several abnormalities reportedly observed in depressed patients (see reviews by Kripke, 1983; Wehr and Goodwin, 1983). These include early acrophases of cortisol and prolactin secretion, early acrophase of oral temperature, and early onset of REM sleep. Several versions of the phase advance hypothesis (Papousek, 1975; Wehr *et al.*, 1979; Kripke, 1981, 1983; Wehr and Wirz-Justice, 1982) have involved a lesser degree of internal dissociation of rhythms, in which a persistent type of misalignment was maintained. While not suggesting complete internal desynchronization, the postulated phase advance of circadian rhythms associated with core temperature in entrained depressed patients was thought to be analogous to phase anomalies observed in healthy, euthymic subjects living for extended periods without time cues, as shown in Figure 5b.

This analogy has raised obvious questions: if an abnormal phase relationship is of causal significance, why haven't the healthy, euthymic subjects become depressed in temporal isolation; and why don't thousands of daily travellers across multiple time zones show depression or mania? Alternative explanations have been presented: (1) a conflict between the abnormal phase relationship and external zeitgebers is necessary; (2) an abnormal phase relationship is necessary but not sufficient for precipitating an affective disorder; and (3) the phase relationship in susceptible individuals has been such that they have slept during a 'depressogenic phase.' Data have accumulated which suggest that substantial phase shifts, either experimental or resulting from air travel, can precipitate mood changes of mild to clinical severity in individuals with a propensity or with previous episodes of affective illness (e.g. Taub and Berger, 1964; Siffre, 1975; Rockwell *et al.*, 1978; Jauhar and Weller, 1982; Surridge-David *et al.*, 1987).

An 'internal coincidence' model of depression (Wehr and Wirz-Justice, 1981), which ascribes clinical state to the simultaneous timing of a critical internal phase with the occurrence of a sleep episode, has been proposed to account for the purported circadian phase abnormalities and also explain the therapeutic effect of a variety of sleep interventions. Recent experiments to test the internal coincidence model suggest that there may not be a specific clock hour during which sleep will induce depression in all cases. In some, but not all, patients who had recovered from depression, a transient recurrence of clinical depression could be produced by imposing a delay in the timing of sleep (Surridge-David *et al.*, 1987; Southmayd and David, 1990). Further, relapse following an antidepressant response to sleep deprivation has been observed to occur at many different time points, and not always during or immediately after a subsequent sleep episode (Knowles *et al.*, 1979; Southmayd *et al.*, 1985; 1990, personal communication).

In addition, empirical tests of the phase advance hypothesis have been complicated, and the results, reviewed in detail elsewhere (Kripke, 1983; Wehr and Goodwin, 1983; Czeisler *et al.*, 1987; Checkley, 1989; Wehr, 1990a), have not been clearcut. Temporal isolation studies have not revealed evidence of circadian phase advance (Pollak *et al.*, 1989a). Some ambulatory recordings of core body temperature in entrained depressed patients appeared to show phase advances, however a great deal of intraindividual variation has been observed from day to day. Several non-circadian sources of core temperature variability, including sleep, are known to complicate data from the ambulatory studies. Therefore, a specific paradigm, known as the 'constant routine', has been used to control the 'masking' sources of temperature fluctuation experimentally in order to sharpen the assessment of the output of the endogenous circadian pacemaker in human subjects (Mills *et al.*, 1978; Minors and Waterhouse, 1984; Czeisler *et al.*, 1985).

We have recently used a 40-h constant routine procedure in the manner of Czeisler *et al.* to study endogenous circadian phase and amplitude in a hospitalized 60-year-old man suffering from severe non-seasonal recurrent major depressive disorder (Anderson *et al.*, 1990b). As shown in Figure 8, this preliminary investigation did not produce evidence of phase advanced circadian rhythms. However, this single case observation remains to be replicated.

7.4.2 Phase delay hypothesis

In contrast to possible phase advances in patients with non-seasonal major depressions, it has also been suggested that the output of the endogenous circadian pacemaker in many autumn/winter seasonal depressives is phase delayed, especially with respect to the timing of the sleep–wake cycle (Lewy *et al.*, 1985). Lewy proposed that patients should undergo a circadian assessment and be 'phase typed' in order to determine the appropriate light therapy regimen for them (Lewy *et al.*, 1985; Lewy and Sack, 1989). Using the time of onset of the nightly melatonin rise, measured in a dim light environment, as an indicator of circadian phase position, Lewy *et al.* concluded that the majority of their winter depression patients were phase delayed. On the basis of the PRC to light, it was held that light therapy should only be efficacious in such patients when given in the morning.

Lewy and colleagues found that early morning light therapy was effective

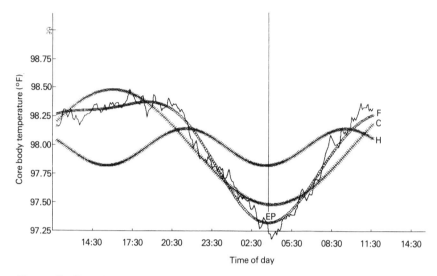

Figure 8 Rectal temperature recorded during a constant routine protocol in the manner of Czeisler *et al.* (1985) in a hospitalized 60-year-old man suffering from severe recurrent major depressive disorder (Anderson *et al.*, 1990b). The procedure of Brown and Czeisler (1985) was used to estimate the time of the circadian temperature minimum and the amplitude of the rhythm from a 24-h data train; one- (C) and two-harmonic (H) best-fit cosine curves and their composite (F) are shown in addition to the actual temperatures obtained. The time of the estimated minimum (04:15) was within the range observed in healthy control subjects of ages 65–73, and the amplitude of the rhythm (0.51°F) was quite robust for a man of this age (see e.g. Dumont *et al.*, 1990).

in treating the depression of these patients and also in advancing the phase of their melatonin rise (Lewy *et al.*, 1987, 1988). The phase delay in the rise time of melatonin rhythms in untreated patients with autumn/winter seasonal depression has been replicated (Terman *et al.*, 1988). In addition, one study using a 27-h constant routine protocol yielded evidence of delays in the phase of the core temperature and hormonal rhythms in depressed autumn/winter seasonal patients prior to phototherapy (Avery *et al.*, 1990; Dahl *et al.*, 1990). This was particularly important, since melatonin rise time has only recently been validated with respect to the tightness of its relationship to the output of the endogenous circadian pacemaker.

New data from healthy, euthymic subjects in a constant routine paradigm have suggested that the time of maximum melatonin secretion is an accurate marker of the output of the endogenous circadian pacemaker (Shanahan, 1990). The time of the fitted maximum of the melatonin curve was highly correlated with the time of the fitted minimum of the core body temperature rhythm, and their *phase angle* (relative timing of two cycling variables to each other, i.e. the amount of time that elapses between a given event on one rhythm and a specific event on the other rhythm) was maintained after large phase shifts induced by a bright light regimen. In contrast, the time of the melatonin rise was more variable with respect to the core body temperature minimum. Therefore, the circadian significance of the observed alterations in melatonin onset time in patients with autumn/winter depression remains to be fully clarified.

The phase delay hypothesis has been very influential. However, most of the early tests by other laboratories have been indirect, in that they were based on comparisons of light therapy treatments administered at different times of day. The results of these treatment studies are still controversial. As discussed below, morning light seems to be most effective overall (see meta-analysis of Terman *et al.*, 1989). However, substantial improvement has been demonstrated after light therapy given at other times of day (James *et al.*, 1985; Rosenthal *et al.*, 1985; Jacobsen *et al.*, 1987; Isaacs *et al.*, 1988; Wirz-Justice *et al.*, 1988; Anderson *et al.*, 1988; also see Wirz-Justice and Anderson, 1990). Moreover, as discussed below, exclusive responsivity to early morning light may not be required theoretically in order to account for improvements following light therapy, even if a phase delay is pathophysiologically important.

The phase delay hypothesis as articulated by Lewy *et al.* has focused on a putative abnormality of the phase angle between the sleep–wake rhythm and the rhythm of core body temperature (Lewy, 1990). The core temperature:sleep–wake phase angle has been implicated in the pathophysiology of non-seasonal depressive disorders (Kripke, 1983), as discussed above. This particular phase angle has not yet been closely tied to the actual symptoms of depressive disorders, and the pathophysiological basis of the proposed circadian phase delay in autumn/winter seasonal depression remains to be established.

7.4.3 Amplitude reduction hypothesis

Although photoperiodism and phase shifting effects of light have been at the centre of attention in recent years, it has long been known that light produces other effects on the circadian timing system as well. The recent unexpected discovery of the role of endogenous-oscillator amplitude in the human PRC to light (Czeisler *et al.*, 1987, 1989) raised the possibility that it is the amplitude enhancing effects of light therapy that are fundamental to its antidepressant efficacy (Czeisler *et al.*, 1987).

Several investigators have reported decreases in circadian amplitude among their non-seasonal depressed patients (e.g. Avery *et al.*, 1982; Lund *et al.*, 1983; Souêtre *et al.*, 1988, 1989; Tsujimoto *et al.*, 1990; see also review by Czeisler *et al.*, 1987). However, these studies measured core temperature in patients who were free to move about and who slept at night. Consequently, it is not clear to what extent the changes measured in their temperature were produced by different physical activities and by the impact of the sleep process and its timing (Czeisler *et al.*, 1987). Depressed subjects studied in temporal isolation had elevated daily core temperatures and plasma cortisol levels, but their circadian waveform and amplitude did not differ from those of control subjects (Pollak *et al.*, 1989b).

Data from our preliminary 40-h constant routine study of endogenous circadian phase and amplitude in a non-seasonally depressed patient, described above (Figure 8), has also failed to demonstrate a decrease in the amplitude of the core temperature rhythm during depression (Anderson *et al.*, 1990). However, this preliminary finding also remains to be confirmed.

7.5 Seasonal affective disorders

Seasonal affective disorders (SAD), known to earlier generations, have recently been rediscovered by Western medicine (Wehr, 1989; Wehr and Rosenthal, 1989). The most extensively studied seasonal pattern consists of recurrent depressive episodes in autumn and winter, alternating with euthymia or hypomania in spring and summer (Rosenthal *et al.*, 1985, 1988b). The autumn/winter SAD occurs in both northern and southern hemispheres (Rosenthal *et al.*, 1985; Wirz-Justice *et al.*, 1986; Boyce and Parker, 1988) and at a range of longitudes (Takahashi, 1989). The autumn/winter seasonal depressive episode is most frequently reflected in excessive fatigue as well as a number of so-called 'atypical' vegetative symptoms: increased sleep and appetite, carbohydrate craving and weight gain.

The seasonal rhythms of mood, sleep and weight changes seen in SAD patients resemble seasonal behaviours such as hibernation, seen in animals (Giedke, 1986). This led to the hypothesis that extension of the photoperiod in winter could lead to simulation of summer behaviour. Bright white light has indeed been found efficacious (Terman *et al.*, 1989), but photoperiod extension not necessary (e.g. see review in Rosenthal *et al.*, 1988b).

Light is a rapid (often within 3–4 days) and powerful treatment for winter depression. Recent work suggests that there is a dose–response relationship (Wirz-Justice *et al.*, 1987; J.S. Terman *et al.*, 1990), and brighter lights have begun to be tested (J.S. Terman *et al.*, 1990). There also appears to be an intensity–duration relationship, with briefer exposure times necessary at higher intensities. Further improvements in efficacy are likely to be forthcoming as the optimal procedural parameters are further clarified.

In addition to the phase delay hypothesis, discussed above, the pathophysiology of autumn/winter seasonal depression has been hypothesized to be related to serotonergic functioning. One of the frequent symptoms of autumn/winter SAD patients is carbohydrate craving (Rosenthal *et al.*, 1985, 1987). High carbohydrate intake can improve mood (Spring *et al.*, 1987), perhaps by increasing serotonin turnover (Wurtman and Wurtman, 1989). The higher carbohydrate intake in autumn/winter seasonal depression has been hypothesized to be an attempt at self-medication. It has been found that light therapy decreases carbohydrate intake (Kräuchi and Wirz-Justice, 1988). In addition, *d*-fenfluramine, a serotonergic releasing drug used to treat carbohydrate-related overeating (Wurtman *et al.*, 1985), has been reported by one laboratory to be as effective as light in treating autumn/winter depression, and in those patients it also decreased carbohydrate consumption (O'Rourke *et al.*, 1987, 1988). Investigations regarding serotonin continue (most recently summarized by Skwerer *et al.*, 1988). However, their relationship to circadian processes remains to be elucidated. Serotonergic innervation of the SCN has been documented, but its function remains unclear. Perhaps one clue to its possible role in the rhythmicity of autumn/winter depression is the observation that carbohydrate craving and consumption by these patients has a diurnal pattern, with most occurring in the second half of the day (Kräuchi *et al.*, 1990).

The effects of melatonin on autumn/winter SAD have also been tested. Originally it was hypothesized that melatonin might mediate symptom formation by functioning as a transducer of photoperiodic information. Given at dusk, melatonin reinstated only some of the symptoms that had previously improved after light (Rosenthal *et al.*, 1985). Furthermore, blockade of melatonin synthesis by systemic atenolol treatment did not generally impove symptoms in a group of patients with autumn/winter seasonal depression (Rosenthal *et al.*, 1988a).

Melatonin has also been tested as a treatment. If patients with autumn/winter seasonal depression have phase delayed circadian rhythms, and if phase advance is the mechanism of therapeutic response, then an advance produced by melatonin treatment might bring concomitant mood improvement. Given in the morning or at night (7 a.m. or 11 p.m.), we have found neither positive (antidepressant) nor negative effects of melatonin in patients with autumn/winter seasonal depression (Wirz-Justice *et al.*, 1990). However, the timing of treatment may not have been optimal. In animals, the circadian window for the phase advancing effects of melatonin is extremely narrow (Armstrong and Chesworth, 1987). The description of a human PRC to melatonin (Lewy *et al.*, 1990; Sack *et al.*, 1990) may be helpful in further studies. Preliminary positive results with light have been found in persons with seasonality of vegetative and mood symptoms that do not reach the severity of a major affective disorder (Kasper *et al.*, 1989; Wirz-Justice *et al.*, 1989; L. Zborowski *et al.*, personal communication). Random sample surveys of the general population in the eastern USA have suggested that about 15% experience some degree of problematic seasonal changes, while roughly 4% seasonally meet criteria for major depression (Rosen *et al.*, 1990). Thus, the full impact of light therapy's benefits may prove to be substantial. However, bright light exposure has *not* been found to improve mood in non-depressed individuals.

The most recent hypotheses regarding autumn/winter seasonal depression have involved putative changes in retinal sensitivity. Basic studies of circadian physiology have demonstrated that phase delays in an entrained rhythm can result from weakening of an entraining zeitgeber. One mechanism for a change in zeitgeber strength is an alteration in the sensitivity of relevant receptor systems. Autumn/winter seasonal depression may be linked to a deficiency in retinal photoreceptor renewal mechanisms, resulting in subsensitivity to light (Remé *et al.*, 1990). However, precisely the opposite has been proposed by Beersma (1990). There is as yet insufficient ophthalmological data in untreated patients to provide firm support for either hypothesis.

The proposed pathophysiological involvement of alterations in retinal sensitivity is not necessarily exclusive of other hypotheses mentioned above regarding autumn/winter seasonal depression, contrary to the suggestion of some authors (e.g. Lewy, 1990). In the multidisciplinary world of neuroscience, it is important to distinguish alternative hypotheses from hypotheses operating at different levels of analysis.

In fact, retinal subsensitivity could reconcile (1) the experimental observations of phase delays in many patients with autumn/winter seasonal depression, with (2) the additional observation that light therapy at many times of day can be effective. While high-intensity morning light exposures appear necessary to produce a substantial advance shift in the phase of the endogenous circadian oscillator, it might be possible to bring about a smaller phase shift in entrained rhythms simply by strengthening the zeitgeber:pacemaker interaction. The photoreceptor renewal hypothesis suggests one mechanism for such a strengthening that does not prescribe only early morning light as a means to achieve it. If phase drifts occur in response to a weakened zeitgeber:pacemaker interaction, with rhythms moving in the direction of their intrinsic period, then any strengthening of the zeitgeber:pacemaker connection might result in movement of the core temperature and melatonin rhythms toward a 24-h period, producing a small apparent advance.

7.6 Chronotherapies

7.6.1 Potential applications

Several potential applications of chronotherapy have already been identified:

Non-seasonal major depression. The success of light therapy for autumn/winter seasonal depression has intensified efforts to treat other affective disorders using phototherapy. Although initial positive reports on light treatment for non-seasonal depression (Kripke *et al.*, 1983a, 1983b) have been followed up (Dietzel *et al.*, 1986; Peter *et al.*, 1986; Wirz-Justice, 1986; Yerevanian *et al.*, 1986; Fleischhauer *et al.*, 1987; Kripke *et al.*, 1987; Asano *et al.*, 1988; Heim, 1988; Prasko, 1988; Schwitzer *et al.*, 1989; Volz *et al.*, 1990), some investigators have reported only a minimal response. This remains a controversial issue (Kripke, 1985).

Investigations of out-patients with atypical depressions, who had many of the same vegetative symptoms as autumn/winter depressed patients but no seasonality, did not find the treatment to be effective (Stewart *et al.*, 1990; B.I. Yerevanian *et al.*, unpublished data). These negative findings in controlled studies of non-seasonal syndromes could constitute evidence for the specificity of light's therapeutic effect to particular forms of affective disorder. Alternatively, it may be that quite different light therapy parameters will be required to treat affective disorders other than autumn/winter seasonal depression.

Shift work. An abundance of gastrointestinal, cardiovascular, behavioural, sleep, mood and marital disturbances have been described in shift workers (e.g. see reviews in Dumont, 1988; Czeisler *et al.*, 1990), some of which appear to persist even for years (Dumont *et al.*, 1988). The disturbances produced by rotating shifts may be reduced in several ways. Rotation schedules can be redesigned to produce less circadian disruption and to facilitate adaptation (e.g. see Turek, 1986). Sleep schedules can be optimized (e.g. see Åkerstedt *et al.*, 1990).

In addition, a strong zeitgeber can be used to facilitate a complete shifting of circadian rhythms. For example, a nurse on weekly rotating shifts came to us complaining of reduced and disturbed sleep and depressive symptoms. We were able to stabilize her rest–activity cycle and improve her mood using 1 h exposure to bright light upon her waking and prior to sleep, a so-called 'skeleton photoperiod' paradigm (A.W.J., unpublished data). Successful circadian adaptation to simulated shift-work schedules have recently been reported by other laboratories using different bright light regimens (Czeisler *et al.*, 1990; Eastman, 1991). Melatonin has also been successfully used with shift workers in a preliminary study (Armstrong *et al.*, 1986).

Jet lag. The speed of jet travel brings not only the transition of cultures, but also the physiological shock of time zone shifts. The use of bright light to re-entrain circadian rhythms after transmeridian flights is an obvious application of the theoretical studies (Daan and Lewy, 1984; Wever, 1985; Armstrong *et al.*, 1986; Redfern, 1989). In addition, double-blind studies of oral melatonin administration after an 8- or 10-h eastward, and 10-h westward time zone shift demonstrated that subjectively-related symptoms of jet lag were minimal in those taking melatonin while remaining significant in those who took placebo. Melatonin was also associated with an improvement in sleep (Arendt *et al.*, 1986; Arendt and Aldhous, 1988; Petrie *et al.*, 1989).

Sleep disorders: delayed or advanced sleep phase syndrome, hypernychthermeral sleep–wake cycle disturbance, and sleep disorders in the blind. Indifference or insensitivity to zeitgeber cues may lead to phase delayed sleep patterns (e.g. unable to sleep before 2–3 a.m., unable to rise easily before noon; Miles *et al.*, 1977). The first description of this syndrome also introduced a novel non-pharmacological treatment: delaying the sleep–wake cycle until the required phase position had been reached (Czeisler *et al.*, 1981a). The success of this approach (Moldofsky *et al.*, 1986) suggested that circadian pathophysiology underlay the symptoms and demonstrated that a circadian manoeuvre could treat it. Light therapy in the morning is currently being evaluated as a phase advance therapy (Rosenthal *et al.*, 1990; A.W.J., unpublished data).

In the Arctic and Antarctic winter darkness, similar sleep disturbances have been observed. Studies have shown that artificial light was also able to resynchronize sleep patterns in those environments (Lingjärde *et al.*, 1985; Arendt and Broadway, 1986). A more rare syndrome is that of advanced sleep phase, for which limited tests of evening light have been conducted (Singer and Lewy, 1989; M. Berger and A. Wirz-Justice, unpublished data).

In addition to the above disorders involving entrainment of the sleep–wake cycle at abnormal phase positions, the disorder known as hypernychthermeral sleep–wake cycle disturbance represents a complete failure of entrainment of the sleep–wake cycle (Kokkoris *et al.*, 1978). Patients with this disorder have a free-running sleep–wake cycle even though exposed to standard 24-h time cues.

Disturbances in the timing of sleep are also often seen in the blind, and have been linked to circadian disturbances (Martens, 1990a; see also review by Martens, 1990b). Melatonin given in the early evening has been used to entrain sleep to an appropriate phase in a preliminary number of blind subjects (Sack and Lewy, 1988; Sarrafzadeh *et al.*, 1990), although it may also provide benefits via non-circadian mechanisms (Folkard *et al.*, 1990). Further studies are required to evaluate the efficacy of melatonin administration at bedtime for sleep (Arendt *et al.*, 1984).

Premenstrual syndrome. In late luteal phase dysphoric disorder (premenstrual syndrome), which also has a strong cyclic pattern, preliminary tests of circadian manipulations including phototherapy and sleep deprivation have been therapeutically successful (Parry and Wehr, 1987; Parry *et al.*, 1987, 1989). The circadian timing system is known to play a role in regulating human reproductive systems, although much remains to be elucidated regarding the mechanisms (see review by Parry, 1989).

Ageing. A pattern of naps during the day and more shallow sleep at night is a general phenomenon in older persons. Circadian studies have suggested that the period of the endogenous pacemaker is decreased in persons over age 65 (Czeisler *et al.*, 1986b). Decreased amplitude of oscillation has also been reported, and in some cases preliminary data suggest that phototherapy can be used to increase circadian amplitude, reset phase and improve sleep timing and quality (Dumont *et al.*, 1990).

7.6.2 Chronopharmacology

Chronobiological studies have demonstrated circadian rhythms in the responsivity of mammalian tissues to light, dark, and psychoactive drugs. The changes over 24 h are not trivial, and in many cases effectively present the pharmacologist with a different substrate for drug action at different times of day. This knowledge can lead to better timing of drug administration so as to reach the target system at its greatest sensitivity, and thus reduce dosage and minimize side-effects. Such applications of chronopharmacology can improve therapy with existing drugs (cf. Reinberg and Smolensky, 1983).

Antidepressant medications are subject to these general chronopharmacological considerations. In addition, it has been discovered that commonly used antidepressant or psychoactive drugs can affect several aspects of circadian rhythmicity. The formulation of circadian hypotheses regarding affective disorders led researchers to test mood stabilizing and antidepressant medications for possible circadian effects. Beginning with investigations of lithium administered to plants (Englemann, 1973), a substantial body of research has developed demonstrating that psychopharmacological agents (also including the monoamine oxidase inhibitor clorgyline, methamphetamine, and benzodiazepines) can modify phase, period or amplitude of circadian oscillations in a host of organisms (Engelmann, 1973; Craig *et al.*, 1981; Friedman and Yocca, 1981; Kafka *et al.*, 1982; McEachron *et al.*, 1982, 1985; Wirz-Justice, 1982, 1983, 1987; Wirz-Justice and Campbell, 1982; Wirz-Justice *et al.*, 1982a, 1982b; Kruse, 1986). Most of the compounds tested to date tend to delay the circadian phase and lengthen the period (see reviews by Wirz-Justice, 1987; Duncan and Wehr, 1988). However, possible effects on the mammalian pacemaker have not been thoroughly tested.

Although the primary site for circadian effects is the circadian pacemaker in the SCN, these drugs may be acting at more than one locus. In particular, all the above mentioned drugs act at the retina to modify the processing of light stimuli (Remé and Wirz-Justice, 1985; M. Terman *et al.*, 1990) and some have been shown to act on a secondary visual pathway to the SCN, via the lateral geniculate nucleus. Methamphetamine, in addition, acts on a food entrainable pacemaker (Honma *et al.*, 1989). Thus, many antidepressant drugs modify circadian timekeeping, or the sensitivity of the organism to light, via actions on the central nervous system.

7.6.3 Novel approaches

Chronobiology highlights the role of environmental variables that had been largely ignored by American and European psychiatry and medicine in this century (Wehr, 1989; Wehr and Rosenthal, 1989). As Wehr has emphasized, their rediscovery can also remind us of other possible environmental and behavioural analyses and interventions. For instance, warm temperatures may provoke some recurrent summer depressions (Wehr *et al.*, 1989a). Temperature manipulations, employed over the centuries in the treatment of certain affective disorders, are being reinvestigated in this context (Wehr, 1989; Wehr and Rosenthal, 1989).

A behavioural variable, diet, may be an adjunct mood elevator. Not only do carbohydrate (CHO)-rich diets increase tryptophan and central nervous system serotonin turnover, but CHO-rich diets can also improve mood and possibly sleep (Rosenthal and Heffernan, 1986; Stohler *et al.*, 1989; Davenne *et al.*, 1990). It is likely that research in the next few years will delineate many syndromes that respond selectively to environmental factors and behavioural manipulations.

7.7 A physiological approach

Finally, whereas modern biological hypotheses about affective disorders have often focused on the synaptic or intracellular rather than the organismic level of analysis (one recent exception being the work of Gold *et al.*, 1989), chronobiology has provided a framework for constructing a *physiological* biological approach. By this, we mean a description of the larger physiological systems associated with these syndromes, an approach which might bridge the gap between synaptic events and the symptoms experienced by depressed individuals.

In particular, physiological systems for energy metabolism and thermo-regulation hold promise for integrating existing information about mood disorders (Anderson, 1991). Such a connection has been touched on by numerous writers over the years (cf. Avery *et al.*, 1982; Rosenthal, 1986; Avery, 1987; Wehr, 1990). Among recognized symptoms of depression are 'fatigue or loss of energy' and 'psychomotor retardation'. Energy can be understood not only phenomenologically, but also at the level of organs, cells, and molecules: biochemical reactions transfer chemical energy from food to vital cellular activities, with a considerable loss of heat energy into the environment. The intricate physiological network by which these reactions are regulated is tied to the endogenous circadian pacemaker and intimately involved with the sleep–wake cycle (e.g. Wehr, 1989, 1990b; Wehr and Rosenthal, 1989; Wehr *et al.*, 1989b). Furthermore, these systems employ a neuroendocrine network that links many of the hormones and neurotransmitters which are known to function abnormally in individuals with depression.

Ongoing discoveries in chronobiological neuroendocrinology promise to flesh out the details of these relationships. For instance, the physiological role of REM sleep is the subject of a recent hypothesis by Wehr (1990b), who has amassed evidence suggesting that REM sleep serves to increase temperature in a small homeothermic core area consisting of the central nervous system and surrounding tissues. This represents one of the most direct examples of recent efforts to approach the chronobiological symptoms of depression in a functional, physiological way, by considering the complex neuroendocrino-logical networks subserving energy metabolism and thermoregulation as an integrative system (e.g. Gao *et al.*, 1989).

Multiple circadian rhythms, with differing strengths of coupling to the output of the endogenous pacemaker, are involved in these neuroendocrine networks. The relationship among these circadian rhythms can be described in part in terms of their phase angles. As we have seen, phase angle abnormalities have been suggested in the past to play a role in affective disorders, but more specific pathophysiological processes have not been identified. Endocrinological research has begun to elucidate the mechanisms by which fine-tuning of metabolic and temperature regulation is possible, in part, to the extent that a number of endogenous substances with different circadian patterns coordinate to affect a given cellular process. This has raised the possibility that disturbances in phase angles of circadian rhythms within the network of energy metabolism and thermoregulation might produce reversible dysfunctions in energy level, appetite, and related processes, and could account for some of their diurnal, catamenial and/or seasonal temporal patterns. Because these systems are so multiply-regulated (including input from gonadal steroids), dysfunctions may begin at different loci in different individuals, but homeostatic mechanisms within these systems could produce a range of compensatory dysfunctions in the network as a whole that would result in considerable overlap in the resulting symptom complexes.

The analysis of biological rhythms and affective disorders has an ancient legacy, but only recently has modern science begun to examine and incorporate its observations. This recent spurt has already produced provocative diagnostic concepts and potentially beneficial new forms of treatment. It also promises to add a powerful new dimension to our theoretical approaches. In particular, as we contemplate further the circadian organization of neuroendocrine networks which serve each day to coordinate diverse physiological activities throughout the body, we may be influenced to construct an integrative and physiological mode of inquiry that can help us to bridge further the conceptual gap between substrate, symptom, and syndrome.

7.8 Summary

Speculations about biological rhythm disturbances in affective disorders have been made repeatedly over the years because these disorders have temporal features, such as diurnal mood variation, changes in sleep architecture and timing, periodicity in the occurrence of episodes, and anomalies in patterns of hormone secretion.

Advances in experimental chronobiology have provided a framework for formulating and evaluating increasingly specific circadian hypotheses of mood disturbances. Studies of the neuroanatomy and neurochemistry of circadian timekeeping, the effects of light and dark on the circadian timing system and the modification of this system by psychoactive drugs, are providing an increasingly firm foundation for clinical investigations. Discoveries in basic circadian neuroscience have already informed the development of non-pharmacological treatment modalities, including light therapy for autumn/

winter seasonal depression and for circadian-related insomnias, melatonin for certain sleep disturbances, and sleep deprivation or shifts in sleep timing for affective disorders. Now, several circadian hypotheses of affective and sleep disorders have been tested using newly available technologies, and additional studies are underway.

The chronobiological approach has also revived intriguing questions regarding the role of inefficiencies and defects in physiological systems for energy metabolism and thermoregulation in the pathophysiology of affective disorders and related conditions. In this way, studies of circadian rhythms have fostered a type of *physiological* approach to the biology of affective disorders, in which larger physiological systems provide a conceptual bridge between events at the synaptic level and actual symptoms experienced by individuals. Although this is necessarily a complex undertaking, the potential to integrate data across a range of techniques and disciplines involved in affective disorders research is one of the most exciting aspects of the chronobiological approach.

Acknowledgements

This review is gratefully dedicated to our colleagues in chronobiology, in particular the patients and other research volunteers who are the unsung heroes and heroines in our joint effort to understand, treat and someday prevent affective disorders.

We greatly appreciate the comments of Drs Margaret F. Jensvold, Elizabeth B. Clark, Karla Moras; and researchers at the Laboratory for Circadian and Sleep Disorders Medicine: Dr James S. Allan, Dr Marie Dumont, Dr Heinz Martens, Ms Megan Jewett and Ms Theresa Shanahan. The Swiss National Science Foundation (SNF No. 3.883-0.83, 3.870-0.85, 3.821-0.86) has generously supported our studies of the clinical applications of light and melatonin. Dr Anderson has been supported by a grant from the Horten Stiftung and a Swiss National Science Foundation exchange fellowship (No. 83NI-028030).

References

Åkerstedt, T., Gillberg, M. & Kecklund, G. (1990) In *Sleep '90* (ed. Horne, J.A.), pp 329–331. Bochum, Pontenagel Press.
Albers, H. & Ferris, C. (1984) *Neurosci. Lett.* **50**, 163–168.
Anderson, J.L. (1991) *5th World Congress of Biological Psychiatry*, Florence, Italy; Symposium 18, Abstract in press.
Anderson, J.L., Rosen, L.N., Mendelson, W.B. *et al.* (1990a) submitted.

Anderson, J.L., Vasile, R.G., Bloomingdale, K.L. & Schildkraut, J.J. (1988) *American Psychiatric Association*, Annual Meeting, Montreal, Canada. New Research Abstract 166.

Anderson, J.L., Wirz-Justice, A., Holsboer-Trachsler, E. *et al.* (1990b) *Society for Light Treatment and Biological Rhythms*, 2nd Annual Meeting, New York, Abstract 31.

Arendt, J. (1989) *Br. J. Psychiatry* **155**, 585–590.

Arendt, J. & Aldhous, M. (1988) *Ann. Rev. Chronopharmacol.* **5**, 53–55.

Arendt, J. & Broadway, J. (1986) *J. Physiol.* **377**, 68P.

Arendt, J. & Broadway, J. (1987) *Chronobiol. Intern.* **4**, 273–282.

Arendt, J., Borbély, A.A., Franey, C. & Wright, J. (1984) *Neurosci. Lett.* **45**, 317–321.

Arendt, J., Aldhous, M. & Marks, V. (1986) *Br. Med. J.* **292**, 1170.

Arendt, J., Broadway, J., Folkard, S. & Marks, M. (1989) In *Seasonal Affective Disorder* (eds Thompson, C. & Silverstone, T.), pp 133–143. London, Clinical Neuroscience.

Armstrong, S.M. (1989) *Pineal Res. Rev.* **7**, 157–202.

Armstrong, S.M. & Chesworth, M.J. (1987) *Colloquium: European Pineal Study Group*, Abstract IV, 26.

Armstrong, S.M., Cassone, V.M., Chesworth, M.J., Redman, J.R. & Short, R.V. (1986) *J. Neural Transm.* **21** (Suppl.), 375–394.

Asano, Y., Honma, K. & Honma, S. (1988) *Collegium Internationale Neuro-Psychopharmacologicum.* Munich, Germany. Abstract 34.07.04.

Aschoff, J. (1979) *Zeitschr. Tierpsychol.* **49**, 225–249.

Aschoff, J. (1981a) In *Handbook of Behavioral Neurobiology* vol. 4 (ed. Aschoff, J.), pp 475–487. New York, Plenum Press.

Aschoff, J. (1981b) In *Handbook of Behavioral Neurobiology* vol. 4 (ed. Aschoff, J.), pp 81–93. New York, Plenum Press.

Aschoff, J. (1981c) In *Handbook of Behavioral Neurobiology* vol. 4 (ed. Aschoff, J.), pp 3–10. New York, Plenum Press.

Aschoff, J. (1983) In *Circadian Rhythms and Psychiatry* (eds Wehr, T.A. & Goodwin, F.K.), pp 33–39. Pacific Grove CA, Boxwood Press.

Aschoff, J. & Wever, R. (1962) *Naturwissenschaften* **49**, 337–342.

Aschoff, J. & Wever, R. (1981) In *Handbook of Behavioral Neurobiology* vol. 4 (ed. Aschoff, J.), pp 311–331. Plenum Press.

Aschoff, J., Gerecke, U. & Wever, R. (1967) *Jpn. J. Physiol.* **17**, 450–457.

Aserinsky, E. & Kleitman, N. (1955) *J. Appl. Physiol.* **8**, 1–10.

Avery, D. (1987) In *Chronobiology and Psychiatric Disorders* (ed. Halaris, A.S.), pp 75–101. New York, Elsevier.

Avery, D.H., Wildschiødtz, G. & Rafaelsen, O.J. (1982) *J. Affective Disord.* **4**, 61–71.

Avery, D.H., Dahl, K., Savage, M. *et al.* (1990) *Biol. Psychiatry.* **27**, 99a.

Badia, P., Boecker, M. & Myers, B. (1990) *European Sleep Research Society, 10th Congress*, Strasbourg, France, Abstract, p. 75.

Bassi, C.J. & Powers, M.K. (1986) *Physiol. Behav.* **38**, 871–877.

Baxter, L.R., Liston, E.M., Schwartz, J.M. *et al.* (1986) *Psychiat. Res.* **19**, 17–23.

Beck-Friis, J., von Rosen, D., Kjellman, B.F., Ljunggren, J.-G. & Wetterberg, L. (1984) *Psychoneuroendocrinology* **9**, 261–277.

Beersma, D.G.M., Daan, S. & van den Hoofdakker, R.H. (1984) *Sleep* **7**, 126–136.

Beersma, D.G.M., Daan, S. & Dijk, D.J. (1987) *Lect. Math. Life Sci.* **19**, 39–62.

Beersma, D.G.M. (1990) *Arch Gen. Psychiatry* **47**, 879–880.

Benoit, O. & Foret, J. (1990) In *Sleep '90* (ed. Horne, J.A.), pp 337–339. Bochum, Pontenagel Press.

Berger, M., Wiegand, M. & Riemann, D. (1990) In *Sleep '90* (ed. Horne, J.A.), Dortmund, Pontenagel Press (in press).

Bohlen, J.G. (1979) *Yearbook of Physical Anthropology* **22**, 47.

Bojkowski, C.J. & Arendt, J. (1988) *Acta Endocrinol.* **117**, 470–478.

Bojkowski, C.J., Aldhous, M.E., English, J. *et al.* (1987) *Horm. Metab. Res.* **19**, 437–440.

Borbély, A.A. (1982) *Hum. Neurobiol.* **1**, 195–204.

Borbély, A.A. (1984) *Schweiz. Aerztezeitung.* **65**, 1606–1613.

Borbély, A.A. (1987) *Pharmacopsychiatry* **20**, 23–29.

Borbély, A.A. & Wirz-Justice, A. (1982) *Hum. Neurobiol.* **1**, 205–210.

Borer, K.T., Johnson, P., Brosammer, M.B., Swaz, U. & Thompson, M.V. (1990) *Society for Research on Biological Rhythms, 2nd Annual Meeting*, Jacksonville FL, Abstract 125, p. 84.

Born, J., Kern, W., Bieber, K., Fehm-Wolfsdorf, G., Schiebe, M. & Fehm, H.L. (1986) *Biol. Psychiatry* **21**, 1415–1424.

Boulos, Z. & Rusak, B. (1982) *J. Comp. Physiol.* **146**, 411–417.

Boyce, P. & Parker, G. (1988) *Am. J. Psychiatry* **145**, 96–99.

Brown, E.N. & Czeisler, C.A. (1985) *Sleep Res.* **14**, 290.

Bünning, E. (1935) *Jahrb. viss Botan.* **8**, 411–418.

Burton, R. (1638) *The Anatomy of Melancholy by Democritus Junior*, 5th edn. Oxford, Henry Cripps.

Buysse, D.J., Jarrett, D.B., Miewald, J.M., Greenhouse, J.B., Kupfer, D.J. & Reynolds, C.F. III. (1990) *European Sleep Research Society, 10th Congress*, Strasbourg, France, Abstract, p. 38.

Campbell, S.S. & Dawson, D. (1990) *Society for Research on Biological Rhythms, 2nd Annual Meeting*, Jacksonville FL, Abstract 67.

Campbell, S.S., Kripke, D.F., Gillin, J.C. & Hrubovcak, J.C. (1988) *Physiol. Behav.* **42**, 141–144.

Carney, P.A., Fitzgerald, C.T. & Monaghan, C. (1989) In *Seasonal Affective Disorder* (eds Thompson, C. & Silverstone, T.), pp 19–27. London, Clinical Neuroscience.

Carpenter, G.A. & Grossberg, S. (1984) *Am. J. Physiol.* **247**, R1067–1082.

Checkley, S. (1989) In *Biological Rhythms in Clinical Practice* (eds Arendt, J., Minors, D.S. & Waterhouse, J.M.), pp 160–183. London, Butterworth.

Cincotta, A.H., Wilson, J.M., de Souza, C.J. & Meier, A.H. (1989) *J. Endocrinol.* **120**, 385–391.

Clodore, M., Foret, J., Aguirre, A., Touitou, Y. & Benoit, O. (1990) *European Sleep Research Society, 10th Congress*, Strasbourg, France, Abstract, p. 71.

Craig, C., Tamarkin, L., Garrick, N. & Wehr, T. (1981) *Soc. Neurosci.* Abstract 719.

Cummings, F.W. (1975) *J. Theor. Biol.* **55**, 455–470.

Czeisler, C.A. & Allan, J.S. (1987) *Sleep Res.* **16**, 605.

Czeisler, C.A., Allan, J.S., Strogatz, S.H. *et al.* (1986a) *Science* **233**, 667–671.

Czeisler, C.A., Brown, E.N., Ronda, J.M., Kronauer, R.E., Richardson, G.S. & Freitag, W.O. (1985) *Sleep Res.* **14**, 295.

Czeisler, C.A., Johnson, M.P., Duffy, J.F., Brown, E.N., Ronda, J.M. & Kronauer, R.E. (1990) *N. Engl. J. Med.* **322**, 1253–1259.

Czeisler, C.A., Rios, C.D., Sanchez, R. *et al.* (1986b) *Sleep Res.* **15**, 268.

Czeisler, C.A., Kronauer, R.E., Allan, J.S. *et al.* (1989) *Science* **244**, 1328–1333.

Czeisler, C.A., Kronauer, R.E., Mooney, J.J., Anderson, J.L. & Allan, J.S. (1987) *Psychiatr. Clin. North Am.* **10**, 687–709.

Czeisler, C.A., Richardson, G.S., Coleman, R.M. *et al.* (1981a) *Sleep* **4**, 1–21.

Czeisler, C.A., Richardson, G.S., Zimmerman, J.C., Moore-Ede, M.C. & Weitzman, E.D. (1981b) *Photochem. Photobiol.* **34**, 239–247.

Czeisler, C.A., Weitzman, E.D., Moore-Ede, M.C., Zimmerman, J.C. & Knauer, R.S. (1980a) *Science* **210**, 1264–1267.

Czeisler, C.A., Zimmerman, J.C., Ronda, J., Moore-Ede, M.C. & Weitzman, E.D. (1980b) *Sleep* **2**, 329–346.

Daan, S. & Lewy, A.J. (1984) *Psychopharmacol. Bull.* **20**, 566–568.

Daan, S., Beersma, D.G.M. & Borbély, A.A. (1984) *Am. J. Physiol.* **246**, R161–R178.

Daan, S., Beersma, D.G.M., Dijk, D.J., Åkerstedt, T. & Gillberg, M. (1988) *Adv. Biosci.* **73**, 183–193.

Dahl, K., Avery, D., Savage, M. *et al.* (1990) *Society for Light Treatment and Biological Rhythms, 2nd Annual Conference*, New York, Abstract 20.

Davenne, D., Francart, A.L. & Renaud, A. (1990) *European Sleep Research Society, 10th Congress*, Strasbourg, France, Abstract, p. 106.

de Mairan, J.J. (1729) *Histoire de l'Académie Royale des Sciences (Paris)* **35**, 35.

Dietzel, M., Saletu, B., Lesch, O.M., Sieghart, W. & Schjerve, M. (1986) *Eur. Neurol.* **25**(Suppl. 2), 93–103.

Dijk, D.J., Visscher, C.A., Bloem, G.M., Beersma, D.G.M. & Daan, S. (1987) *Neurosci. Lett.* **73**, 181–186.

Dijk, D.J., Beersma, D.G.M., Daan, S. & Lewy, A.J. (1989) *Am. J. Physiol.* **256**, R106–R111.

Dinges, D.F., Graeber, R.C., Carskadon, M.A., Czeisler, C.A. & Dement, W.C. (1989) *Science* **245**, 342.

Dumont, M. (1988) Doctoral dissertation. University of Montreal.

Dumont, M., Montplaisir, J. & Infante-Rivard, C. (1988) *Sleep Res.* **17**, 371.

Dumont, M., Richardson, G.S. & Czeisler, C.A. (1990) *Society for Research on Biological Rhythms, 2nd Annual Meeting*, Jacksonville FL, Abstract.

Duncan, W.C. Jr. & Wehr, T.A. (1988) In (eds Reinberg, A., Smolensky, M. & Labrecque, G.) *Ann. Rev. Chronopharmacol.* **4**, 137–170.

Earnest, D. & Turek, F. (1985) *Proc. Natl Acad. Sci. USA* **82**, 4277–4281.

Eastman, C.I. (1991) *Perspectives in Biology and Medicine*, **34**, 181–195.

Ellis, G.B., McKlveen, R.E. & Turek, F.W. (1982) *Am. J. Physiol.* **242**, R44–R50.

Elsenga, S. & van den Hoofdakker, R.H. (1985) *Sleep Res.* **14**, 326.

Engelmann, W. (1973) *Z. Naturforsch. C.* **28**, 733–736.

Engelmann, W., Himer, W. & Giedke, H. (1985) *J. Interdiscipl. Cycle Res.* **16**, 167.

Fleischhauer, J., Glauser, G. & Hofstetter, P. (1987) *World Psychiatric Association Meeting*, Abstract 070.

Folkard, S., Arendt, J., Aldhous, M. & Kennett, H. (1990) *Neuroscience Lett.* **113**, 193–198.

Friedman, E. & Yocca, F.D. (1981) *J. Pharmacol. Exp. Ther.* **219**, 121–124.

Gao, B., Duncan, W. & Wehr, T. (1989) *Sleep Res.* **18**, 52.

Georgi, F. (1947) *Schweiz. Med. Wochenschr.* **49**, 1276–1280.

Giedke, H. (1986) *Pharmacopsychiatry* **19**, 192–193.

Giedke, H. (1988) In *Sleep '86* (eds Kölla, W.P., Obál, F., Schulz, H. & Visser, P.), pp 451–453. Stuttgart, Gustav Fischer Verlag.

Gillberg, M. & Åkerstedt, T. (1982) *Sleep* **5**, 378–388.

Gold, P.W., Goodwin, F.K. & Chrousos, G.P. (1989) *N. Engl. J. Med.* **319**, 413–420.

Götze, U. & Tölle, R. (1981) *Psychiatr. Clin.* **14**, 129–149.

Gwinner, E. (1981) In *Handbook of Behavioral Neurobiology* vol. 4 (ed. Aschoff, J.), pp 391–410. New York, Plenum Press.

Hajek, M., Meier-Ewert, K., Wirz-Justice, A., Brosig, B. & Tobler, I. (1987) *Sleep Res.* **16**, 345.

Halberg, F. (1959) *Z. Vitimin. Hormon. Ferment. Forsch.* **10**, 225–296.

Halberg, F. (1968) In *Cycles Biologiques et Psychiatrie* (ed. Ajuriaguerra, J.). pp 73–126. Paris, Georg Geneve Masson.

Hastings, J.W. & Sweeney, B.M. (1958) *Biol. Bull.* **115**, 440.

Heim, M. (1988) *Psychiat. Neurol. Med. Psychol. Leipzig* **40**, 269–277.

Holsboer-Trachsler, E., Wiedemann, K. & Holsboer, F. (1988) *Neuropsychobiology* **19**, 73–78.

Honma, K.-I., Honma, S. & Wada, T. (1987a) *Experientia* **43**, 572–574.

Honma, K.-I., Honma, S., Wada, T. (1987b) In *Biological Sciences in Space 1986* (eds Watanabe, S., Mitarai, G. & Mori, S.), pp 121–128. Tokyo, Myu Research.

Honma, S., Honma, K.-I. & Hiroshige, T. (1989) *Physiol. Behav.* **45**, 1057–1065.

Hume, K.I. & Mills, J.N. (1977) *Waking Sleeping* **1**, 291–296.

Illnerová, H. (1988) *Pineal Res. Rev.* **6**, 173–217.

Illnerová, H., Zvolský, P. & Vaněček, J. (1985) *Brain Res.* **328**, 186–189.

Illnerová, H., Vaněček, J. & Hoffmann, K. (1989) *J. Biol. Rhythms* **4**, 187–200.

Isaacs, G., Stainer, D.S., Sensky, T.E., Moor, S. & Thompson, C. (1988) *J. Affective Disord.* **14**, 13–19.

Jacobsen, F.M., Wehr, T.A., Skwerer, R.A., Sack, D.A. & Rosenthal, N.E. (1987) *Am. J. Psychiatry* **144**, 1301–1305.

James, S.P., Wehr, T.A., Sack, D.A., Parry, B.L. & Rosenthal, N.E. (1985) *Br. J. Psychiatry* **147**, 424–428.

Jauhar, P. & Weller, M.P.I. (1982) *Br. J. Psychiatry* **140**, 231–235.

Jewett, M.E., Kronauer, R.E. & Czeisler, C.A. (1991) *Nature* **350**, 59–62.

Kafka, M.S., Wirz-Justice, A., Naber, D., Marangos, P.J., O'Donohue, T.L. & Wehr, T.A. (1982) *Neuropsychobiology* **8**, 41–50.

Kasper, S., Rogers, S.L.B., Yancey, A., Schulz, P.M., Skwerer, R.G. & Rosenthal, N.E. (1989) *Arch. Gen. Psychiatry* **46**, 837–844.

Klein, D.C., Smoot, R., Weller, J.L. *et al.* (1983) *Brain Res. Bull.* **10**, 647–652.

Knörchen, R., Gundlach, E.M. & Hildebrandt, G. (1976) In *Biologische Rhythmen und Arbeit* (ed. Hildebrandt, G.), pp 43–53. Vienna, Springer Verlag.

Knowles, J.B., Southmayd, S.E., Delva, N., MacLean, A.W., Cairns, J. & Letemendia, F.J. (1979) *Br. J. Psychiatry* **135**, 403–410.

Kokkoris, C.P., Weitzman, E.D., Pollack, C.P., Spielman, A.J., Czeisler, C.A. & Bradlow, H. (1978) *Sleep* **1**, 177–190.

Kräuchi, K. & Wirz-Justice, A. (1988) *Psychiatry Res.* **25**, 323–338.

Kräuchi, K., Wirz-Justice, A. & Graw, P. (1990) *J. Affective Disord.* **20**, 43–53.

Kripke, D.F. (1981) In *Biological Psychiatry 1981* (eds Perris, C., Struwe, G. & Jansson, B.), pp 1249–1252. Amsterdam, Elsevier/North-Holland Biomedical Press.

Kripke, D.F. (1983) In *Circadian Rhythms in Psychiatry* (eds Wehr, T.A. & Goodwin, F.K.), pp 41–69. Pacific Grove CA, Boxwood Press.

Kripke, D.F. (1985) *Ann. N.Y. Acad. Sci.* **453**, 270–281.

Kripke, D.F. & Gregg, L.W. (1990) In *Medical Monitoring in the Home and Work Environment* (eds Miles, L.E. & Broughton, R.J.), pp 187–195. New York, Raven Press.

Kripke, D.F., Mullaney, D.J., Atkinson, M. & Wolf, S. (1978) *Biol. Psychiatry* **13**, 335–351.

Kripke, D.F., Risch, S.C. & Janowsky, D. (1983a) *Psychiatry Res.* **10**, 105–111.

Kripke, D.F., Risch, S.C. & Janowsky, D.S. (1983b) *Psychopharm. Bull.* **19**, 526–530.

Kripke, D.F., Gillin, J.C., Mullaney, D.J., Risch, S.C. & Janowsky, D.S. (1987) In *Chronobiology and Psychiatric Disorders* (ed. Halaris, A.S.), pp 207–218. New York, Elsevier.

Kruse, J.S. (1986) *Soc. Neurosci.* **12**, Abstract 210.

Kuhs, H. & Tölle, R. (1986) *Fortschr. Neurol. Psychiatr.* **54**, 341–355.

Lacoste, V. & Wirz-Justice, A. (1989) In *Seasonal Affective Disorders and Phototherapy* (eds Rosenthal, N.E. & Blehar, M.C.), pp 167–229. New York, Guilford Press.

Lewy, A.J. (1990) *Chronobiol. Int.* **7**, 15–21.

Lewy, A.J. & Sack, R.L. (1989) *Chronobiol. Int.* **6**, 93–102.

Lewy, A.J., Wehr, T.A., Goodwin, F.K., Newsome, D.A. & Markey, S.P. (1980) *Science* **210**, 1267–1269.

Lewy, A.J., Sack, R.L. & Singer, C.M. (1985) *Psychopharmacol. Bull.* **21**, 368–372.

Lewy, A.J., Sack, R.L., Miller, L.S. & Hoban, T.M. (1987) *Science* **235**, 352–354.

Lewy, A.J., Sack, R.L., Singer, C.M., White, D.M. & Hoban, T.M. (1988) *J. Biol. Rhythms* **3**, 121–134.

Lewy, A.J., Sack, R.L. & Latham, J.M. (1990) *Society for Light Treatment and Biological Rhythms, 2nd Annual Meeting*, New York, Abstract 22.

Lingjärde, O., Bratlid, T. & Hansen, T. (1985) *Acta Psychiatr. Scand.* **71**, 506–512.

Lund, R. (1974) *Kongress der deutschen Gesellschaft für Psychologie*, Regensburg, **1**, 391–392.

Lund, R., Kammerloher, A. & Dirlich, G. (1983) In *Circadian Rhythms in Psychiatry* (eds Wehr, T.A. & Goodwin, F.K.), pp 77–88. Pacific Grove CA, Boxwood Press.

Lund, R., Schulz, H. & Berger, M. (1984) In *Klinische Psychologie. Psychophysiologische Merkmale Klinischer Symptome*, vol. 2, Depression und Schizophrenie (eds Ferstl, R., Rey, E.R. & Vaitl, D.), p. 49. Weinheim, Beltz.

McCarley, R. (1982) *Am. J. Psychiatry* **139**, 565–570.

McEachron, D.L., Kripke, D.F., Hawkins, R., Haus, E., Pavlinac, D. & Deftos, L. (1982) *Neuropsychobiology* **8**, 12–29.

McEachron, D.L., Kripke, D.F., Sharp, F.R., Lewy, A.J. & McClellan, D.E. (1985) *Brain Res. Bull.* **15**, 347–350.

McIntyre, I.M., Norman, T.R., Burrows, G.D. & Armstrong, S.M. (1989) *J. Pineal Res.* **6**, 149–156.

Martens, H. (1990a) *Sleep Res.* **19**, 398.

Martens, H. (1990b) Thesis, in preparation.

Maywood, E.S., Buttery, R.C., Vance, G.S., Herbert, J. & Hastings, M.H. (1990) *Biol. Reprod.* **43**, 174–182.

Meier, A.H. & Cincotta, A.H. (1990) *Society for Research on Biological Rhythms, 2nd Annual Meeting*, Jacksonville FL, Abstract 12, p. 27.

Meier, A.H., Martin, D.D.R. & MacGregor, I. (1971) *Science* **173**, 1240–1242.

Meijer, J.H. & Rietveld, W.J. (1989) *Physiol. Rev.* **69**, 671–707.

Mendelson, W.B. (1989) In *Slow Wave Sleep: Physiological, Pathophysiological, and Functional Aspects* (eds Wauquier, A., Dugovic, C. & Radulovacki, M.), pp 155–165. New York, Raven Press.

Menninger-Lerchenthal, E. (1960) *Periodizität in der Psychopathologie*. Vienna, Wilhelm Maudrich.

Miles, L.E.M., Raynal, D.M. & Wilson, M.A. (1977) *Science* **198**, 421–423.

Mills, J.N., Minors, D.S. & Waterhouse, J.M. (1974) *J. Physiol.* **240**, 567.

Mills, J.N., Minors, D.S. & Waterhouse, J.M. (1978) *J. Physiol.* **285**, 455–470.

Minors, D.S. & Waterhouse, J.M. (1981) *Circadian Rhythms in the Human*. Bristol, Wright and Sons.

Minors, D.S. & Waterhouse, J.M. (1984) *Chronobiol. Int.* **1**, 205–216.
Mistlberger, R. & Rusak, B. (1986) *Neurosci. Lett.* **72**, 357–362.
Moldofsky, H., Musisi, S. & Phillipson, E.A. (1986) *Sleep* **9**, 61–65.
Moore, R.Y. (1983) *Fed. Proc.* **42**, 2783–2789.
Moore-Ede, M. (1986) *Am. J. Physiol.* **250**, R735–R752.
Moore-Ede, M.C. & Czeisler, C.A. (1984) *Mathematical Models of Circadian Sleep-Wake Cycles.* New York, Raven Press.
Moore-Ede, M., Sulzman, F. & Fuller, C. (1982) *The Clocks that Time Us: Physiology of the Circadian Timing System.* Cambridge MA, Harvard University Press.
Mrosovsky, N. (1988) *J. Biol. Rhythms* **3**, 189–207.
Mrosovsky, N. & Salmon, P.A. (1987) *Nature* **330**, 372–373.
Okudaira, N., Kripke, D.F. & Webster, J.B. (1983) *Am. J. Physiol.* **245**, R613–R615.
O'Rourke, D., Wurtman, J. & Brzezinski, A. (1987) *Psychopharmacol. Bull.* **23**, 3.
O'Rourke, D., Wurtman, J.J. & Wurtman, R.J. (1988) In *The Psychobiology of Bulimia Nervosa.* (eds Pirke, K.M., Vandereycken, W. & Ploog, D.), pp 13–17. Berlin, Springer-Verlag.
Papousek, M. (1975) *Fortschr. Neurol. Psychiatr.* **43**, 381–440.
Parry, B.L. (1989) *Psychiat. Clin. North Am.* **12**, 207–220.
Parry, B.L. & Wehr, T.A. (1987) *Am. J. Psychiatry* **144**, 808–810.
Parry, B.L., Rosenthal, N.E., Tamarkin, L. & Wehr, T.A. (1987) *Am. J. Psychiatry* **144**, 762–766.
Parry, B.L., Berga, S.L., Mostofi, N., Sependa, P.A., Kripke, D.F. & Gillin, J.C. (1989) *Am. J. Psychiatry* **146**, 1215–1217.
Peter, K., Räbiger, U. & Kowalik, A. (1986) *Psychiatr. Neurol. Med. Psychol. Leipzig* **38**, 384–390.
Petrie, K., Conaglen, J.V., Thompson, L. & Chamberlain, K. (1989) *Br. Med. J.* **298**, 705.
Pflug, B. & Tölle, R. (1971) *Int. Pharmacopsychiatry* **6**, 187–196.
Pflug, B., Johnsson, A. & Martin, W. (1983) In *Circadian Rhythms in Psychiatry* (eds Wehr, T.A. & Goodwin, F.K.), pp 71–76. Pacific Grove CA, Boxwood Press.
Pickard, G.E., Ralph, M.R. & Menaker, M. (1987) *J. Biol. Rhythms* **2**, 35–56.
Pittendrigh, C.S. (1960) *Cold Spring Harbor Symp. Quant. Biol.* **25**, 159–184.
Pittendrigh, C.S. (1974) In *The Neurosciences: Third Study Program* (eds Schmitt, F.O. & Worden, F.G.), pp 437–458. Cambridge MA, MIT Press.
Pittendrigh, C.S. (1979) In *Biological Rhythms and their Central Mechanisms* (eds Suda, M., Hayaishi, O. & Nakagawa, H.), pp 3–12. Amsterdam, Elsevier/North-Holland Biomedical Press.
Pittendrigh, C.S. (1981) In *Handbook of Behavioural Neurobiology* vol. 4, (ed. Aschoff, J.), pp 95–124. New York, Plenum Press.
Pittendrigh, C.S. (1988) *J. Biol. Rhythms* **3**, 173–188.
Pittendrigh, C.S. & Bruce, V.G. (1957) In *Rhythmic and Synthetic Processes in Growth* (ed. Rudnick, D.), pp 75–109). Princeton NJ, Princeton University Press.
Pollak, C.P., Alexopoulos, G.S., Moline, M.L. & Wagner, D.R. (1989a) *Sleep Res.* **18**, 436.
Pollak, C.P., Alexopoulos, G.S., Moline, M.L. & Wagner, D.R. (1989b) *Sleep Res.* **18**, 437.
Prasko, J. (1988) *Collegium Internationale Neuro-Psychopharmacologicum.* Munich, Germany. Abstract 34.07.13.
Rapp, P. (1987) *Prog. Neurobiol.* **29**, 261–273.
Redfern, P.H. (1989) *Hum. Psychopharmacol.* **4**, 159–168.

Redman, J., Armstrong, S. & Ng, K.T. (1983) *Science* **219**, 1080–1081.
Reinberg, A. & Smolensky, M. (1983) *Biological Rhythms and Medicine*. New York, Springer-Verlag.
Reinink, E., Bouhuys, A.L., Gordijn, M.C.M. & van den Hoofdakker, R.H. (1990a) *European Sleep Research Society, 10th Congress*, Strasbourg, France, Abstract.
Reinink, E., Bouhuys, N., Wirz-Justice, A. & van den Hoofdakker, R. (1990b) *Psychiatry Res.* **32**, 113–124.
Remé, C. & Wirz-Justice, A. (1985) In *Circadian Rhythms in the Central Nervous System* (eds Redfern, P.H., Campbell, I.C., Davies, J.A. & Martin, K.F.), pp 135–146. London, Macmillan.
Remé, C., Terman, M. & Wirz-Justice, A. (1990) *Arch. Gen. Psychiatry* **47**, 878–879.
Remé, C., Wirz-Justice, A. & Terman, M. (1991) *J. Biol. Rhythms* **6**, 1–25.
Reppert, S.M., Weaver, D.R., Rivkees, S.A. & Stopa, E.G. (1988) *Science* **242**, 78–81.
Reynolds, C.F. III. (1987) *Psychiatr. Clin. North Am.* **10**, 583–591.
Reynolds, C.F. III. & Kupfer, D.J. (1987) *Sleep* **10**, 199–215.
Riemann, D., Wiegand, M. & Berger, M. (1990) In *Sleep '90* (ed. Horne, J.A.), pp 323–334. Bochum, Pontenagel Press.
Rietveld, W.J. & Wirz-Justice, A. (1986) *Ann. Rev. Chronopharmacol.* **3**, 33–36.
Rockwell, D.A., Winget, C.M., Rosenblatt, L.S., Higgins, E.A. & Hetherington, N.W. (1978) *J. Nerv. Ment. Dis.* **166**, 851.
Roenneberg, T. & Aschoff, J. (1990a) *J. Biol. Rhythms* **5**, 195–216.
Roenneberg, T. & Aschoff, J. (1990b) *J. Biol. Rhythms* **5**, 217–240.
Rosen, L.N., Targum, S.D., Terman, M. *et al.* (1990) *Psychiatry Res.* **31**, 131–144.
Rosenthal, N.E. (1986) *Arch. Gen. Psychiatry* **43**, 188–189.
Rosenthal, N.E. & Heffernan, M.M. (1986) In *Nutrition and the Brain* (eds Wurtman, R.J. & Wurtman, J.J.), pp 139–166. New York, Raven Press.
Rosenthal, N.E., Sack, D.A., James, S.P. *et al.* (1985) *Ann. N.Y. Acad. Sci.* **453**, 260–269.
Rosenthal, N.E., Genhart, M., Jacobsen, F.M., Skwerer, R.G. & Wehr, T.A. (1987) *Ann N.Y. Acad. Sci.* **499**, 216–230.
Rosenthal, N.E., Jacobsen, F.M., Sack, D.A. *et al.* (1988a) *Am. J. Psychiatry* **145**, 52–56.
Rosenthal, N.E., Sack, D.A., Skwerer, R.G., Jacobsen, F.M. & Wehr, T.A. (1988b) *J. Biol. Rhythms* **3**, 101–120.
Rosenthal, N.E., Joseph-Vanderpool, J.R., Levendosky, A.A. *et al.* (1990) *Sleep* (in press).
Rosenwasser, A. & Adler, N. (1986) *Neurosci. Biobehav. Rev.* **10**, 431–448.
Rusak, B. (1989) *J. Biol. Rhythms* **4**, 121–134.
Rusak, B. & Zucker, I. (1979) *Physiol. Rev.* **59**, 449–526.
Sack, D.A., Nurnburger, J., Rosenthal, N.E., Ashburn, E. & Wehr, T.A. (1985) *Am. J. Psychiatry* **142**, 606–608.
Sack, D.A., Duncan, W.C. Jr., Rosenthal, N.E., Mendelson, W.E. & Wehr, T.A. (1988) *Acta Psychiatr. Scand.* **77**, 219–224.
Sack, R.L. & Lewy, A.J. (1988) *Sleep Res.* **17**, 396.
Sack, R.L., Lewy, A.J., Latham, J. & Blood, M. (1990) *Society for Research on Biological Rhythms, 2nd Annual Meeting*, Jacksonville FL, Abstract 94, p. 69.
Saletu, B., Dietzel, M., Lesch, O.M., Musalek, M., Walter, H. & Grünberger, J. (1986) *Eur. Neurol.* **25** (Suppl. 2), 82–92.
Sarrafzadeh, A., Wirz-Justice, A., Arendt, J. & English, J. (1990) In *Sleep '90* (ed. Horne, J.A.), pp 51–54. Bochum, Pontenagel Press.
Schilgen, B. & Tölle, R. (1980) *Arch. Gen. Psychiatry* **37**, 267–271.
Schulte, W. (1959) *Med. Klin.* **20**, 969–973.

Schulz, H. & Lund, R. (1985) *Psychiatry Res.* **16**, 65–77.

Schwitzer, J., Neudorfer, C., Schifferle, I. *et al.* (1989) *Neuropsychiatrie*

Sewitch, D.E., Dinges, D.F., Kribbs, N.B., Powell, J.W., Orne, E.C. & Orne, M.T. (1990) *Sleep Res.* **19**, 406.

Shanahan, T.L. (1990) Undergraduate thesis, Boston College.

Siffre, M. (1975) *Nat. Geogr.* **147**, 426.

Singer, C.M. & Lewy, A.J. (1989) *Sleep Res.* **18**, 445.

Skwerer, R.G., Jacobsen, F.M., Duncan, C.C. *et al.* (1988) *J. Biol. Rhythms* **3**, 135–154.

Souêtre, E., Salvati, E., Pringuey, D., Plasse, Y., Savelli, M. & Darcourt, G. (1987) *J. Affective Disord.* **12**, 41–46.

Souêtre, E., Salvati, E., Wehr, T.A., Sack, D.A., Krebs, B. & Darcourt, G. (1988) *Am. J. Psychiatry* **145**, 1133–1137.

Souêtre, E., Salvati, E., Belugou, J.-L. *et al.* (1989) *Psychiatry Res.* **28**, 263–278.

Southmayd, S.E. & David, M. (1989) *Sleep Res.* **18**, 378.

Southmayd, S.E. & David, M. (1990) *Sleep Res.* **19**, 356.

Southmayd, S.E., Delva, N.J., Cairns, J. *et al.* (1985) *Sleep Res.* **14**, 258.

Spring, B., Chiodo, J. & Bowen, D.J. (1987) *Psychol. Bull.* **102**, 234–256.

Stewart, J.W., Quitkin, F.M., Terman, M. & Terman, J.S. (1990) *Psychiatry Res.* **33**, 121–128.

Stohler, R., Kräuchi, K., Wirz-Justice, A., Ulrich, K., van der Werf, H. & Brunner, M. (1989) *Sleep Res.* **18**, 156.

Strogatz, S.H. (1990) *J. Biol. Rhythms* **5**, 169–174.

Sulzman, F.M., Ellman, D., Fuller, C.A., Moore-Ede, M.C. & Wassmer, G. (1984) *Science* **225**, 232–234.

Surridge-David, M., MacLean, A., Coulter, M. & Knowles, J. (1987) *Psychiatry Res.* **22**, 149–158.

Takahashi, K. (1989) *Society for Light Treatment and Biological Rhythms Newsletter* **1**, 6–7.

Tamarkin, L., Baird, C.J. & Almeida, O.F.X. (1985) *Science* **227**, 714–720.

Taub, J.M. & Berger, R.S. (1964) *Psychosom. Med.* **36**, 164.

Terman, J.S., Terman, M., Schlager, D. *et al.* (1990a) *Psychopharmacol. Bull.* **26**, 3–11.

Terman, M. & Terman, J. (1985) *Ann. N.Y. Acad. Sci.* **453**, 147–161.

Terman, M., Terman, J.S., Quitkin, F.M. *et al.* (1988) *J. Neural Transm.* **72**, 147–165.

Terman, M., Terman, J.S., Quitkin, F.M., McGrath, P.J., Stewart, J.W. & Rafferty, B. (1989) *Neuropsychopharmacology* **2**, 1–22.

Terman, M., Remé, C. & Wirz-Justice, A. (1990b) *J. Biol. Rhythms* **6**, 27–44.

Thompson, C. (1989) In *Seasonal Affective Disorder* (eds Thompson, C. & Silverstone, T.), pp 1–17. London, Clinical Neuroscience.

Tsujimoto, T., Yamada, N., Shimoda, K., Hanada, K. & Takahasi, S. (1990) *J. Affective Disord.* **18**, 199–210.

Turek, F.W. (1985) *Ann. Rev. Physiol.* **47**, 49–64.

Turek, F.W. (1986) *Am. J. Physiol.* **251**, R636–R638.

Turek, F.W. (1989) *J. Biol. Rhythms* **4**, 135–147.

Tzischinsky, O. & Lavie, P. (1990) *European Sleep Research Society, 10th Congress*, Strasbourg, France, Abstract, p. 97.

van den Hoofdakker, R.H. & Beersma, D.G.M. (1985) *Psychiatry Res.* **16**, 155–163.

van den Hoofdakker, R.H., Bouhuys, A.L. & Beersma, D.G.M. (1990) *European Sleep Research Society, 10th Congress*, Strasbourg, France, Abstract, p. 39.

Van Reeth, O. & Turek, F.W. (1989) *Nature* **339**, 49–51.

Vogel, G.W., Vogel, F., McAbee, R. *et al.* (1980) *Arch. Gen. Psychiatry* **37**, 247–253.

Volz, H.P., Mackert, A. & Stieglitz, R.D. (1990) *J. Affective Disord.* **19**, 15–21.

von Zerssen, D. (1987) In *Chronobiology and Psychiatric Disorders* (ed. Halaris, A.), pp 159–179. New York, Elsevier.

Wehr. T.A. (1988) In *Biological Rhythms and Mental Disorders* (eds Kupfer, D.J., Monk, T.H. & Barchas, J.D.), pp 143–175. New York, Guilford Press.

Wehr, T.A. (1989a) In *Seasonal Affective Disorders and Phototherapy* (eds Rosenthal, N.E. & Blehar, M.C.), pp 11–32. New York, Guilford Press.

Wehr, T.A. (1990a) *Chronobiol. Int.* **7**, 11–14.

Wehr, T.A. (1990b) In *Sleep and Biological Rhythms* (eds Montplaisir, J. & Godbout, R.) pp 42–86. London, Oxford Press.

Wehr, T.A. & Goodwin, F.K. (1983) In *Circadian Rhythms in Psychiatry* (eds Wehr, T.A. & Goodwin, F.K.), pp 129–184. Pacific Grove CA, Boxwood Press.

Wehr, T.A. & Rosenthal, N.E. (1989) *Am J. Psychiatry* **146**, 829–839.

Wehr, T.A. & Wirz-Justice, A. (1981) In *Sleep 1980* (ed. Kölla, W.), pp 26–33. Basle, Karger.

Wehr, T.A. & Wirz-Justice, A. (1982) *Pharmacopsychiatry* **15**, 31–39.

Wehr, T.A., Wirz-Justice, A., Goodwin, F.K., Duncan, W. & Gillin, J.C. (1979) *Science* **206**, 710–713.

Wehr, T.A., Goodwin, F.K., Wirz-Justice, A., Breitmaier, J. & Craig, C. (1982) *Arch. Gen. Psychiatry* **39**, 559–565.

Wehr, T.A., Sack, D.A. & Rosenthal, N.E. (1987) *Am. J. Psychiatry* **144**, 201–204.

Wehr, T.A., Rosenthal, N.E. & Sack, D.A. (1988) *Acta Psychiatr. Scand.* **77** (Suppl. 341), 44–52.

Wehr, T.A., Giesen, H., Schulz, P.M. *et al.* (1989a) In *Seasonal Affective Disorders and Phototherapy* (eds Rosenthal, N.E. & Blehar, M.C.), pp 55–63. New York, Guilford Press.

Wehr, T.A., Joseph-Vanderpool, J.R. & Kasper, S. (1989b) *Sleep Res.* **18**, 381.

Weitzman, E.D., Nogeire, C., Perlow, M. *et al.* (1974) *J. Clin. Endocrinol. Metab.* **38**, 1018–1030.

Wever, R.A. (1975) *Int. J. Chronobiol.* **3**, 19–55.

Wever, R. (1979) *The Circadian System of Man: Results of Experiments under Temporal Isolation.* New York, Springer Verlag.

Wever, R.A. (1985) *Ann. N.Y. Acad. Sci.* **453**, 282–304.

Wever, R.A. (1989) *J. Biol. Rhythms* **4**, 161–185.

Wever, R.A., Polasek, J. & Wildgruber, C.M. (1983) *Pflügers Arch.* **396**, 85–87.

Wiegand, M., Berger, M., Zulley, J., Lauer, C. & von Zerssen, D. (1987) *Biol. Psychiatry* **22**, 389–392.

Winfree, A.T. (1980) *The Geometry of Biological Time*, Biomathematics, vol. 8. New York, Springer Verlag.

Winfree, A.T. (1987) *The Timing of Biological Clocks*, Scientific American Libraries, vol. 19. New York, Scientific American Books.

Wirz-Justice, A. (1982) In *Basic Mechanisms in the Action of Lithium* (eds Emrich, H.M., Aldenhoff, J.B. & Lux, H.D.), pp 249–258. Amsterdam, Excerpta Medica.

Wirz-Justice, A. (1983) In *Circadian Rhythms and Psychiatry* (eds Wehr, T.A. & Goodwin, F.K.), pp 255–264. Pacific Grove CA, Boxwood Press.

Wirz-Justice, A. (1986) *Psychopathology* **19** (Suppl. 2), 136–141.

Wirz-Justice, A. (1987) *Prog. Neurobiol.* **29**, 219–259.

Wirz-Justice, A. & Anderson, J.L. (1990) *Psychopharmacology Bull.* **26**.

Wirz-Justice, A. & Campbell, I.C. (1982) *Experientia* **38**, 1301–1309.

Wirz-Justice, A. & Pringle, C. (1987) *Sleep* **10**, 57–61.

Wirz-Justice, A., Pühringer, W. & Hole, G. (1979) *Am. J. Psychiatry* **136**, 1222–1223.

Wirz-Justice, A., Groos, G. & Wehr, T.A. (1982a) In *Vertebrate Circadian Systems: Structure and Physiology* (eds Aschoff, J., Daan, S. & Groos, G.), pp 183–193. Heidelberg, Springer Verlag.

Wirz-Justice, A., Kafka, M.S., Naber, D. *et al.* (1982b) *Brain Res.* **241**, 115–122.

Wirz-Justice, A., Wever, R.A. & Aschoff, J. (1984) *Naturwissenschaften* **71**, 316–319.

Wirz-Justice, A., Bucheli, C., Graw, P., Kielholz, P., Fisch, H.-U. & Woggon, B. (1986) *Acta Psychiatr. Scand.* **74**, 193–204.

Wirz-Justice, A., Schmid, A.C., Graw, P. *et al.* (1987) *Experientia* **43**, 574–576.

Wirz-Justice, A., Graw, P., Jochum, A. *et al.* (1988) *Psychopharmacology* **96** (Suppl.), 114.

Wirz-Justice, A., Graw, P., Bucheli, C. *et al.* (1989) In *Seasonal Affective Disorder* (eds Thompson, C. & Silverstone, T.), pp 69–76. London, Clinical Neuroscience.

Wirz-Justice, A., Graw, P., Kräuchi, K. *et al.* (1990) *J. Psychiatr. Res.* **24**, 129–137.

Wu, J.C. & Bunney, W.E. (1990) *Am. J. Psychiatry* **147**, 14–21.

Wurtman, J.J., Wurtman, R.J., Mark, S., Tsay, R., Gilbert, W. & Growdon, J. (1985) *Int. J. Eat. Disord.* **4**, 89–99.

Wurtman, R.J. & Wurtman, J.J. (1989) *Sci. Am.* **260**, 68–75.

Yerevanian, B.I., Anderson, J.L., Grota, L.J. & Bray, M. (1986) *Psychiatry Res.* **18**, 355–364.

Zatz, M. & Herkenham, M. (1981) *Brain Res.* **212**, 234–238.

Zucker, I. (1988) *J. Biol. Rhythms* **3**, 209–223.

Zulley, J. (1990) In *Sleep '90* (ed. Horne, J.A.), pp 319–323. Bochum, Pontenagel Press.

Zulley, J., Wever, R. & Aschoff, J. (1981) *Pflügers Arch.* **391**, 314–318.

_____ CHAPTER 8 _____

MANIA

Trevor Silverstone

Medical College of St Bartholomew's Hospital, University of London, London EC1, UK

Table of Contents

BIOLOGICAL ASPECTS OF AFFECTIVE DISORDERS
ISBN 0-12-356510-3

Mania is a serious psychiatric illness which affects almost 1% of the population at some time in their lives. It tends to begin early in adult life and is often recurrent. In most patients mania alternates with depressive episodes, but in others it recurs without any intervening depression. Whether or not depressive episodes occur the illness is referred to as bipolar affective disorder, which is a subcategory of what Kraepelin (1921) originally called manic-depressive insanity.

Bipolar disorder has been recognized world-wide in many diverse ethnic groups (Silverstone and Romans-Clarkson, 1989). As well as causing great distress to the sufferer, it can have disastrous social and economic consequences, and is associated with an increased mortality rate (Tsuang and Woolson, 1977; Goodwin and Jameson, 1984).

This chapter will examine the evidence relating to the psychobiological changes described in manic patients, evaluate certain physical and pharmacological precipants of relapse, assess treatment strategies, and discuss critically some current theories which have been advanced to explain bipolar disorder in biological terms.

8.1 Clinical features

Mania is characterized by an elevated or irritable mood, overactivity, and increased talkativeness ('pressure of speech'), accompanied by a reduced need for sleep, racing thoughts, distractability leading to 'flight of ideas', an inflated self-regard sometimes amounting to grandiose delusions, and extravagant, disinhibited behaviour (Winokur *et al.*, 1969).

Hypomania is a term used to describe less severe episodes of mania which do not cause marked impairment in social or occupational functioning.

If a patient has only hypomanic attacks the condition is referred to as bipolar II disorder, in distinction to bipolar I which requires at least one attack of frank mania. Some consider hypomania to differ in kind as well as intensity from mania (Coryell *et al.*, 1987) but most authorities do not distinguish between the two when discussing biological factors, a practice which will be followed here.

While the presence of strictly defined Schneiderian first-rank symptoms does not preclude the diagnosis of mania, they are uncommon in otherwise clear-cut manic episodes (O'Grady, 1990); the same applies to schizophrenic type thought disorder (Jampala *et al.*, 1989).

Following an initial manic episode, recurrences occur in over 75% of cases (Silverstone and Romans-Clarkson, 1989). In our series of 21 patients admitted with a first episode of mania, 50% relapsed within 2 years (N. Hunt and T. Silverstone, unpublished data). Having had a previous depressive episode and being aged 30 or more at the time of the first manic episode worsened the short-term prognosis.

The relapse frequency often increases over the years; when it reaches four episodes per year the pattern is referred to as one of 'rapid cycling' (Dunner *et al.*, 1977; Roy-Byrne *et al.*, 1984).

8.1.1 Seasonality

Kraepelin (1921) in his classical account of the condition noted that some of his patients showed a clear-cut seasonal pattern to their illness, with many becoming depressed in the autumn and winter and getting better in the summer. A careful statistical analysis by Slater (1938) of Kraepelin's original data revealed a marked summer peak of admissions for manic-depressive illness. Admission rates for mania in the British Isles show an excess of admissions in the summer months (Walter, 1977; Myers and Davies, 1978; Carney *et al.*, 1988).

Data from other countries also show a seasonal variation in admission rates for mania. It appears as if in more temperate climes, such as in the United

Kingdom, Ireland and New Zealand (Mulder *et al.*, 1990), or where there is little seasonal variation in temperature, as in Hawaii (Brewerton and McClaughlin, 1986), the peak of manic admissions occurs in summer. In places with greater temperature swings, such as Hungary (Rihmer, 1980), Yugoslavia (Demirovic and Zec, 1986), Greece (Frangos *et al.*, 1980) and Australia (Parker and Walter, 1982), the peak occurs in spring. These differences are unlikely to be due simply to differences in latitude, as in Ontario, which spans the latitudes of much of Europe, no seasonal variation was seen in admission rates for mania (Eastwood and Stiasny, 1978). It is not known whether it is day length, the rate of temperature change, the amount of sunlight, air ionization, or relative humidity which is the critical variable in determining seasonal variation.

Rosenthal *et al.* (1984) coined the term 'seasonal affective disorder' (SAD) to describe a series of 29 patients who regularly became depressed in the autumn or winter, with their mood lifting the following spring or summer, some becoming mildly manic. Is SAD a variant of bipolar disorder? The high frequency of clear-cut bipolar episodes, with manic episodes occurring in the summer, would suggest that it is. However, SAD patients who also fulfil the diagnostic criteria for bipolar disorder are more likely, when depressed, to display atypical features, such as hypersomnia and increased appetite, than other bipolar patients (Thompson and Isaacs, 1988). While nine (23%) out of one series of 39 bipolar patients experienced seasonal changes (Rosenthal *et al.*, 1984), it is uncertain how many bipolar patients can be classified as suffering from SAD, and how many show regular seasonal variation in symptoms. Further longitudinal studies of unselected bipolar patients are required to resolve this issue, which is a potentially important one from the biological perspective.

8.1.2 Secondary mania

The term 'secondary mania' originates with Krauthammer and Klerman (1978) who used it to describe an episode of mania, in a patient with no previous history of affective disorder, which follows and is possibly precipitated by physical illness or by drugs. From the psychiatric point of view, the clinical features differ little from 'primary mania' although the age of onset is generally greater. A positive family history is less common than in primary mania. Of particular relevance are those cases of mania following brain injury; these are considered in some detail below.

8.2 Brain structure and function

In recent years a number of techniques have been developed for examining the structure, and function of the human brain in the living subject. These include computerized tomography (CT), magnetic resonance imaging (MRI), single photon emission tomography (SPET) and positron emission tomography (PET). Such methods are difficult to apply in the frankly manic patient, as a satisfactory record usually requires the patient to keep still for a period of several minutes. Nevertheless, some studies have been undertaken, necessarily in less severe cases or when the patient had returned to a euthymic state.

8.2.1 Computerized tomography (CT)

Early CT studies suggested that there was ventricular enlargement in the brains of bipolar patients (Nasrallah *et al.*, 1982, Reider *et al.*, 1983; Pearlson *et al.*, 1984), but the differences were not always striking. In one series the cerebral ventricles were larger than in matched control subjects in only three out of 24 bipolar patients (Nasrallah *et al.*, 1982). In another study (Reider *et al.*, 1983), the bipolar patients were older than the controls, thereby making interpretation difficult. The patients were not always representative of bipolar patients in general. In the study by Pearlson *et al.* (1984), they were at the more severe end of the spectrum, with a past history of delusions and hallucinations; and within this severe group those with dilated ventricles had had more hospital admissions than those with smaller ventricles. Another recent series of bipolar patients with psychotic symptoms also showed some dilatation of the lateral ventricles, but not the third ventricle (Harvey *et al.*, 1990). By contrast Dewan *et al.* (1988a) found differences only in the width of the third ventricle in bipolar patients. There is little abnormality at the onset of illness, with enlargement of the third ventricle being seen in only one out of 17 psychotic bipolar patients, and no difference in lateral ventricle size from control subjects (Iacono *et al.*, 1988). The normal cerebral asymmetry, in which the frontal part of the brain on the right is larger than that on the left while the occipital portion is larger on the left, is maintained in bipolar disorder, in contrast to schizophrenia, where it is reversed (Dewan *et al.*, 1987).

In general the CT scan abnormalities seen in patients with bipolar disorder would appear to be slight, certainly less than in schizophrenia, and when they do occur the clinical picture is more schizoaffective.

275

8.2.2 Magnetic resonance imaging (MRI)

Two studies have failed to show any difference in brain size, and in particular the size of the temporal lobes, in bipolar patients as compared with normals, whereas both found a reduced brain size in schizophrenia (Johnstone *et al.*, 1989; Dupont *et al.*, 1989). However, a more recent report describes a reduction in brain size in bipolar patients with psychotic features (Coffman *et al.*, 1990). Abnormalities in the subcortical areas of the brain have been observed. In one series of 20 bipolar patients, 19 showed subcortical signal hyperintensities, with frontal lobe involvement in seven (Dupont *et al.*, 1990). As with the patients with enlarged ventricles, those with the hyperintensities had had a greater number of hospitalizations than those without. The significance of these abnormalities is unclear. They have also been observed in older bipolar patients (McDonald *et al.*, 1990).

8.2.3 Electroencephalogram (EEG)

EEG power spectra analyses have indicated that patients with bipolar disorder are likely to have increased activity in the right frontal area (Flor-Henry, 1979). More recent EEG studies have revealed a high frequency of abnormalities among bipolar patients, occurring in 12 out of 26 in one series (Dewan *et al.*, 1988b). None of the six patients who had a dilated third ventricle in the CT scan had an abnormal EEG, prompting the suggestion that there may be two distinct subgroups of bipolar patients: those with subcortical pathology who have a normal EEG, and those with an abnormal EEG indicating cortical pathology. Combined MRI and EEG should help to clarify this point. Patients with EEG abnormalities are less likely to have a positive family history than those with a normal EEG, again suggesting at least two subtypes of bipolar illness, the acquired (with an abnormal EEG) and the inherited (Cook *et al.*, 1986).

8.2.4 Single photon emission tomography (SPET)

In the few measurements of cerebral blood flow using SPET which have been undertaken in manic patients, little difference from normal controls has been seen, either when manic or euthymic (Silfverskiöld and Risberg, 1989; Delvenne *et al.*, 1989). While one might expect increased cerebral blood flow in a condition characterized by generalized overactivity, the more overactive patients almost certainly would have been excluded from SPET studies because they are unable to co-operate sufficiently or because they have been sedated, a procedure which is likely to attenuate any manic-related increase in cerebral blood flow.

8.2.5 Positron emission tomography (PET)

In a small series of five manic patients, whole brain glucose utilization rates were similar to those of normal control subjects and were greater than those seen during a depressive episode (Baxter *et al.*, 1985). By contrast Cohen *et al.* (1989) describe the PET scans of patients with bipolar disorder as being similar to those of schizophrenics during an auditory performance task; but as only two hypomanic patients and no manics were studied in their series these findings must be regarded as tentative. The number of manic patients studied thus far with PET is far too small to allow any conclusions to be drawn.

8.2.6 Brain injury

Studying patients who develop mania after a focal brain lesion should reveal the localization of the brain sites most closely related to the pathogenesis of mania.

Patients who become manic after a cerebrovascular lesion are more likely to have a right-sided lesion (Robinson *et al.*, 1988). Cummings and Mendez (1984) emphasize that in the majority of cases where a focal brain lesion is associated with mania, the lesion is in the right basal forebrain region. However, only a minority of patients who have a right-sided lesion become manic (Starkstein and Robinson, 1989). Those that do are more likely to have a positive family history of affective disorder, suggesting that a genetic predisposition is an additional factor in determining whether or not a given patient becomes manic after a right-sided stroke. In a recent series of 93 patients who had a right-sided lesion nearly half had no significant mood change, 28 (30%) were depressed, and 19 (20%) showed undue cheerfulness, a proportion being frankly manic (Starkstein *et al.*, 1989).

Head injury has been followed by mania in a number of cases (Clark and Davison, 1987; Shukla *et al.*, 1987; Yatham *et al.*, 1988; Zwil *et al.*, 1990). According to Nizamie *et al.* (1988), such patients tend to have dysfunction of the right hemisphere rather than the left. Mania following head injury is more likely to be characterized by irritability than euphoria (Shukla *et al.*, 1987). In contrast to post-stroke mania, most patients are less likely to have positive family histories.

In keeping with the association of secondary mania with right-sided brain lesions is the report by Barczak *et al.* (1988) of three cases of hypomania occurring as an interictal phenomenon in patients with complex partial seizures originating on the right.

Thus, there appears to be general agreement that lesions of the right-side of the brain, possibly involving the right basal forebrain, are prone to cause mania. This naturally suggests that the, as yet unknown, pathological changes which underlie the development of primary mania are likely to be found in this part of the brain.

8.3 Neurochemistry

According to the monoamine hypothesis of affective disorders, mania is due to a functional excess of monoamine transmitter activity at certain sites in the brain (Schildkraut, 1965). There have been many attempts to explore this hypothesis and to determine which, if any, of the currently recognized neurotransmitters might be implicated. These include noradrenaline, dopamine, 5-hydroxytryptamine (5-HT), acetylcholine and γ-aminobutyric acid.

Direct studies of neurotransmitter activity within the brain of manic patients is not possible. We have instead to rely on the examination of neurotransmitter metabolites in the cerebrospinal fluid (CSF), blood or urine. Such indirect measures can only give a crude approximation, at best, of what is happening within the brain, and give no indication of where any changes are taking place. Platelets allow measurement of transport mechanisms, particularly of 5-HT, which might reflect what is happening within the brain as the platelet membrane is similar to that of neurones and derives from the same embryonic origin (see Chapter 4). The observed changes in platelet activity in mania may not be fully representative of similar changes in neural activity, particularly in view of the confounding effects of motor activity.

8.3.1 Noradrenaline (NA)

The principal brain metabolite of NA is 3-methoxy-4-hydroxyphenyl glycol (MHPG). In the CSF, MHPG may be higher in mania than in depression, but not higher than in normal controls. (Annitto and Shopsin, 1979; Post, 1980). By contrast, a rise in CSF MHPG in mania has been reported by Swann et al. (1988), but this could be secondary to an increase in motor activity.

Levels of NA itself were higher in the CSF of six manic patients than in the majority of neurological 'controls' or depressed patients (Post et al., 1978). This was not thought to be secondary to overactivity.

Dopamine β-hydroxylase (DBH) is the enzyme which converts dopamine (DA) to NA and could therefore be a marker of CNS NA function. CSF DBH appears to be reduced in mania, but the significance of this finding is unclear (Post et al., 1984). CSF levels of cyclic AMP are normal in mania (Post et al., 1977).

DA and NA-sensitive adenylate cyclases in the brain and periphery are thought to be associated with post-synaptic receptors. Plasma levels of c-AMP are raised in mania and low in depression (Lykouras *et al.*, 1978). Although physical activity increases plasma levels of c-AMP, the levels in affective disorder correlate more closely with mood than with activity (Lykouras *et al.*, 1979). The plasma levels of c-AMP in mania fall during treatment with neuroleptic drugs (Lykouras *et al.*, 1978) or lithium (Arato *et al.*, 1980).

Early reports of reduced β-adrenoceptor activity on lymphocytes in mania (Extein *et al.*, 1979; Pandey *et al.*, 1979) have not been confirmed (Berrettini *et al.*, 1988).

Although a majority of the published studies report an elevation of urinary MHPG in mania, at least in comparison to depression, most relate to few patients. While some insist that longitudinal studies of individual patients 'consistently demonstrate higher urinary MHPG in mania as compared to depression' (Post, 1980), others can find no clear-cut trend (Annitto and Shopsin, 1979). The level of NA itself has been found to be raised in those manic episodes which appear to have been triggered by an environmental event, but not in those in which the onset was more autonomous (Swann *et al.*, 1989).

In two manic-depressive patients plasma MHPG was elevated in the manic phases; it fell slowly to normal after remission (Halaris, 1978).

In summary, there are no systematic changes in NA or its metabolites that are consistently associated with mania.

8.3.2 Dopamine

The activity of brain DA pathways has been studied by measuring the levels in the CSF of the major metabolite of DA, homovanillic acid (HVA). However, this metabolite is thought mainly to reflect DA turnover within the corpus striatum, and may thus only indirectly be related to mania. In the majority of the investigations of CSF HVA in manic patients no elevation has been detected (Post and Goodwin, 1978; Post, 1980). However, Sedvall (unpublished observations quoted by Annitto and Shopsin, 1979) has reported that CSF HVA as measured by mass spectrophotometry was elevated in mania, and that the level fell to normal when the symptoms abated following treatment with lithium. Bunney *et al.* (1977) describe a patient in whom there was a slow increase in CSF HVA before the switch from depression into mania occurred.

8.3.3 5-Hydroxytryptamine (serotonin; 5-HT)

5-Hydroxyindoleacetic acid (5-HIAA) is the primary metabolite of 5-HT; and its levels in lumbar CSF give an indication of the turnover of 5-HT in the brain. Although motor activity may lead to an increased CSF level of 5-HIAA, most studies have found normal or reduced levels in mania (Post, 1980; Tandon *et al.*, 1988).

Manic patients showed no deficiency in their ability to transport L-tryptophan (LTP) into the CSF or metabolize it to 5-HIAA in lumbar CSF (Ashcroft *et al.*, 1973). Normal CSF levels of LTP were found in mania (Bech *et al.*, 1978).

Wirz-Justice *et al.* (1975) demonstrated a significant rise in free plasma LTP levels accompanying improvement in a small series of manic patients. In platelets the uptake of 5-HT is increased early in the illness, reverting to normal on effective treatment with antipsychotic drugs (Meagher *et al.*, 1990). 5-HT-induced platelet aggregation is also increased in mania. The role of 5-HT receptor subtypes in the pathogenesis of mania remains completely unknown.

Brain 5-HT (Carlsson *et al.*, 1980) and the uptake of 5-HT by platelets (Wirz-Justice and Richter, 1979; Swade and Coppen, 1980) show seasonal variations, in keeping with the seasonal pattern of relapse discussed earlier. Furthermore, a 5-HT releasing compound, *d*-fenfluramine, was found more effective than placebo in improving the depressed mood in patients with seasonal affective disorder (O'Rourke *et al.*, 1989).

8.3.4 Calcium

Calcium ions have pronounced effects on neurotransmitter activity, and changes in Ca^{2+} concentration and uptake in mania may be related to the occurrence of a relapse. Ca^{2+} acts via a series of binding proteins, the most important of which is calmodulin.

Earlier reports indicating a slightly reduced Ca^{2+} level in the CSF in mania (Jimerson *et al.*, 1979) have not been confirmed by more recent studies (Bowden *et al.*, 1988). Moreover, the report of a reduced plasma level of Ca^{2+} during manic episodes, which is reflected in a lowering of the intraplatelet Ca^{2+} concentration (Bowden *et al.*, 1988), has been criticized on methodological grounds by Dubovsky *et al.* (1989), who found an increase of Ca^{2+} in platelets but not in plasma. The relevance of such changes in the peripheral blood to what is going on in the brain of manic patients is at best uncertain.

The transport of Ca^{2+} through neuronal membranes is controlled by calcium channels; Ca^{2+}-activated K^+ conductance governs the rate of action potential generation, and thus the rate of neurotransmitter release. It is of interest, therefore, that calcium channel blockers such as verapamil can ameliorate the symptoms of mania (Dinan *et al.*, 1988). As such drugs become active only in situations where normal Ca^{2+}-activated K^+ conductance is impaired, it has been suggested that in mania there is an abnormality in this conductance which can be reversed by calcium channel blockers (Dinan, 1989).

8.4 Pharmacology

8.4.1 Drugs affecting NA neurotransmission

The great majority of the currently available antidepressant drugs, including all the tricyclic compounds, block the reuptake of NA (and/or 5-HT) from the synaptic cleft into the presynaptic neurone.

There have been a considerable number of case reports of mania being precipitated by monoamine reuptake inhibitors (MARI), with the overall risk being estimated at almost 9% (Wehr and Goodwin, 1987). Bipolar patients appear to be particularly susceptible (Prien et al., 1973). Of 26 bipolar patients being treated with MARI, 18 became manic and five developed a pattern of rapid cycling (Wehr and Goodwin, 1979). Others have questioned the relationship of relapse to treatment with antidepressants, suggesting instead that such relapses would have occurred whether or not antidepressant drugs had been taken (Lewis and Winokur, 1982; Angst, 1985). Nevertheless, it does seem that, in some patients at least, manic episodes are triggered by MARI treatment.

Mania can also be triggered by stopping MARI (Mirin et al., 1981). This might be related to an anticholinergic withdrawal syndrome (Dilsaver et al., 1987).

Yohimbine, a presynaptic α_2-adrenoceptor blocking drug, which has the net effect of increasing central noradrenergic neurotransmission, has been reported to precipitate a manic episode in three patients (Price et al., 1984). While such a finding is strongly suggestive of a role for NA in the pathogenesis of mania, the numbers studied are few; the finding needs to be replicated.

Fusaric acid is a specific inhibitor of dopamine β-hydroxylase, the enzyme which converts DA to NA. When given to four patients exhibiting symptoms of moderate to severe mania, it caused a pronounced worsening in three (Sack and Goodwin, 1974). This was accompanied by a rise in the level of HVA in the CSF and a fall in MHPG, confirming that the drug was reducing NA synthesis while probably increasing that of DA. Such a finding is consistent with the view that overactivity of DA rather than NA neurotransmitter pathways are involved in mania.

Clonidine, which reduces NA transmission by a direct agonist action on the presynaptic α_2-adrenoceptors, has been reported to ameliorate mania in a few patients in uncontrolled studies. Unfortunately the only double-blind placebo-controlled trial failed to confirm the antimanic activity of clonidine (see below). The role of NA in the pathogenesis of mania thus remains unresolved.

8.4.2 Drugs affecting DA neurotransmission

DA neurotransmission can be increased by precursor loading using L-dopa (Bunney *et al.*, 1972), by increasing the release of preformed DA using amphetamine (Carlsson, 1970), or by direct stimulation of DA receptors by bromocriptine (Corrodi *et al.*, 1972).

L-Dopa, when given to nine patients presenting with a bipolar depressive illness, precipitated mania in eight, whereas only one of 13 patients with unipolar depression became manic (Murphy, 1972).

Dextro-amphetamine (*d*-AMP) has also been found to precipitate mania in bipolar but not unipolar depression (Gerner *et al.*, 1976).

Oral *d*-AMP in single 10 mg and 20 mg doses increases mood and arousal in a dose-related manner in normal subjects (Silverstone *et al.*, 1983), giving rise to a picture suggestive of mild mania (Jacobs and Silverstone, 1986). *d*-AMP-induced arousal and euphoria in man is likely to be mediated through a dopaminergic mechanism, as it is attenuated by pimozide (Jonsson, 1972; Silverstone *et al.*, 1980).

Piribedil, a DA receptor agonist which acts directly on the receptors, when given to a patient suffering from bipolar depression led to mania after 12 days of treatment (Gerner *et al.*, 1976).

Another DA receptor agonist, bromocriptine (BMC) can lead to mania when given to depressed patients (Nordin *et al.*, 1981), when given to suppress lactation during the puerperium (Brook and Cookson, 1978; Vlissides *et al.*, 1978), and in patients with pituitary tumours (Turner *et al.*, 1984). BMC appears to be particularly effective in the treatment of bipolar depression; Colonna *et al.* (1979) have reported that six out of eight bipolar depressed patients responded well to BMC. We have also found BMC to be more effective in patients with bipolar depression than in those with unipolar depression; of five bipolar patients given BMC, all improved (two becoming manic), whereas none of the five unipolar patients did so (Silverstone, 1984). In a double-blind trial of BMC in depressive illness, the one bipolar patient given BMC responded well (Waehrens and Gerlach, 1981).

Antipsychotic drugs, which all share the pharmacological property of blocking DA receptors, are the most effective treatment for acutely disturbed manic patients (Prien *et al.*, 1972). The relatively specific DA receptor blocking drug, pimozide, is particularly effective (Cookson *et al.*, 1981), a finding in keeping with the view that it is the DA receptor blocking action which is important in the antimanic action of antipsychotic drugs. This is supported by the observation that the *cis*-isomer of clopenthixol, which possesses DA receptor blocking properties, is an effective antimanic drug, whereas *trans*-clopenthixol, which has no DA receptor blocking activity, is clinically ineffective in mania (Nolen, 1983a).

During treatment with pimozide (Cookson *et al.*, 1982) and haloperidol (Silverstone and Cookson, 1983), we found a close correspondence between the time-course of clinical response and that of the rise in serum prolactin, further supporting the involvement of DA in mania. Which DA receptor (D1 or D2) is involved is uncertain. The selective D2 receptor blocking drug, remoxipride, has been found by some (Chouinard and Steiner, 1986) but not by others (Cookson, 1986) to ameliorate mania. Christie *et al.* (1988) reported that sulpiride, another selective D2 receptor blocker, was better than lithium in reducing manic symptoms, but the trial was not double-blind. Resolution of this matter awaits further research.

8.4.3 Drugs affecting 5-hydroxytryptamine

There is something of a paradox in that the precursors of 5-HT, LTP and 5-hydroxytryptophan can precipitate mania (Meltzer and Lowy, 1987) and may also be effective antimanics (Prange *et al.*, 1974). However, a double-blind placebo-controlled trial revealed no benefit from LTP (Chambers and Naylor, 1978).

It has recently been shown that lithium (Cowen *et al.*, 1988) and carbamazepine (Elphick *et al.*, 1990), both of which are effective in the treatment of mania (see below), enhance 5-HT neurotransmission in normal subjects as measured by LTP-induced release of prolactin.

8.4.4 Drugs affecting acetylcholine

Janowski *et al.* (1972) described 'reversal of manic symptoms' by the cholinesterase inhibitor physostigmine given intravenously to three patients in a double-blind study including placebo; in two patients depressive symptoms developed. The acetylcholine receptors involved were thought to be muscarinic, since injection of atropine was found partially to counteract the improvement.

Carroll *et al.* (1973) confirmed that physostigmine produced a rapid reduction in motor activity and speech in two manic patients but observed no change in the thought content, which remained grandiose. In a further series of eight manic patients (Janowski *et al.*, 1973), intravenous physostigmine was compared, under double-blind conditions, with neostigmine, a cholinesterase inhibitor that does not cross the blood–brain barrier. Manic symptoms diminished after physostigmine but not after placebo or neostigmine. Improvement was observed in ratings of elation, grandiosity and flight of ideas, as well as in motor activity and pressure of speech. Davis *et al.* (1978) reported similar results.

Consistent with acetylcholine playing a role in the pathogenesis of mania is the report that the addition of lecithin (a precursor of brain acetylcholine), was more beneficial than the addition of placebo to the concurrent medication in five out of six patients exhibiting symptoms of mania (Cohen *et al.*, 1980).

8.4.5 Drugs affecting γ-aminobutyric acid (GABA)

The possible involvement of GABA in mania originated from the finding that the anticonvulsant drug, valproate, which is thought to act by increasing the availability of GABA in the brain, was more effective than placebo in relieving manic symptoms (Emrich *et al.*, 1980).

Another anticonvulsant drug, carbamazepine, has also been used successfully in treatment of mania (see Silverstone, 1990, for review), but it is uncertain how carbamazepine works.

In keeping with a role for GABA in the pathogenesis of mania are two reports that withdrawal of baclofen, a GABA agonist having an inhibitory effect on mesolimbic DA neurones, can lead to mania (Arnold *et al.*, 1980; Kirubakaran *et al.*, 1984). Similarly, clonazepam, a benzodiazepine used mainly for its anticonvulsant properties, which are assumed to be GABA-mediated, has been reported as being effective in mania (Chouinard *et al.*, 1983).

8.5 Neuroendocrinology

As the release of hormones from the pituitary gland is under the control of hypothalamic releasing factors, which in turn are regulated by central neurotransmitter systems, the study of the neuroendocrine changes accompanying manic episodes may throw light on the changes taking place within these neurotransmitter pathways.

8.5.1 Hypothalamic–pituitary–adrenocortical (HPA) system

In milder cases of mania, plasma cortisol may be low (Carroll, 1979a; Joyce *et al.*, 1987a). When the manic symptoms become more severe the plasma cortisol is elevated, with a blunting of the circadian rhythm (Sachar, 1975;

Akesode *et al.*, 1976; Cookson *et al.*, 1985; Joyce *et al.*, 1987a; Whalley *et al.*, 1989).

In our own series of 25 manic patients all but three had raised midnight cortisol levels, with 11 also having raised levels at 9 a.m. (Cookson *et al.*, 1985). During treatment with the DA receptor blocking drug, pimozide, cortisol levels returned towards normal, with a time-course parallel to that of clinical improvement (Cookson *et al.*, 1980). Since DA is not thought to be involved in the normal control of adrenocorticotrophic hormone (ACTH) and cortisol secretion, other neurotransmitter pathways activated in mania must be concerned in the rise in cortisol. Normal suppression of cortisol by dexamethasone in manic patients has been reported by Schlesser *et al.* (1980), but in another series of 50 manic patients, 46% showed an abnormal lack of suppression; ratings of severity of mania did not distinguish suppressors from non-suppressors (Graham *et al.*, 1982).

Exogenous corticosteroids can precipitate a manic episode in patients with no previous psychiatric history (Krauthammer and Klerman, 1978). The same is true of anabolic steroids taken by body-builders, where over 10% may experience a clear-cut manic episode (Pope and Katz, 1988).

8.5.2 Thyroid

The free thyroxine index in manic patients has been reported as no different from that of normal controls (Kirkegaard *et al.*, 1978; Rinieris *et al.*, 1978), whereas free tri-iodothyronine (T_3) and free T_3 index were significantly lower than in depressed patients or normal controls matched for age in one series of manic patients (Kirkegaard *et al.*, 1978), but similar in another (Bech *et al.*, 1978).

Basal thyrotrophin (TSH) levels are in the normal range in mania (Takahashi *et al.*, 1975; Kirkegaard *et al.*, 1978), although the TSH response to thyrotrophin-releasing hormone (TRH) has been found to be decreased (Kirkegaard *et al.*, 1978; Extein *et al.*, 1980; Gold *et al.*, 1980; Beasley *et al.*, 1988; Kiriike *et al.*, 1988). However, Coppen *et al.* (1980) could not confirm the decreased TSH response in mania. The results may be confounded by prior treatment with lithium, as TSH response to TRH may be reduced even 3 weeks after lithium therapy is stopped (Gold *et al.*, 1977).

In the few manic patients studied, the levels of TRH in the CSF were normal; this is in contrast to depression, where they were raised (Banki *et al.*, 1988). In general, there would appear to be no marked or consistent change in thyroid function during a manic episode.

Rapid cycling is said by some (Cowdry *et al.*, 1983; Bauer *et al.*, 1990), but not by others (Joffe *et al.*, 1988), to be more frequent in bipolar patients with impaired thyroid function. In contrast to normal subjects, rapid cyclers show no nocturnal surge in TSH (Sack *et al.*, 1988). Treatment with thyroxine is of benefit when TSH levels are raised, but not when they are within normal limits (Kusalic, 1988). They may thus be two types of rapid cyclers: those who are hypothyroid and respond to thyroid treatment, and those who are euthyroid, who do not benefit from thyroid treatment but who may benefit from carbamazepine. Generally, bipolar patients with impaired thyroid function do not respond well to treatment until they are rendered euthyroid (Cookson, 1988).

In view of the seasonal variation in the admission rates for mania, it is of interest that thyroid function also shows seasonal changes in normal subjects (Smals *et al.*, 1977; McLellan *et al.*, 1979).

8.5.3 Growth hormone (GH)

Plasma levels of GH in a series of 11 manic patients did not differ significantly from levels found during treatment with pimozide, or after recovery (Cookson *et al.*, 1982).

The apomorphine-induced rise in GH, a measure of DA receptor sensitivity in the hypothalamus, has been reported as being the same in manic patients as in normal controls (Casper *et al.*, 1977), and Meltzer *et al.* (1984) have suggested that hypothalamic DA synapses controlling GH secretion function relatively normally in mania. However, Hirschowitz *et al.* (1986) and Annseau *et al.* (1987) report a blunted GH response to apomorphine. The latter authors also found a similarly blunted response to the α_2-noradrenergic receptor agonist clonidine in seven drug-free manic subjects. They suggest that their negative results undermine the catecholamine hypothesis of affective disorder as, contrary to prediction, their findings point to impaired noradrenergic and dopaminergic neurotransmission in mania.

8.5.4 Prolactin

Untreated manic patients have plasma levels of prolactin (PRL) within the normal range Cookson *et al.* (1982). In patients being treated with pimozide or haloperidol, the level of prolactin rose with a time course that corresponded closely to that of clinical improvement (Cookson *et al.*, 1982; 1985). By contrast, in schizophrenia clinical response lagged behind the rise in prolactin (Silverstone and Cookson, 1983). Such observations suggest that the therapeutic activity of antipsychotic drugs in mania is more closely linked to DA receptor blockade than it is in schizophrenia.

Plasma levels of prolactin in the afternoon were found to be lower in bipolar than in unipolar depression (Joyce *et al.*, 1988). Bipolar depressed patients were also more sensitive to the DA antagonist metoclopramide (Joyce *et al.*,

1987b). This is in keeping with the heightened sensitivity in bipolar depression to the DA agonist bromocriptine (Silverstone, 1984), and contrary to the blunted growth hormone response to apomorphine reported by Hirschowitz *et al.* (1986).

8.5.5 Melatonin

Melatonin is a methylated indole, secreted from the pineal gland by β-adrenoceptor stimulation. The circadian rhythm and nocturnal secretion of melatonin is thought to be controlled by the suprachiasmatic nucleus of the hypothalamus, and bright light suppresses the secretion. This is of interest in view of the seasonal pattern of relapse which occurs in some bipolar patients. Melatonin levels may be increased in mania (Kennedy *et al.*, 1989), possibly due to the phase shift in certain circadian rhythms that occurs in manic-depressive illness (Wehr, 1984). Such phase shifts might be secondary to an increase in the responsiveness of melatonin suppression to light in bipolar patients (Lewy *et al.*, 1981; Nurnberger *et al.*, 1988). However, Lam *et al.* (1990) failed to find any such supersensitivity in eight bipolar patients; if anything, their responsiveness was less than that of the normal control subjects. This inconsistency awaits further clarification.

8.5.6 Gonadotrophins

A rise in the plasma level of luteinizing hormone (LH) has been observed in young men (but not women) during a manic episode (Whalley *et al.*, 1985). This persists after recovery and is accompanied by an increased LH response to luteinizing hormone releasing hormone (LHRH) (Whalley *et al.*, 1987). These authors attribute their findings to an increase in the responsiveness of the pituitary secondary to LHRH release, which might be a consequence of an increase in central noradrenergic activity.

It is of interest, in view of the analogy between amphetamine-induced arousal and mild mania (Jacobs and Silverstone, 1986), that low-dose amphetamine also causes a rise in plasma LH in young male volunteers (Jacobs *et al.*, 1989).

8.5.7 Puerperal psychosis

A high proportion of manic and schizomanic illnesses (about 50%) is found among patients admitted for mental illnesses that begin within 2 weeks after delivery (Brockington *et al.*, 1981; Dean and Kendell, 1981; Katona, 1982; Meltzer and Kumar, 1985). Such manic episodes have a better prognosis than non-puerperal mania, with fewer breakdowns in the next 3 years. In one series of 51 patients, 38 (75%) experienced only the single illness (Dean et al., 1989). This distinguishes puerperal psychosis from bipolar disorder unrelated to childbirth, which has a worse prognosis. By contrast, Platz and Kendell (1988) remarked on the similarity in outcome between patients who became manic in the puerperium and those who became manic at other times. It is thus uncertain whether puerperal psychoses are 'simply affective disorders precipitated by the as yet unspecified stresses associated with parturition', as Platz and Kendell believe. Female bipolar patients are especially vulnerable in the puerperium, with a high rate of breakdown (20–40%) occurring at that time (Reich and Winokur, 1970; Targum et al., 1979; Katona, 1982). It may be that systemic changes follow delivery and constitute a trigger for a manic syndrome to which genetically predisposed manic-depressives are especially vulnerable.

After delivery, circulating oestrogen levels fall dramatically. It is therefore relevant to the DA hypothesis of mania that studies in animals reveal interactions between circulating oestrogen and brain dopamine pathways; in both the pituitary and the striatum, oestrogen reduces responses to DA (Cookson, 1981). In addition, chronic oestradiol treatment leads to an increase in spiroperidol-binding sites (DA receptors) in the striatum (Di Paola et al., 1981). Thus, oestrogens resemble antipsychotic drugs in their ability to antagonize the effects of dopamine and to induce the formation of more dopamine receptors. Puerperal mania might therefore be explained in terms of the DA hypothesis, with the fall in oestrogen after delivery exposing supersensitive DA receptor systems in the mesolimbic system. In keeping with this view is the report of eight patients with a recent puerperal psychosis who had recovered but who relapsed shortly before the onset of the first menstrual period after delivery, a time of falling oestrogen (Brockington et al., 1988).

8.5.8 Aldosterone and Na-K-ATPase

Intracellular sodium (Na^+) concentrations were found to be raised in mania (Coppen et al., 1966). Intracellular water volume was also increased. Such findings indicate either an increased influx of Na^+ into the cells or a deficiency in active transport of Na^+ out of cells; the latter might be caused by a deficiency in Na-K-ATPase, the membrane enzyme system for the sodium pump, or by alterations in the hormone control of fluid and electrolyte balance.

Early reports indicated a lowering of Na-K-ATPase activity in red cells in mania compared with recovery (Naylor et al., 1980). However, more recent studies in acutely manic patients have found Na-K-ATPase activity to be raised (Wood et al., 1989). There remains considerable doubt about the relevance of peripheral cell ATPase activity to the cerebral changes in affective disorders (Whalley et al., 1980).

Since vanadate ions inhibit Na-K-ATPase, it was proposed that mania may be caused by raised levels of vanadium (Naylor and Smith, 1981). However, no clear-cut relationship has been found between serum vanadium levels and mood changes in bipolar patients, and there is no convincing evidence that raised vanadium levels lead to mania (Chiu and Rimon, 1988).

Aldosterone stimulates sodium transport and Na-K-ATPase in some circumstances. Plasma levels of aldosterone in mania are higher than in controls and fall during treatment (Hendler, 1975; Akesode et al., 1976). The mechanisms responsible for such an increase in aldosterone levels are unknown; it could be related to a deficit in the renin–angiotensin–aldosterone system (Hullin et al., 1977).

8.6 Treatment

There is a range of drugs available for the treatment of acute mania. Which one to use depends largely on the severity of the manic state to be treated, as well as the response to the standard treatments.

8.6.1 Antipsychotic drugs

For the more disturbed patient, antipsychotic drugs such as chlorpromazine or haloperidol are the treatment of choice, being more effective than lithium (Prien et al., 1972, 1973). We have found the selective DA receptor blocking drug, pimozide, to be as effective as chlorpromazine in controlling manic symptoms (Cookson et al., 1981). By contrast, in a population of patients designated as psychotic, pimozide was reported as being less effective in controlling manic symptoms than lithium, but better in reducing delusions and hallucinations (Johnstone et al., 1988). However, in this study many of the patients allocated to receive lithium as a sole treatment had also received adjuvant antipsychotic treatment.

8.6.2 Lithium

Cade's (Cade, 1949) seminal finding that lithium is effective in mania has been amply confirmed. Four double-blind clinical trials have shown it to be superior to placebo, at least for cases of mild to moderate severity (for reviews, see Goodwin and Zis, 1979; Coxhead and Silverstone, 1987). If, however, as has already been pointed out, the manic symptoms are florid, then antipsychotic drugs are more effective. In less severe cases lithium produces just as good results with fewer untoward side-effects, although it takes longer to act, becoming effective in about 7–10 days.

Some 70–80% of patients treated with lithium respond (Black et al., 1988). Predictors of a favourable response include a short episode duration, older age of onset, and little psychiatric or medical co-morbidity. Looking at neurotransmitter metabolites in the CSF, Bowden et al. (1990) found that those patients in whom there was a close correspondence between MHPG and 5-HIAA did better. Treatment with lithium can lead to a lowering of CSF MHPG, which is more marked in non-responders (Swann et al., 1987).

The mode of action of lithium is unknown but there are a number of possibilities. It competes with calcium at the neuronal membrane, acting as a calcium channel blocker, it reduces the activity of adenylate cyclase, the second messenger system for D1 receptors, and it affects the turnover of inositol phosphate, another second messenger system (Goodwin, 1988). In normal subjects it enhances central 5-HT neurotransmission (Cowen et al., 1988).

During lithium administration careful monitoring of the plasma concentration is required to avoid toxicity, which usually begins when the lithium concentration exceeds 1.5 mmol/litre, but toxic symptoms such as nausea and vomiting may occur at a lower level. The presence of such symptoms demands immediate withdrawal of lithium until the plasma level has been ascertained and any elevation dealt with appropriately.

8.6.3 Carbamazepine

In recent years, carbamazepine has come to be accepted as an effective alternative to lithium. While there have been relatively few placebo-controlled studies, those that have been undertaken suggest that carbamazepine is better than placebo (Goncalves and Stoll, 1985; Post et al., 1987b). In two studies, carbamazepine was compared with lithium; in one it did slightly less well (Lerer et al., 1987), in the other the response to the two drugs was similar (Okuma, 1988). Comparing carbamazepine to antipsychotics it was found to be equal in efficacy to chlorpromazine (Okuma et al., 1979; Grossi et al., 1984) and to haloperidol (Stoll et al., 1986; Brown et al., 1989). However, as with lithium, the more severe cases require antipsychotic medication, at least to start with, because carbamazepine takes some 10 days to become effective. Another limiting factor is the frequency of a rash which occurs in some 15% of bipolar patients treated with carbamazepine (Elphick et al., 1988). The mode of action of carbamazepine remains largely unknown (Silverstone, 1990). Although it is an anticonvulsant, there is no convincing evidence to link its prophylactic efficacy to this action. Like lithium, carbamazepine enhances central 5-HT neurotransmission in normal subjects (Elphick et al., 1990).

8.6.4 Sodium valproate

Following encouraging reports from Germany of the value of another anticonvulsant, sodium valproate, in the treatment of mania (Emrich *et al.*, 1980), several open uncontrolled clinical trials have yielded a response rate of some 60% (Ballenger, 1990). In a series of 55 rapid cyclers largely resistant to lithium, sodium valproate was effective in alleviating manic symptoms, but less so for depression (Calbrese and Delucchi, 1990). Side-effects include gastrointestinal symptoms, tremor, ataxia and alopecia.

8.6.5 Clonazepam

The benzodiazepine anticonvulsant clonazepam has been reported as being of benefit in the management of acute mania by Chouinard *et al.* (1983) and Victor *et al.* (1984). In sharp contrast, Aronson *et al.* (1989) found clonazepam to be of no benefit in five lithium-resistant bipolar patients. It is unclear whether clonazepam, when it is effective, is so merely because of its sedative properties or because it has an additional primary antimanic effect.

8.6.6 Clonidine

Initial uncontrolled trials of the α_2-adrenoceptor agonist, clonidine indicated an antimanic effect (Giannini *et al.*, 1983; Zubenko *et al.*, 1984; Hardy *et al.*, 1986). Unfortunately, the only double-blind placebo-controlled study to date failed to confirm these promising results (Janicak *et al.*, 1989). Few of the 21 manic or mixed bipolar patients improved significantly on either clonidine (two patients) or placebo (one patient). Four patients on clonidine failed to complete, two because of an unacceptable fall in blood pressure and two because of a rash. Thus the value of clonidine in the treatment of mania is as yet unproven.

8.6.7 Verapamil

As stated previously, calcium transport regulates the release of neurotransmitters from presynaptic neurones. Thus interference with this neuronal transport system by drugs which block calcium channels could well influence brain function and psychopathology. The calcium channel blocker verapamil, which crosses the blood–brain barrier, given to three manic patients for 3 weeks improved the clinical state, which worsened on placebo substitution (Dubovsky and Franks, 1983). We gave verapamil to six manic patients, five of whom improved during the first 2 weeks of treatment, but one of these relapsed in the third week (Dinan *et al.*, 1988). Verapamil also compared favourably with antipsychotic drugs in an uncontrolled comparison in 36 manic patients (Hoschl and Kozeny, 1989). Finally, in a four-way, between-patient, controlled clinical trial of verapamil, nifedipine, lithium and placebo, involving 60 manic patients (15 on each treatment), the proportion improving on verapamil (60%), nifedipine (67%) and lithium (67%) was greater than on placebo (31%) (Vohra *et al.*, 1989). Calcium channel blockers thus appear to be a promising new treatment for mania.

8.7 Prevention of relapse

8.7.1 Lithium

Following its success in the management of acute manic episodes, lithium was introduced as a prophylactic treatment for bipolar illness. Evidence from a number of controlled clinical trials has confirmed that it can significantly reduce the risk of relapse in bipolar illness (Baastrup *et al.*, 1970; Coppen *et al.*, 1971; Prien *et al.*, 1984; Bunney and Gurland-Bunney, 1987).

Despite this, in one catchment area in Scotland, only a bare majority of those taking lithium were thought to be reaping any worthwhile benefit (McCreadie *et al.*, 1985). Furthermore, admission rates in Edinburgh over the period 1970–1981 failed to reflect any impact of the availability of lithium prophylaxis, with the number of admissions for manic episodes actually rising threefold during these 12 years (Dickson and Kendell, 1986), Nevertheless, on balance it appears that lithium has a definite potential to reduce the rate of recurrences in many patients with bipolar illness. Some 20–50% of patients fail, however, to respond to lithium prophylaxis (Dunner *et al.*, 1976; Carroll, 1979b; Kukopulos and Reginaldi, 1980; Maj *et al.*, 1984). The only reliable predictor of the outcome for individual patients is their past experience with lithium (Carroll, 1979b; Kocsis and Stokes, 1979). Patients with four or more recurrences a year, so-called 'rapid cyclers', are generally recognized as being unlikely to do well on lithium (Dunner *et al.*, 1976; Misra and Burns, 1977; Carroll, 1979b; Kukopulos and Reginaldi, 1980; Abou-Saleh and Coppen, 1986). A positive family history for bipolar disorder may or may not influence response. Some say it does (Maj *et al.*, 1984; Abou-Saleh and Coppen, 1986); others not (Dunner *et al.*, 1976; Mander, 1986).

Neither the age of the onset of the illness, the age at starting lithium nor gender affect the long-term outcome (Dunner *et al.*, 1976; Kocsis and Stokes, 1979; Maj *et al.*, 1984; Abou-Saleh and Coppen, 1986; Mander, 1986; Goodnick *et al.*, 1987). Nor, according to some reports, do social circumstances

(Kocsis and Stokes, 1979; Maj *et al.*, 1984). Personality variables may play some part, with anxious patients doing less well (Maj *et al.*, 1984; Abou-Saleh and Coppen 1986). Sudden cessation of lithium can lead to a rapid recurrence of mania (Mander and Loudon, 1988). This has been termed a lithium withdrawal reaction (Greil and Schmidt, 1988).

A common endocrinological consequence of long-term treatment with lithium is a lowering of thyroid function which occurs in 15–25%, more frequently in women (Transbol *et al.*, 1978; Lazarus *et al.*, 1981). This may have an effect on relapse frequency (see section 8.5.2).

8.7.2 Carbamazepine

As with lithium, initial success in the treatment of manic episodes led to carbamazepine being tried as a prophylactic for bipolar disorder. In the first placebo-controlled clinical trial involving 12 patients in Japan, the relapse rate was more than halved by carbamazepine (Okuma *et al.*, 1981). A similarly gratifying response to carbamazepine was seen by Ballenger and Post (1980) in six bipolar patients.

Since then a number of double-blind prospective clinical trials comparing carbamazepine to lithium have been carried out in representative samples of patients (Placidi *et al.*, 1986; Watkins *et al.*, 1987; Lusznat *et al.*, 1988; Silverstone *et al.*, 1989). All show therapeutic equivalence, with carbamazepine causing fewer side-effects. Rapid cyclers tend to respond better to carbamazepine than to lithium (Joyce, 1988). The combination of lithium and carbamazepine is sometimes better than either drug alone (Lipinski and Pope, 1982; Nolen, 1983b; Post *et al.*, 1987a; Desai *et al.*, 1989).

8.7.3 Depot antipsychotics

Although antipsychotic drugs are used widely in the management of acute mania (see above), they have been little studied as prophylactics, particularly in the depot form. The addition of depot fluphenazine or flupenthixol to lithium has been shown to reduce the frequency of manic episodes (Naylor and Scott, 1980), as has flupenthixol alone (Ahlfors *et al.*, 1981). However, a placebo-controlled trial failed to show any advantage of adding flupenthixol to lithium (Esparon *et al.*, 1986). This is surprising in the light of clinical experience, where the use of depot antipsychotics has been found to help significantly in the management of the more unstable bipolar patients (Lowe and Batchelor, 1986). Depot antipsychotics have the potential disadvantage of causing tardive dyskinesia (Mukherjee *et al.*, 1986). In our series of bipolar patients who had received prophylactic antipsychotics, 48% exhibited signs of tardive dyskinesia (N. Hunt and T. Silverstone, unpublished data).

8.8 Theoretical considerations

Mania appears to be a genetically heterogeneous condition which runs an episodic course. Recurrences can be influenced by seasonal variation, by drug treatment, and by change in endocrine status. Some patients respond to lithium, others to carbamazepine, and some to neither. Thus, no one hypothesis is likely to suffice for all cases of mania.

8.8.1 Monoamine hypothesis

This is the most venerable of the current theories of affective disorder (Schildkraut, 1965). In its original form, mania was thought to be due to an excess of monoamine neurotransmitter activity. Despite having received many buffetings over the years, the monoamine hypothesis has survived, at least in qualified form.

We have seen that there is good pharmacological evidence to implicate dopamine in the pathogenesis of mania (Silverstone, 1985): drugs increasing DA neurotransmission can precipitate mania in predisposed individuals, while drugs blocking DA receptors ameliorate it. An action on DA does not, however, explain the efficacy of lithium or carbamazepine. 5-HT may play a role, as both drugs have been shown to enhance central 5-HT neurotransmission. Also, brain 5-HT shows a seasonal variation, as do the admission rates for mania. In animal studies, 5-HT can influence DA neuronal activity; it may therefore be an imbalance in the activities of the DA and the 5-HT neurotransmitter systems which underlies the pathogenesis of bipolar disorder.

8.8.2 'Kindling'

Post et al. (1984b) have pointed out that in some patients with bipolar disorder the frequency of relapse increases with the number of episodes, with later episodes having a more precipitous onset and the impact of psychological factors being less prominent. They liken this to the phenomenon of 'kindling' in experimental animals, whereby the eventual development of a major motor seizure can result from intermittent electrical stimulation of the brain with a current originally insufficient to produce overt behavioural effects. Kindling is generated more easily within the limbic system than in the cortex and reflects a long-lasting, possibly permanent, change in neuronal excitability which gives rise both to spontaneous and to stress-related seizures. This could explain the efficacy of anticonvulsant drugs such as carbamazepine in reducing the frequency of relapse in bipolar disorder. However, as they themselves admit, bipolar disorder cannot be considered clinically as a seizure disorder in any sense of the term (Post and Weiss, 1989). They regard kindling simply as 'a non-homologous model for only some aspects of the longitudinal course of manic-depressive illness'. Adamec (1990) is more sceptical of the value of kindling as a model for mania, emphasizing that there is hardly any evidence that it occurs in humans.

8.8.3 Behavioural sensitization

This is the name given to the phenomenon by which repeated applications of a low dose of a psychomotor stimulant, such as cocaine or amphetamine, leads to increasing behavioural effects, with an ever-decreasing latency. It is thought to be mediated by DA pathways (Post and Weiss, 1989). According to this view, changes in susceptibility to relapse in bipolar disorder might reflect alterations in the sensitivity of DA neurones. It is an hypothesis compatible with the idea presented above, that relapse is related to an imbalance between DA and 5-HT neurotransmitter systems.

8.8.4 Sleep deprivation

Wehr *et al.* (1987) believe that reduction of sleep forms the final common pathway in the pathogenesis of mania. They argue that many of the factors implicated as causes of manic episodes, such as psychosocial stresses, post-partum changes and administration of various drugs and hormones, may all be associated with interference with sleep. In support of this hypothesis, when bipolar patients are deprived of sleep for a night they frequently become manic (Wehr *et al.*, 1982). It is also in keeping with the finding from London Airport that patients arriving with a manic illness are more likely to have been deprived of sleep by having flown overnight from west to east than going in the other direction (Jauhar and Weller, 1982). It is also compatible with the observation that in genetically predisposed men with a past history of mania the risk of relapse is high in the 'postpartum' period, presumably because the new baby keeps them awake at night (Wehr *et al.*, 1987). However we have failed to confirm any such association in a series of men with bipolar disorder (T. Silverstone, N. Hunt, H. McPherson & S. Romans-Clarkson, unpublished observations).

8.9 Conclusion

Mania, with its exhausting overactivity, bellicose self-confidence, racing thoughts and flight of ideas, is clearly the consequence of a serious disturbance of function within the brain. It looks as if this might occur mainly in the right frontal-temporal region, an area which includes the limbic system. Both dopaminergic and serotoninergic neurotransmitter pathways are likely to be involved, but others may be as well. While a number of neuroendocrine changes have been observed in mania, most are probably secondary epiphenomena, although a pathogenic role for endogenous or exogenous steroids cannot be ruled out. The puerperium is a time of increased risk for women, perhaps related to an increased sensitivity of dopamine receptors.

All these mechanisms may play a part in the pathogenesis of mania, with some being more significant in certain patients than in others. It is likely that the relative benefits of a particular treatment in a given patient are determined by which neurological system is most affected in that patient.

References

Abou-Saleh, M.T. & Coppen, A. (1986) *J. Affective Disord.* **10**, 115–125.

Adamec, R.E. (1990) *Biol. Psychiatry* **27**, 249–279.

Ahlfors, U.G., Baastrup, P.C., Dencker, S.J. & Elgen, K. (1981) *Acta Psychiatr. Scand.* **64**, 226–237.

Akesode, A., Hendler, N. & Konarski, A.A. (1976) *Psychoneuroendocrinology* **1**, 419–426.

Angst, J. (1985) *Psychopathology* **18**, 140–154.

Annitto, W. & Shopsin, B. (1979) In *Manic Illness* (ed. Shopsin, B.), pp 105–162. New York, Raven Press.

Annseau, M., von Frenckell, R., Cerfontaine, J.-L. *et al.* (1987) *Psychiatry Res.* **22**, 193–206.

Arato, M., Rihmer, Z. & Felszeghy, K. (1980) *Biol. Psychiatry* **15**, 319–322.

Arnold, E.S., Rudd, S.N. & Kirschner, H. (1980) *Am. J. Psychiatry* **137**, 1446–1447.

Aronson, T.A., Shukla, S. & Hirschowitz, J. (1989) *Am. J. Psychiatry* **146**, 77–80.

Ashcroft, G., Crawford, T., Cundall, R. *et al.* (1973) *Psychol. Med.* **3**, 326–332.

Baastrup, P.C., Poulson, J.C., Schou, M., Thomsen, K. & Amdisen, A. (1970) *Lancet* **ii**, 326–330.

Ballenger, J.C. (1990) *Int. Clin. Psychopharmacol.* **5** (Suppl. 1), 1–7.

Ballenger, J.C. & Post, R.M. (1980) *Am. J. Psychiatry* **137**, 782–790.

Banki, C., Bisette, G., Arato, M. & Nemeroff, C. (1988) *Am. J. Psychiatry* **145**, 1526–1531.

Barczak, P., Edmunds, E. & Betts, T. (1988) *Br. J. Psychiatry* **152**, 137–139.

Bauer, M.S., Whybrow, P. & Winokur, A. (1990) *Arch. Gen. Psychiatry* **47**, 427–432.

Baxter, L.R., Phelps, M.E., Mazziotta, J.C. *et al.* (1985) *Arch. Gen. Psychiatry* **42**, 441–447.

Beasley, C., Magnusson, M. & Garver, D. (1988) *Biol. Psychiatry* **24**, 423–431.

Bech, P., Kirkengaard, C., Bock, E., Johanesson, M. & Rafaelson, O. (1978) *Neuropsychobiology* **4**, 99–112.

Berrettini, W., Hoehe, M., Lontes, K. *et al.* (1988) *Psychopharmacology* **96** (Suppl.), 66.

Black, D., Winokur, G., Hulbert, J. & Nasrallah, A. (1988) *Biol. Psychiatry* **24**, 191–198.

Bowden, C., Huang, L., Javors, M. *et al.* (1988) *Biol. Psychiatry* **23**, 367–376.

Bowden, C., Rush, A.J. & Swann, A. (1990) *Biol. Psychiatry* **27**, 144A.

Brewerton, T.D. & McClaughlin, D. (1986) Paper presented at the *IVth World Congress of Biological Psychiatry*, Philadelphia, Abstract 528.3

Brockington, I.F., Cernik, K., Schofield, E., Downing, A., Francis, A. & Keelan, C. (1981) *Arch. Gen. Psychiatry* **38**, 829–833.

Brockington, I.F., Kelly, A., Hall, P. & Deakin, W. (1988) *J. Affective Disord.* **14**, 287–292.

Brook, W.M. & Cookson, Z.B. (1978) *Br. Med. J.* **2**, 510.

Brown, D., Silverstone, T. & Cookson, J. (1989) *Int. Clin. Psychopharmacol.* **4**, 229–238.

Bunney, W.E. & Garland-Bunney, B.L. (1987) In *Psychopharmacology: The Third Generation of Progress* (ed. Meltzer, H.Y.), pp 553–565. New York, Raven Press.

Bunney, W.E., Gershon, E., Murphy, D. & Goodwin, F.K. (1972) *J. Psychiatr. Res.* **9**, 207–226.

Bunney, W., Wehr, T. & Gillin, J. (1977) *Ann. Intern. Med.* **87**, 319–335.

Cade, J.F. (1949) *Med. J. Aust.* **2**, 349–353.

Calbrese, J.R. & Delucchi, G.A. (1990) *Am. J. Psychiatry* **147**, 431–434.

Carlsson, A. (1970) In *Amphetamine and Related Compounds* (eds Costa, E. & Garattani, S.), pp 289–300. New York, Raven Press.

Carlsson, A., Svennerholm, L. & Winblad, B. (1980) *Acta Psychiatr. Scand.* **61** (Suppl. 280), 75–83.

Carney, P.A., Fitzgerald, C.T. & Monaghan, C. (1988) *Br. J. Psychiatry* **152**, 820–823.

Carroll, B.J. (1979a) In *Manic Illness* (ed. Shopsin, B.), pp 163–176. New York, Raven Press.

Carroll, B.J. (1979b) *Arch. Gen. Psychiatry* **36**, 870–878.

Carroll, B.J., Frazer, Schless, A. & Mendels, J. (1973) *Lancet*, **i**, 427.

Casper, R., Davis, J., Pandey, G., Garver, D. & Dekirmenjian, H. (1977) *Psychoneuroendocrinology* **2**, 105–113.

Chambers, C.A. & Naylor, G.J. (1978) *Br. J. Psychiatry* **132**, 555–559.

Chiu, L.P.W. & Rimon, R. (1988) *Hum. Psychopharmacol.* **3**, 159–169.

Chouinard, G. & Steiner, W. (1986) *Biol. Psychiatry* **21**, 1429–1433.

Chouinard, G., Young, S.N. & Annable, L. (1983) *Biol. Psychiatry* **18**, 451–466.

Christie, J., Whalley, L., Hunter, R., Bennie, J. & Fink, G. (1988) *J. Affective Disord.* **16**, 115–120.

Clark, A.F. & Davison, K. (1987) *Br. J. Psychiatry* **150**, 841–844.

Coffman, J.A., Bornstein, R.A., Olson, S., Schwarzkoff, S. & Nasrallah, H. (1990) *Biol. Psychiatry* **27**, 1188.

Cohen, B., Miller, A.L., Lipinski, J.P. & Pope, H.G. (1980) *Am. J. Psychiatry* **137**, 242–243.

Cohen, R., Semple, W., Gross, M. *et al.* (1989) *Neuropsychopharmacology* **2**, 241–254.

Colonna, L., Petit, M. & Lepine, J.P. (1979) *J. Affective Disord.* **1**, 173–177.

Cook, B.L., Shukla, S. & Hoff, A.L. (1986) *J. Affective Disord.* **11**, 147–149.

Cookson, J.C. (1981) *Br. J. Psychiatry* **139**, 365–366 (letter).

Cookson, J.C. (1986) Paper presented at Collegium Internationale Neuro-Psychopharmacologicum Meeting, Puerto Rico.

Cookson, J.C. (1988) *Psychopharmacology* **96** (Suppl.), 63.

Cookson, J., Silverstone, T., Besser, G.M. & Williams, S. (1980) *Neuropharmacology* **10**, 1234–1244.

Cookson, J., Silverstone, T. & Wells, B. (1981) *Acta Psychiatr. Scand.* **64**, 381–397.

Cookson, J.C., Silverstone, T. & Rees, L. (1982) *Br. J. Psychiatry* **140**, 274–279.

Cookson, J.C., Silverstone, T., Williams, S. & Besser, G.M. (1985) *Br. J. Psychiatry* **146**, 498–502.

Coppen, A., Shaw, D., Malleson, A. & Costain, R. (1966) *Br. Med. J.* **1**, 71–75.

Coppen, A., Noguera, R., Bailey, J. *et al.* (1971) *Lancet* **ii**, 275–279.
Coppen, A., Rao, V., Bishop, M., Abou-Saleh, M. & Wood, K. (1980) *J. Affective Disord.* **2**, 317–320.
Corrodi, H., Farnebo, L. & Fuxe, K. (1972) *Eur. J. Pharmacology* **20**, 195–204.
Coryell, W., Andreasen, N., Endicott, J. & Keller, M. (1987) *Am. J. Psychiatry* **144**, 309–315.
Cowdry, R.W., Wehr, T.A., Zis, A.P. & Goodwin, F.F. (1983) *Arch. Gen. Psychiatry* **40**, 414–424.
Cowen, R., McCance, S., Friston, K., Julier, D. & Gelder, M. (1988) Paper presented at the Royal College of Psychiatry, Brighton, July.
Coxhead, N. & Silverstone, T. (1987) In *Depression and Mania. Modern Lithium Therapy* (ed. Johnson, F.N.), pp 31–34. Oxford, IRL Press.
Cummings, J.L. & Mendez, M. (1984) *Am. J. Psychiatry* **141**, 1084–1087.
Davis, K.L., Berger, P.A., Hollister, L.E. & Defraites, E. (1978) *Arch. Gen. Psychiatry* **35**, 119–122.
Dean, C. & Kendell, R.E. (1981) *Br. J. Psychiatry* **139**, 128–133.
Dean, C., Williams, R.J. & Brockington, I.F. (1989) *Psychol. Med.* **19**, 637–647.
Delvenne, V., Delecluse, F., Hubain, P., Schoutens, A., DeMaertelaer, V. & Mendlewicz, J. (1989) *8th World Congress of Psychiatry, Athens.* Excerpta Medica, International Congress Series **899**, Abstract 832 p. 222.
Demirovic, V. & Zec, N. (1986) Paper presented at the *IVth World Congress of Biological Psychiatry*, Philadelphia, Abstract 10, 528.5.
Desai, N., Gangadhar, B., Channabasavanna, S. & Shetty, K. (1989) In *New Directions In Affective Disorders* (eds Lerer, B. & Gershon, S.). Berlin, Springer-Verlag.
Dewan, M., Haldipur, C., Lane, E., Donelly, M., Boucher, M. & Major, L. (1987) *Biol. Psychiatry* **22**, 1058–1066.
Dewan, M.J., Haldipur, C., Lane, E., Ispahani, A., Boucher, M. & Major, L. (1988a) *Acta Psychiatr. Scand.* **77**, 670–676.
Dewan, M., Haldipur, C.V., Boucher, M., Ramachandran, T. & Major, L. (1988b) *Acta Psychiatr. Scand.* **77**, 677–682.
Dickson, W.E. & Kendell, R.E. (1986) *Psychol. Med.* **16**, 521–530.
Dilsaver, S.C., Greden, J.F. & Snider, R.M. (1987) *Int. Clin. Psychopharmacol.* **2**, 1–19.
Dinan, T.G. (1989) *Hum. Psychopharmacol.* **4**, 139–144.
Dinan, T.G., Silverstone, T. & Cookson, J.C. (1988) *Int. Clin. Psychopharmacol.* **3**, 151–156.
Di Paola, T., Poyet, P. & Labrie, F. (1981) *Eur. J. Pharmacol.* **73**, 105–106.
Dubovsky, S.L. & Franks, R.D. (1983) *Biol. Psychiatry* **18**, 781–797.
Dubovsky, S.L., Christiano, J., Daniell, L.C. *et al.* (1989) *Arch. Gen. Psychiatry* **46**, 632–638.
Dunner, D.L., Fleiss, J.L. & Fieve, R.R. (1976) *Br. J. Psychiatry* **129**, 40–44.
Dunner, D.L., Patrick, V. & Fieve, R.R. (1977) *Compr. Psychiatry* **18**, 561–566.
Dupont, R., Jernigan, T., Gillin, C., Heaton, R., Zisook, S. & Braff, D. (1989) Paper presented at the American College of Neuropsychopharmacology, Hawaii.
Dupont, R., Jernigan, T., Butters, N. *et al.* (1990) *Arch. Gen. Psychiatry* **47**, 55–59.
Eastwood, M.R. & Stiasny, S. (1978) *Arch. Gen. Psychiatry* **35**, 769–771.
Elphick, M., Lyons, F. & Cowen, P. (1988) *J. Psychopharmacol.* **2**, 1–4.
Elphick, M., Yang, J.-D. & Cowen, P.J. (1990) *Arch. Gen. Psychiatry* **47**, 135–140.
Emrich, H.M., Zerssen, D. & Kissling, W. (1980) *Arch. Psychiatr. Nervenkr.* **229**, 1–6.
Esparon, J., Kolloori, J., Naylor, G.J., McHarg, A.M., Smith, A.H.W. & Hopwood, S.E. (1986) *Br. J. Psychiatry* **148**, 723–725.

Extein, I., Taliman, J., Smith, C.C. & Goodwin, F.K. (1979) *Psychiatry Res.* **1**, 191–197.

Extein, I., Pottash, A.L.C., Gold, M.S. *et al.* (1980) *Psychiatry Res.* **2**, 199–204.

Flor-Henry, P. (1979) *Biol. Psychiatry* **14**, 677–698.

Frangos, A., Athanassenas, G., Tsitourides, S. *et al.* (1980) *J. Affective Disord.* **2**, 239–247.

Gerner, R.H., Post, R.M. & Bunney, W.E. (1976) *Am. J. Psychiatry* **133**, 1177–1180.

Giannini, A., Extein, I. & Gold, M. (1983) *Drug Dev. Res.* **3**, 101–103.

Gold, M.S., Pottash, A.L.C., Ryan, N., Sweeney, D.R., Davies, R.K. & Martin, R.M. (1980) *Psychoneuroendocrinology* **5**, 147–155.

Gold, P., Goodwin, F., Wehr, T. & Rebar, R. (1977) *Am. J. Psychiatry* **134**, 1028–1031.

Goncalves, N. & Stoll, K. (1985) *Nervenarzt* **56**, 43–47.

Goodnick, P.J., Fieve, R.R., Schleger, A. & Baxter, N. (1987) *Am. J. Psychiatry* **144**, 367–369.

Goodwin, F.K. & Jamison, K.R. (1984) In *Neurobiology of Mood Disorders* (eds Post, R.M. & Ballenger, J.C.), pp 20–38. Baltimore, Williams & Wilkins.

Goodwin, F. & Zis, A. (1979) *Arch. Gen. Psychiatry* **36**, 840–846.

Goodwin, G. (1988) *Curr. Opin. Psychiatry* **1**, 72–75.

Graham, P.M., Booth, J., Boranga, G. *et al.* (1982) *J. Affective Disord.* **4**, 201–211.

Greil, W. & Schmidt, S. (1988) In *Lithium* (ed. Birch, N.), pp 149–153. Oxford, IRL Press.

Grossi, E., Sallhetti, E., Vita, A. *et al.* (1984) In *Anticonvulsants in Affective Disorders* (eds Emrich, H.M., Okuma, T. & Muller, A.A.), pp 177–187. Amsterdam, Excerpta Medica.

Halaris, A.E. (1978) *Am. J. Psychiatry* **135**, 493–494.

Hardy, M.-C., Lecrubier, Y. & Widlocher, D. (1986) *Am. J. Psychiatry* **143**, 1450–1453.

Harvey, I., Williams, M., Toone, B.K., Lewis, S.W., Turner, S.W. & McGuffin, P. (1990) *Psychol. Med.* **20**, 55–62.

Hendler, N. (1975) *J. Nerv. Ment. Disord.* **161**, 49–54.

Hirschowitz, J., Zemlan, F., Hitzemann, R., Fleischmann, R. & Garver, D. (1986) *Biol. Psychiatry* **21**, 445–454.

Hoschl, C. & Kozeny, Y. (1989) *Biol. Psychiatry* **25**, 128–140.

Hullin, R.P., Jerram, T.C., Lee, M.R., Levell, M.J. & Tyrer, S.P. (1977) *Br. J. Psychiatry* **131**, 575–581.

Iacono, W.G., Smith, G.N., Moreau, M. *et al.* (1988) *Am. J. Psychiatry* **145**, 820–824.

Jacobs, D. & Silverstone, T. (1986) *Psychol. Med.* **16**, 323–329.

Jacobs, D., Silverstone, T. & Rees, L. (1989) *Int. Clin. Psychopharmacol.* **4**, 135–148.

Jampala, V.C., Taylor, M.C. & Abrams, R. (1989) *Am. J. Psychiatry* **146**, 459–463.

Janicak, P., Sharma, R., Easton, M., Omaty, J. & Davis, J. (1989) *Psychopharmacol. Bull.* **25**, 243–245.

Janowski, D., El-Yousef, M. & Davis, J. (1972) *Lancet* **ii**, 632–635.

Janowski, D.S., El-Yousef, M. & Davis, J.M. (1973) *Arch. Gen. Psychiatry* **28**, 542–547.

Jauhar, P. & Weller, M.P.I. (1982) *Br. J. Psychiatry* **140**, 231–235.

Jimerson, D.C., Post, R.M., Carman, J.S. *et al.* (1979) *Biol. Psychiatry* **14**, 37–51.

Joffe, R.T., Kutcher, S. & MacDonald, C. (1988) *Psychiatry Res.* **25**, 117–121.

Johnstone, E., Crow, T., Frith, C. & Owens, D. (1988) *Lancet* **ii**, 119–125.

Johnstone, E., Owens, D., Crow, T. *et al.* (1989) *J. Neurol. Neurosurg. Psychiatry* **52**, 736–741.

Jonsson, L.E. (1972) *Eur. J. Clin. Pharmacol.* **4**, 206–211.

Joyce, P.R. (1988) *Int. Clin. Psychopharmacol.* **3**, 123–129.

Joyce, P.R., Donald, R.A. & Elder, P.A. (1987a) *J. Affective Disord.* **12**, 1–5.

Joyce, P.R., Donald, R.A., Livesey, J.H. & Abbott, R.M. (1987b) *Biol. Psychiatry* **22**, 508–512.

Joyce, P., Sellman, J., Donald, R., Livesey, J. & Elder, P. (1988) *J. Affective Disord.* **14**, 189–193.

Katona, C.L.E. (1982) *Br. J. Psychiatry* **141**, 447–452.

Kennedy, S.H., Tighe, S., McVey, G. & Brown, G. (1989) *J. Nerv. Ment. Disord.* **177**, 300–303.

Kiriike, N., Izumiya, Y., Nishiwaki, S., Maeda, Y., Nagata, T. & Kawakita, Y. (1988) *Biol. Psychiatry* **24**, 415–422.

Kirkegaard, C., Bjoeum, N., Cohn, D. *et al.* (1978) *Arch. Gen. Psychiatry* **35**, 1017–1021.

Kirubakaran, V., Mayfield, D. & Rengachary, S. (1984) *Am. J. Psychiatry* **141**, 692–693.

Kocsis, J.H. & Stokes, P.E. (1979) *Am. J. Psychiatry* **136**, 563–566.

Kraepelin, E. (1921) *Manic-Depressive Insanity and Paranoia* (Trans. Barclay, R.M.), Edinburgh, E. & S. Livingstone.

Krauthammer, C. & Klerman, G.L. (1978) *Arch. Gen. Psychiatry* **35**, 1333–1339.

Kukopulos, A. & Reginaldi, D. (1980) In *Handbook of Lithium Therapy* (ed. Neil Johnson, F.), pp 109–117. Lancaster, MTP Press.

Kusalic, M. (1988) *Psychopharmacology* **96** (Suppl.), 291.

Lam, R., Berkowitz, A., Berga, S., Clark, C., Kripke, E. & Gillin, J. (1980) *Biol. Psychiatry* **27**, 151A.

Lazarus, J.H., John, R., Bennie, E.H., Chalmers, R.J. & Crockett, G. (1981) *Psychol. Med.* **11**, 85–92.

Lerer, B., Moore, N., Meyendorf, E., Cho, S.R. & Gershon, S. (1987) *J. Clin. Psychiatry* **48**, 89–93.

Lewis, J.L. & Winokur, G. (1982) *Arch. Gen. Psychiatry* **39**, 303–306.

Lewy, A., Wehr, T., Goodwin, F., Newsome, D. & Rosenthal, N. (1981) *Lancet* **i**, 383–384.

Lipinski, J.F. & Pope, H.G. (1982) *Am. J. Psychiatry* **139**, 948–949.

Lowe, M.R. & Batchelor, D.H. (1986) *Int. Clin. Psychopharmacol.* **1** (Suppl. 1), 53–62.

Lusznat, R.M., Murphy, D.P. & Nunn, C.M.H. (1988) *Br. J. Psychiatry* **153**, 198–204.

Lykouras, E., Varsau, E. & Garelis, E. (1978) *Acta Psychiatr. Scand.* **57**, 447–453.

Lykouras, E., Garelis, E. & Varsau, E. (1979) *Am. J. Psychiatry* **136**, 540–542.

McCreadie, R.G., McCormid, M. & Morrison, D.P. (1985) *Br. J. Psychiatry* **146**, 74–80.

McDonald, W., Krishnan, R., Doraiswamy, M. & Blazer, D. (1990) *Biol. Psychiatry* **27**, 162A.

McLennan, G.H., Riley, W.J. & Davies, C.P. (1979) *Lancet* **i**, 883–884.

Maj, M., Del Vecchio, M., Starace, F., Pirozzi, R. & Kemali, D. (1984) *Acta Psychiatr. Scand.* **69**, 37–44.

Mander, A. (1986) *J. Affective Disord.* **11**, 35–41.

Mander, A.J. & Loudon, J.B. (1988) *Lancet* **ii**, 15–17.

Meagher, J., O'Halloran, A., Carney, P. & Leonard, B. (1990) *J. Affective Disord.* **19**, 191–196.

Meltzer, E.S. & Kumar, R. (1985) *Br. J. Psychiatry* **147**, 647–654.

Meltzer, H.Y. & Lowy, M.T. (1987) In *Psychopharmacology: The Third Generation of Progress* (ed. Meltzer, H.Y.), pp 513–526. New York, Raven Press.

Meltzer, H., Kolakowska, T., Fang, V. *et al.* (1984) *Arch. Gen. Psychiatry* **41**, 512–519.

Mirin, S.M., Schatzberg, A.F. & Creasey, D.E. (1981) *Am. J. Psychiatry* **138**, 87–89.

Misra, P.C. & Burns, B.H. (1977) *Acta Psychiatr. Scand.* **55**, 32–40.

Mukherjee, S., Rosen, A., Caracci, G. & Shukla, S. (1986) *Arch. Gen. Psychiatry* **43**, 342–346.

Mulder, R.T., Cosgriff, J.P., Smith, A.M. & Joyce, P.R. (1990) *Aust. N.Z. J. Psychiatry* **24**, 187–190.

Murphy, D.L. (1972) In Neurotransmitters. Research Publications of the Association of Research into Nervous and Mental Diseases, (Ed. J.J. Koplin) **50**, 472–493.

Myers, D.H. & Davies, P. (1978) *Psychol. Med.* **8**, 433–440.

Nasrallah, H.A., McCalley-Whitters, M. & Jacoby, C.G. (1982) *J. Affective Disord.* **4**, 15–19.

Naylor, G. & Scott, C. (1980) *Br. J. Psychiatry* **136**, 105.

Naylor, G.J. & Smith, A.H.W. (1981) *Psychol. Med.* **11**, 249–256.

Naylor, G.J., Smith, A.H.W., Dick, E.G., Dick, D.A.T., McHarg, A.M. & Chambers, C.A. (1980) *Psychol. Med.* **10**, 521–525.

Nizamie, S., Nizamie, A., Borde, M. & Sharma, S. (1988) *Acta Psychiatr. Scand.* **77**, 637–639.

Nolen, W.A. (1983a) *J. Affective Disord.* **5**, 91–96.

Nolen, W.A. (1983b) *Acta Psychiatr. Scand.* **67**, 218–225.

Nordin, C., Siwers, B. & Bertilsson, L. (1981) *Acta. Psychiat. Scand.* **64**, 25–33.

Nurnberger, J., Berlettini, W., Tamarkin, L., Hamovit, J., Norton, J. & Gershon, E. (1988) *Neuopsychopharmacology* **1**, 217–223.

O'Grady, J.C. (1990) *Br. J. Psychiatry* **156**, 496–500.

Okuma, T. (1988) *Psychopharmacology* **96** (Suppl.), 102.

Okuma, T., Inanaga, K., Otsuki, S. *et al.* (1979) *Psychopharmacology* **66**, 211–217.

Okuma, T., Inanga, K. & Otsuki, S. (1981) *Psychopharmacology* **73**, 95–96.

O'Rourke, D., Wurtman, J.J., Wurtman, R.J., Chebli, R. & Gleason, R. (1989) *J. Clin. Psychiatry* **50**, 343–347.

Pandey, G.N., Dysken, M., Garver, D. & Davis, J. (1979) *Am. J. Psychiatry* **136**, 675–678.

Parker, G. & Walter, S. (1982) *Br. J. Psychiatry* **140**, 626–632.

Pearlson, G., Garbacacz, D., Tomkins, R., Ahn, H., Veroff, A. & Depaulo, J. (1984) *Am. J. Psychiatry* **141**, 253–256.

Placidi, G.F., Lenzi, A., Lazzerini, F., Cassano, G.B. & Akiskal, H.S. (1986) *J. Clin. Psychiatry* **47**, 490–494.

Platz, C. & Kendell, R.E. (1988) *Br. J. Psychiatry* **153**, 90–94.

Pope, H.G. & Katz, D.L. (1988) *Am. J. Psychiatry* **145**, 487–490.

Post, R.M. (1980) In *Mania* (ed. Belmaker, R.H. & van Praag, H.M.), pp 217–265. Lancaster, MTP Press.

Post, R. & Goodwin, F. (1978) In *Handbook of Psychopharmacology*, vol. 13 (eds Iversen, L., Iversen, S. & Snyder, S.), pp 147–185. New York, Plenum Press.

Post, R.M. & Weiss, S.R.B. (1989) In *The Clinical Relevance of Kindling* (eds Bolwig, T.G. & Trimble, M.R.), pp 209–230. Chichester, John Wiley.

Post, R.M., Cramer, H. & Goodwin, F. (1977) *Psychol. Med.* **7**, 599–605.

Post, R., Lake, C., Jimerson, D. *et al.* (1978) *Am. J. Psychiatry* **135**, 907–912.

Post, R., Jimerson, D., Ballenger, J., Lake, C.R., Uhde, T. & Goodwin, F. (1984a) In *Neurobiology of Mood Disorders* (eds Post, R.M. & Ballenger, J.C.), pp 539–553. Baltimore, Williams & Wilkins.

Post, R.M., Rubinow, D.R. & Ballenger, J.C. (1984b) In *Neurobiology of Mood Disorders* (eds Post, R.M. & Ballenger, J.C.), pp 432–466. Baltimore, Williams & Wilkins.

Post, R.M., Kramlinger, K.G. & Uhde, T.W. (1987a) *Int. Drug Ther. Newslett.* **22**, 5–8.

Post, R.M., Uhde, T.W., Roy-Byrne, P.P. & Joffe, R.T. (1987b) *Psychiatry Res.* **21**, 71–83.

Prange, A.J., Wilson, I.C., Lynn, C.W., Alltop, L.B. & Stikeleather, R.A. (1974) *Arch. Gen. Psychiatry* **30**, 52–62.

Price, L.H., Charney, D.S. & Heninger, G.R. (1984) *Am. J. Psychiatry* **141**, 1267–1268.

Prien, R.F., Caffey, E.M. & Klett, C.J. (1972) *Arch. Gen. Psychiatry* **26**, 146–153.

Prien, R.F., Klett, C.J. & Caffey, E.M. (1973) *Arch. Gen. Psychiatry* **29**, 420–425.

Prien, R., Kupfer, D., Mansky, P. *et al.* (1984) *Arch. Gen. Psychiatry* **14**, 1096–1104.

Reich, T. & Winokur, G. (1970) *J. Nerv. Ment. Dis.* **151**, 60–68.

Reider, R.O., Mann, L.S., Weinberger, D.R., Van Kammen, D.S. & Post, R.M. (1983) *Arch. Gen. Psychiatry* **40**, 735–739.

Rihmer, Z. (1980) *Psychiatry Res.* **3**, 247–251.

Rinicris, P., Christodoulu, G., Souvatzoglou, A., Koutras, D. & Stefanis, C. (1978) *Compr. Psychiatry* **19**, 561–564.

Robinson, R.G., Boston, J.D., Starkstein, S.E. & Price, T.R. (1988) *Am. J. Psychiatry* **145**, 172–178.

Rosenthal, N.E., Sack, D.A., Gillin, J.C. *et al.* (1984) *Arch. Gen. Psychiatry* **41**, 72–80.

Roy-Byrne, P., Joffe, R. & Uhde, T. (1984) *Br. J. Psychiatry* **145**, 543–550.

Sachar, E.J. (1975) In *Biology of the Major Psychoses*, Vol. 54 (ed. Freeman, D.X.), pp 347–357. New York, Raven Press.

Sack, R.L. & Goodwin, F.K. (1974) *Arch. Gen. Psychiatry* **31**, 649–654.

Sack, D., James, S.P., Rosenthal, N. & Wehr, T. (1988) *Psychiatry Res.* **23**, 179–191.

Schildkraut, J.J. (1965) *Am. J. Psychiatry* **122**, 509–522.

Schlesser, M., Winokur, G. & Sherman, B. (1980) *Arch. Gen. Psychiatry* **37**, 737–743.

Shukla, S., Cook, B.L. & Mukherjee, S. (1987) *Am. J. Psychiatry* **144**, 93–96.

Silfverskiold, P. & Risberg, J. (1989) *Arch. Gen. Psychiatry* **46**, 253–259.

Silverstone, T. (1984) *Lancet* **i**, 903–904.

Silverstone, T. (1985) *J. Affective Disord.* **8**, 225–231.

Silverstone, T. (1990) In *Reviews in Contemporary Pharmacotherapy* (eds Johnson, S. & Johnson, F.N.), pp 115–123. Lancaster, Marius Press.

Silverstone, T. & Cookson, J. (1983) *Neuropharmacology* **22**, 539–541.

Silverstone, T. & Romans-Clarkson, S. (1989) *Br. J. Psychiatry* **154**, 321–335.

Silverstone, T., Fincham, J., Wells, B. & Kyriakedes, M. (1980) *Neuropharmacology* **19**, 1235–1237.

Silverstone, T., Wells, B. & Trenchard, E. (1983) *Psychopharmacology* **79**, 242–245.

Silverstone, T., Coxhead, N. & Cookson, J. (1989) 8th World Congress of Psychiatry, Athens. Excerpta Medica, International Congress Series **899**, Abstract 1205.

Slater, E. (1938) *Z. Gesamte Neurol. Psychiatr.* **162**, 794–801.

Smals, A.G.H., Ross, H.A. & Kloppenborg, P.W. (1977) *J. Clin. Endocrinol. Metab.* **44**, 998–1001.

Starkstein, S. & Robinson, R. (1989) *Br. J. Psychiatry* **154**, 170–182.

Starkstein, S., Robinson, R.G., Honig, M., Parikh, R., Joselyn, J. & Price, T. (1989) *Br. J. Psychiatry* **155**, 79–85.

Stoll, K., Bisson, H.E., Fischer, E. *et al.* (1986) In *Biological Psychiatry* (eds Shagass, C. *et al.*), pp 332–334. Amsterdam, Elsevier.

Swade, C. & Coppen, A. (1980) *J. Affective Disord.* **2**, 249–255.

Swann, A.C., Koslow, S.H., Katz, M.M. *et al.* (1987) *Arch. Gen. Psychiatry* **44**, 345–354.

Swann, A., Secunda, S., Koslow, S., Maas, J. & Davis, J. (1988) In *Progress in Catecholamine Research*, part C (eds Belmaker, R., Sandler, M. & Dahlstrom, A.), pp 217–221. New York, Alan R. Liss.

Swann, A., Secunda, S., Stokes, P. *et al.* (1989) Meeting of the American College of Neuropsychopharmacology held in Maui, Hawaii.

Takahashi, R., Kondo, H., Yashimura, M. & Ochi, Y. (1975) *Folia Psychiatr. Neurol. Jpn.* **29**, 231–237.

Tandon, R., Channabasavanna, S. & Greden, J. (1988) *Acta Psychiatr. Scand.* **78**, 289–297.

Targum, S.D., Davenport, Y.B. & Webster, M.J. (1979) *J. Nerv. Ment. Dis.* **167**, 572–574.

Thompson, C. & Isaacs, G. (1988) *J. Affective Disord.* **14**, 1–11.

Transbol, I., Chriastiansen, C. & Baastrup, P.C. (1978) *Acta Endocrinol.* **87**, 759–767.

Tsuang, M.T. & Woolson, R.F. (1977) *Br. J. Psychiatry* **130**, 162–166.

Turner, T., Cookson, J., Waas, J., Drury, P., Price, R. & Besser, M. (1984) *Br. Med. J.* **289**, 1101–1103.

Victor, B.S., Link, N.A., Binder, R.L. & Bell, I.R. (1984) *Am. J. Psychiatry* **141**, 1111–1112.

Vlissides, D.N., Gill, D. & Castelow, J. (1978) *Br. Med. J.* **2**, 510.

Vohra, A., Gupta, A. & Puri, D. (1989) *8th World Congress of Psychiatry*, Athens. Excerpta Medica, International Congress Series **899**, Abstract 1207.

Waehrens, J. & Gerlach, J. (1981) *J. Affective Disord.* **3**, 193–202.

Walter, S.D. (1977) *Br. J. Psychiatry* **131**, 345–350.

Watkins, S., Callender, K., Thomas, D.R., Tidmarsh, S.F. & Shaw, D.M. (1987) *Br. J. Psychiatry* **150**, 180–182.

Wehr, T.A. (1984) In *Neurobiology of Mood Disorders* (eds Post, R.M. & Ballenger, J.C.), pp 190–206. Baltimore, Williams & Wilkins.

Wehr, T.A. & Goodwin, F.K. (1979) *Arch. Gen. Psychiatry* **36**, 555–559.

Wehr, T.A. & Goodwin, F.K. (1987) *Am. J. Psychiatry* **144**, 1403–1411.

Wehr, T.A., Sack, D.A. & Rosenthal, N.E. (1987) *Am. J. Psychiatry* **144**, 201–204.

Wehr, T.A., Wirz-Justice, A. & Goodwin, F.K. (1982) *Arch. Gen. Psychiatry* **39**, 559–565.

Whalley, L.J., Scott, M., Reading, H.W. & Christie, J. (1980) *Br. J. Psychiatry* **137**, 343–345.

Whalley, L.J., Christie, J.E., Bennie, J. *et al.* (1985) *Br. Med. J.* **290**, 99–102.

Whalley, L., Kutcher, S., Blackwood, D., Bennie, J., Dick, H. & Fink, G. (1987) *Br. J. Psychiatry* **150**, 682–684.

Whalley, L.J., Christie, J., Blackwood, D. *et al.* (1989) *Br. J. Psychiatry* **155**, 455–461.

Winokur, G., Clayton, P.J. & Reich, T. (1969) *Manic Depressive Illness*. St. Louis, C.V. Mosby.

Wirz-Justice, A. & Richter, R. (1979) *Psychiatry Res.* **1**, 53–60.

Wirz-Justice, A., Puhringer, W., Hale, G. & Menzie, R. (1975) *Pharmacopsychiatry* **8**, 310–317.

Wood, A.J., Aronson, J.K., Cowen, P.J. & Grahame-Smith, D.G. (1989) *Br. J. Psychiatry* **155**, 501–504.

Yatham, L., Benbow, J.C. & Jeffers, A. (1988) *Acta Psychiatr. Scand.* **77**, 359–360.

Zubenko, G.S., Cohen, B.M., Lipinski, J.F. & Jonas, J.M. (1984) *Am. J. Psychiatry* **141**, 1617–1618.

Zwil, A., McCallister, T. & Raimo, E. (1990) *Biol. Psychiatry* **27**, 55A.

_____ CHAPTER 9 _____

GENETIC ASPECTS OF AFFECTIVE DISORDERS

Larry Rifkin and Hugh Gurling
Molecular Psychiatry Laboratory, Academic Department of Psychiatry, University College and Middlesex School of Medicine, Riding House Street, London W1P 7PN, UK

Table of Contents

9.1 Introduction

The aim of this chapter is to give an introduction to the genetic methods that can be applied to the study of affective disorders and to give an overview of

BIOLOGICAL ASPECTS OF AFFECTIVE DISORDERS
ISBN 0-12-356510-3

what has been achieved with them. Fortunately, there have been many recent advances in our knowledge about genes and their effects and also about how the brain works. As a result, it seems likely that we are on the threshold of identifying mechanisms for some of the more strongly genetic affective disorder syndromes. There are, however, specific problems that genetic investigations of affective disorders must cope with. Perhaps the most prominent of these is the fact that affective disorders are very common and on an intuitive basis must have many different causes. The geneticist has approached this problem by choosing to study manic depression and related unipolar depression rather than the more common and less easy to define types of affective disorders.

Enough convincing genetic work has been carried out to confirm the hypothesis that genetic factors play a role in the cause of certain subtypes of the affective disorders. The strongest genetic evidence is for bipolar affective disorder (manic depression) which has been shown to have a susceptibility gene on the X chromosome in a minority of families. The evidence that genes play an important role in the less severe and much more frequent subtypes of depression, such as neurotic depression, is not strong. However, most non-psychotic forms of depression have not been studied with genetic methodology in great detail.

Recombinant DNA technology offers the potential to transform psychiatric genetics because of the systematic approach that can be utilized to screen chromosomes for susceptible genes. Such technology should eventually lead to the identification of gene defects at the level of abnormal nucleotide sequence. As progress towards an understanding of the foundations of subtypes of affective illness is made at a molecular level, there is the prospect of unmasking the interplay between genes and the environment in ways that have the potential for new treatment and preventive strategies.

9.2 Methodology in human genetics: some basic concepts

The genes of each individual are contained in supercoiled DNA sequences that constitute the chromosomes present in every nucleus. DNA sequences encode for proteins or non-coding regions of the human genome. Approximately 95% of the genomic (chromosomal) DNA is non-coding sequence. Any sequence of human genomic DNA, including non-functional interspersed DNA or DNA from coding or control regions of a gene, may exist in different versions, due to variation in the sequence of nucleic acids. In some instances this variation will affect the function of a gene negatively and is a disease mutation. Other types of variation will be neutral or have minor effects. Any variant sequence of DNA is known as an allele; different forms (alleles) of the gene or DNA sequence can be inherited from parents. If different alleles at the same locus on homologous chromosomes are simultaneously inherited by an individual, then this individual is called heterozygous for the particular locus.

An individual, therefore, has a genotype which is the assortment of alleles inherited from both parents. Information stored in the DNA is transported to the extranuclear part of the cell by messenger RNA (mRNA), which contains information complementary to genomic DNA. The mRNA can then be translated to the amino acid sequence comprising the protein, with triplets of nucleotides coding each amino acid being arranged in a sequence specific for the protein. mRNA can be reverse transcribed into complementary DNA (cDNA), which has the same sequence as the genomic DNA from which it was originally derived, except that all non-coding DNA is no longer represented. It is therefore possible to identify genes using libraries of genomic DNA clones which are produced directly from genomic DNA, or from libraries of cDNA clones derived from the expressed mRNA within a tissue. This technology is relevant to the affective disorder because clones of potentially relevant genes, such as those that encode the proteins for brain neurotransmitter receptors or enzymes that are expressed in the brain, can be employed in experiments to test specific hypotheses concerning genetic effects. For example, molecular cloning techniques have shown that there are three subtypes of dopamine receptor, D1, D2 and D3 (Bunzow et al., 1988; Sokoloff et al., 1990; Sunahara et al., 1990), and several types of 5-hydroxytryptamine (5-HT) receptor (Kobilka et al., 1987; Forgin et al., 1988; Julius et al., 1988). The advances in this area are explored later in this chapter.

The traditional approach in behaviour genetics has consisted of twin, family, adoption and half sib studies. All of these methods have limitations which preclude the precise estimation of the amount of genetic and environmental variance that is present (Feldman and Cavalli-Sforza, 1979; Cavalli-Sforza and Feldman, 1981). However, an overall impression of the relative contributions of genetic and environmental effects can be gained if all of these methods are used in a variety of different environments at different times. The statistical methods employed either derive from the use of variance, the correlation coefficient (path analysis) or from log linear statistics to deal with categorical data (Falconer, 1985). All the methods suffer from the limitation that genes and environment may not be perfectly separated in the experimental design. In addition, there may be secular (time-related or cohort) effects on assortative mating or the expressivity of the illness which disturb some of the fundamental assumptions on which the genetic analyses are based. The twin method has limitations caused by the special case of twins producing unexpected correlations (Gurling et al., 1985). Analyses of family data which seek to estimate genetic effects by correlating genetic relatedness with the presence or absence of disorder in relatives may also be misleading if assortative mating is taking place in the population as a whole and this is not taken into account (Henderson, 1982).

Until such time as genetic markers become available, estimates of recurrence in twins, adoptees and family studies on their own can do little more than suggest the presence or absence of a genetic effect and cannot determine a specific mode of inheritance. On the other hand, segregation analysis of family data can provide evidence for a particular mode of transmission (i.e. recessive, dominant, multifactorial, polygenic). This can be computed from single, large or many small kindreds but has limitations imposed by incomplete penetrance and reduced fertility. Lastly, linkage analysis can localize genes involved in the affective disorders by specifying chromosomal regions that have markers which happen to be close to a disease susceptibility gene. This last approach is the most favoured investigation for the affective disorders in recent years and is generally considered to be the most useful and powerful approach to the elucidation of genetic mechanisms in human diseases.

9.3 Family, twin and adoption studies of the affective disorders

The affective disorders (Weissman and Myers, 1978; Weissman et al., 1984a) are a spectrum of clinical phenotypes describing disturbances of mood, cognition and physiological functioning. The population prevalence of all types of affective disorder is anywhere up to 20% of the population, according to the definition used (Blehar et al., 1988). The affective disorders have been classified variously in terms of clinical symptoms, the course of the disorder, or putative aetiology (see Chapter 1). For research purposes, structured operational diagnostic criteria, such as Research Diagnostic Criteria (Spitzer et al., 1978), Present State Examination and associated CATEGO algorithms (Wing et al., 1974), and DSM-III-R (American Psychiatric Association, 1980), have been developed. These systems, while sharing a high degree of inter-rater reliability and allowing for comparisons between studies, do not solve the problems of clinical heterogeneity within a given subtype of affective disorder or the lack of any external validity for the diagnosis.

In general, all the current systems of classification overlap and have shortcomings in terms of aetiological relevance, treatment goals and prognosis. Genetic classification might eventually be superior to other classifications because it could simultaneously lead to advances in all three areas. At the present stage in genetic research employing genetic linkage analysis there is no external validation of diagnosis that can be used in order to avoid the inclusion of false-positive (i.e. non-genetic) cases or phenocopies. Unfortunately, linkage analysis is particularly sensitive to this type of error. If an individual has a non-genetic form of affective disorder within a family selected for having a number of severe bipolar cases, then the inclusion of such an individual as a genetic case in linkage analysis will appear as a genetic recombinant (see below) and will weaken the evidence for linkage.

The most commonly employed system in recent family (Andreasen, 1977) and genetic linkage studies is the Research Diagnostic Criteria (RDC; Spitzer et al., 1978). Several related diagnoses are recognized by his system. Major Depressive Disorder (MDD) comprises eleven categories of disturbed (depressed) mood, biological symptoms of depression, depressive thought content and impairment of social functioning. There have been proposals to use clinical covariates of severity so that the probability of correctly identifying a true genetic case from a non-genetic case (a phenocopy) is increased (Rice et al., 1987; Cox et al., 1989). Bipolar (BP) illness requires that in addition to the depressive episodes there are manic (BP I) or hypomanic (BP II) episodes. Hypomania implies that the delusions found in mania are not present and that the intensity and duration is less than in a manic episode. The problem here for genetic studies is that much history-taking to establish a lifetime diagnosis is carried out retrospectively. In general, there is the problem of inaccurate recall, as well as the fact that a period of normal functioning against a background of depression might be misinterpreted as a hypomanic episode (Endicott, 1984). A further major category is Schizoaffective Disorder (SA), in which some features of both depression and schizophrenia occur. In the RDC, SA is subdivided into manic and depressed subtypes. It has been found to occur in the relatives of both schizophrenic and bipolar probands and probably shares the aetiology of both of these disorders (Baron et al., 1982; Endicott et al., 1986). The existence of a true schizoaffective disorder that does not share the aetiology of either schizophrenia or manic depression is currently the subject of investigation. Finally, Cyclothymia is defined as a disorder in which there are rapid mood swings which occur frequently and which do not meet the criteria for MDD or Manic Disorder.

9.3.1 Family studies

Much of the early evidence for the importance of genetic factors in the affective disorders is derived from family studies. In the family method the morbid risk (adjusted prevalence) of the illness is determined within families, and rates of recurrence for the different classes of relatives are compared with those of the general population.

The family method is also able to provide information that can lead to aetiological classifications. An important early advance in genetic studies was the diagnostic distinction of Leonhard (1959) between two types of disorder: Bipolar (BP) Illness, characterized by episodes of both mania and depression, and Unipolar (UP) Illness, characterized by depressive episodes only (see Chapter 1). Work on the affective disorders was continued in the 1960s by Winokur et al. (1966), Winokur and Clayton (1967), Angst (1966) and Perris (1966a, 1966b). Despite differences in methodology and illness definitions, these studies provided support for Leonhard's Bipolar/Unipolar subtypes and evidence that affective disorder recurred in families more than would be expected by chance. In the 1970s, further studies confirmed these results (Gershon et al. 1975b; James and Chapman, 1975; Johnson and Leeman, 1977); however, research up to this time was conducted prior to the methodological advances of the 1980s, which have enhanced family studies. These include the development of structured interviews (Endicott and Spitzer, 1977, 1978), well-defined diagnostic criteria (Spitzer et al., 1978) and the availability of new methods of genetic analysis.

The pooled results from a large number of studies re-analysed by McGuffin and Katz (1989b) and by Rice et al. (1987) show the morbid risk for BP illness in the relatives of BP and UP probands (Table 1).

The results demonstrate that the risk of developing BP illness in the first-degree relatives of BP probands is very significantly elevated (6.8%), whilst the first-degree relatives of UP probands (0.7%) have a risk for BP

Table 1   BP illness in the first-degree relatives of BP and UP probands.

Study	No. at risk	Morbid risk of BP disorder
BP probands		
Rice *et al.* (1987)	2500	5.8
McGuffin and Katz (1989b)	3170	7.8
UP probands		
Rice *et al.* (1987)	2314	0.8
McGuffin and Katz (1989b)	2319	0.6
General population		<1.0

Pooled data of seven studies from Rice *et al.* (1987) and 12 studies from McGuffin and Katz (1989b).

disorder no higher than the general population. The morbid risk rates for UP depression found in the first-degree relatives of BP probands have ranged from a high of 22.4% to a low of 0.5%. Gershon *et al.* (1982) cite 10.2% as the average rate of UP depression among relatives of BP probands and 6.5% as the average rate of UP depression amongst relatives of UP probands. The pooled data of McGuffin and Katz (1989b) demonstrates the morbid risk of UP illness in first-degree relatives of BP and UP probands to be 11.5% and 9.1% respectively. It is worth noting that the above data show the combined rates for affective illness to be higher in the relatives of BP probands than in the relatives of UP probands.

Two recent family studies of depression have been conducted as part of the National Institute of Mental Health Collaborative study of the psychobiology of depression. Weissman *et al.* (1984b) studied 2003 first-degree relatives of 335 probands, and Andreasen *et al.* (1987) studied 3423 first-degree relatives of 616 probands. These studies employed standardized diagnostic criteria and modern methodological techniques. Both studies demonstrated significantly increased rates of UP illness in relatives of UP and BP probands and an increased risk of BP illness in the relatives of BP probands. These observations are generally consistent with previous studies. In addition, Andreasen and co-workers (1987) found that, while 1.1% of relatives of BP II probands have BP I disorder, 8.2% have BP II disorder, thus suggesting that BP II disorder may be partially independent. They also demonstrated that relatives of probands with the RDC bipolar form of schizoaffective disorder had relatively high rates of BP I disorder, whilst rates of schizophrenia were not elevated (Coryell *et al.*, 1984, 1985). In contrast, the probands with the depressed subtype of SA disorder had a very low prevalance of BP I disorder and a relatively high rate of schizophrenia. These findings are consistent with the possibility that the SA/BP subtype is more closely related to BP I and that the SA/depressed subtype is related to schizophrenia. This is consistent with the evidence of Baron *et al.* (1982). However, several previous studies have attempted to clarify the status of SA disorder without clear results. This work is comprehensively reviewed by Levitt and Tsuang (1988).

Family studies provide an approach to identifying valid subgroups within manic depression and the spectrum of affective disorders. Such subgroups may have specific genetic aetiologies. Weissman and her colleagues (1986a, 1986b) reported that early age of onset of depression (less than 30 years) or major depression with an anxiety disorder or secondary alcoholism were related independently to an increased risk of major depression in relatives. They showed no significant increase in familial aggregation of endogenous as compared with non-endogenous depression. This last finding was echoed by Andreasen *et al.* (1986) in a study of 2942 first-degree relatives of probands with UP illness. They used four different definitions of endogenous depression and concluded that 'in general no matter which definition was used, the relatives of the patients with endogenous illness did not have higher rates of depression than the non-endogenous group'.

In the past it has been assumed that depression arising for no apparent reason was more 'genetic' than depression following stress or adverse life-events. A study by Pollitt (1972) found a morbid risk rate of 21% in relatives of probands with no obvious precipitant for the depression, as compared with 6–12% in the relatives of probands whose depression followed some form of psychological or physical stress. However, McGuffin and Katz (1989a) studied the relatives of a mixed group of 83 affective disorder probands who were consecutive registrations at a London hospital. They followed the terminology of Brown and Harris (1978) to assess life events. They found no significant difference in the frequency of depression in the relatives of probands who had a significant life event as compared with the relatives of probands where depression was not associated with a life event. A surprising finding of this study was that the first-degree relatives of depressed probands had a highly significant increase in the rate of life events when compared with a control community sample. This remained so when potentially confounding events were taken into account.

McGuffin and Katz (1989b) also reviewed the results of their own and previous studies of affective disorder in relatives of depressive neurosis probands. A wide range of morbid risk from 5 to 25% was found but could largely be explained by methodological differences. All these studies found higher rates of affective illness in relatives of probands with neurotic depression than in the normal population.

A genetic approach to the subtyping of the affective disorders was proposed by Winokur (1979). He distinguished between 'Pure Depressive Disorder', which did not have strong familial co-morbidity with other psychiatric disorders, and 'Depressive Spectrum Disease', which presented mainly as alcoholism and antisocial behaviour in the male relatives of probands and as depression in the female relatives. However this concept has not received strong support from other family studies or statistical analyses (Cloninger et al., 1979). Nevertheless the idea that depression and alcoholism are intimately linked in some individuals is widespread amongst clinicians and there is ample evidence for such co-morbidity in epidemiological and family studies. Estimates of the strength of association between the two disorders confirm this (Merikangas et al., 1985; Schuckit 1986). A co-twin control study of alcoholism concluded that depression was both primary and secondary to alcoholism (Gurling et al., 1984). In conclusion, there is evidence from the family studies to confirm two broad observations: one is that family members of UP probands show an increased frequency of UP disorder but not a great increase in BP disorder (Baron et al., 1982; Gershon et al., 1982; Winokur *et al.*, 1982; Weissman *et al.*, 1984b; Andreasen *et al.*, 1987); the second is that relatives of BP probands show elevated rates of BP disorder as well as elevated rates of UP disorder (Angst, 1966; Perris *et al.*, 1966a, 1966b; Winokur and Clayton, 1967; Weissman *et al.*, 1984b; Andreasen *et al.*, 1987).

9.3.2 Twin studies

Twin studies compare concordance rates for illness in pairs of monozygotic (MZ) and dizygotic twins (DZ). The central assumption of these studies is that monozygotic twins share the same genes, whilst dizygotic twins have on average 50% of their genes in common. Prenatal and postnatal familial environmental factors are assumed to be a constant in both sets of twins. Twin studies can give information about the effects of shared (family) environment as well as non-shared (unique, specific) environment. One problem for the twin method is that exposure to the same family environment may have differential effects on MZ twins as compared with DZ twins. In addition, MZ twins share the same placental circulation.

The first significant twin study of affective disorders and neurosis was conducted by Bertelsen (1979). One hundred and ten same sex twin pairs, where at least one member of each pair suffered from a BP or UP disorder requiring hospitalization, were identified by the Danish Twin Study Register. The concordance for the 55 MZ twins was 67%, whilst that for the 52 DZ pairs was 20%. In addition, the concordance for MZ over DZ twins was four times higher if the proband had BP disorder. If the proband had UP disorder then the concordance in MZ twins was only twice the rate found in DZ twins. There was a tendency for the twin pairs to have the same subtype of affective disorder but overlap was noted with seven pairs of concordant MZ twins having one twin with UP and the other with BP disorder. Bertlesen (1987) later reviewed eight other twin studies and the combined strict concordance (UP to UP and BP to BP) was 59% for MZ and 18% for DZ twins. Gershon *et al.* (1975a) combined the results of six studies and found 60% of MZ twins concordant, whereas only 13.3% of DZ twins were concordant. Two series of twins selected on the basis of BP disorder probands have been the most thoroughly investigated over a particularly long time. These are the twins investigated by Bertelsen and those at the Maudsley hospital. A recent reassessment of the Maudsley twins has now shown that the concordance for all subtypes of affective disorder in the co-twins is 100% (A. Reveley, 1990, personal communication). Bertelsen (1988, personal communication) has also followed up his series of twins and if a diagnosis of suicide is counted as a case then the concordance amongst MZ twins is also 100%. It seems plausible, therefore, that the genetic predisposition to BP and related UP disorders is highly penetrant once age-related risk is taken into account. Baron (1980)

313

has analysed concordance data from the published twin studies by testing multiple threshold models. He found that the multifactorial polygenic model could be rejected and that the autosomal single major locus provided an acceptable fit. This evidence therefore tends to support the hypothesis that the genetic susceptibility to BP and related UP affective disorder is highly penetrant.

Twin studies of neurotic depression by Slater and Shields (1969) and Torgersen (1986) show similar concordance for MZ and DZ twin pairs, whilst demonstrating concordance rates higher than the rate in the population. This suggests familial rather than genetic influences. Shapiro (1970) found markedly higher concordance rates in MZ than DZ twins for neurotic depression but the affective disorders that were studied in this twin sample were quite severe. McGuffin and Katz (1989a, 1989b) analysed data from three twin studies and estimated the relative contributions to the variance in liability to develop depression. They divided the variance into that attributed to genes, common family environment and non-shared (unique, specific) environment. Their model assumed a multifactorial liability threshold in which 'liability' to develop the disorder is normally distributed in the population. Their results provide support for the view that BP illness is largely determined by genetic factors, 'manic depressive' UP illness occupies an intermediate position and neurotic depression is predominantly of non-genetic origin.

9.3.3 Adoption studies

Adoption and cross-fostering studies seek to clarify further the respective contributions of genes and environment. A drawback is that the biological parents of adopted children are known to be more deviant, with a higher rate of psychiatric disorder, alcoholism and criminality than ordinary parents (Bohman, 1978). On the other hand adoptive parents are usually carefully screened to ensure good parental health. One might therefore expect to find a generalized increase in psychiatric disorder in adopted children compared with controls.

There have not been many adoption studies investigating the affective disorders. However three out of four studies have provided evidence for the hypothesis that there are genetic mechanisms in depression. Mendlewicz and Rainer (1977) compared the psychiatric diagnosis of parents of 29 BP and 22 normal adult adoptees (all adopted in infancy) with those of parents of 31 non-adopted BP individuals and 20 people with poliomyelitis, chosen to control for the effects of an ill child on parents. They showed a 31% incidence in the biological parents of BP adoptees as opposed to a 2% prevalance in the biological parents of normal adoptees. They found a broad spectrum of affective disorders. Adoptive parents of BP adoptees had a rate of 12% in comparison with a 10% prevalence in the adoptive parents of both normal adoptees and the poliomyelitis group.

Another adoption study (Cadoret and Gath, 1978) also supports the role of genetic factors in affective illness, with little evidence for the role of family associated environmental factors in AD. However, the adoption study by Van Knorring *et al.* (1983) found no evidence of an elevated rate of affective illness in biological or adoptive parents of adoptees with affective disorders.

Wender and Kety (1986) investigated the psychiatric status of biological and adopted relatives of 71 adult adoptees and 71 well-matched control subjects. The adult adoptees had a wide range of affective disorders. An increased frequency of affective spectrum disorders was found among the biological relatives of affectively ill adoptees. This included a highly significant eightfold increase in the rate of UP depression and a fifteenfold increase in suicide amongst the biological relatives of affectively ill adoptees compared with adoptive relatives and relatives of matched control adoptees.

9.3.4 Overview of family, twin and adoption studies

The family, twin and adoption studies are highly suggestive of genetic transmission in the affective disorders. They provide evidence for a greater genetic contribution in BP as compared with UP disorders, neurotic depression showing little evidence of a significant genetic component. There is also evidence that whilst Leonard's UP/BP distinction is to some extent confirmed, important differences appear to exist between the two. Thus BP and UP disorders can be both discrete entities but can also be transmitted within families, where they presumably share the same aetiology. Although information about disease recurrence for the affective disorders from family, twin and adoption studies can contribute to an understanding about the extent of genetic effects, such methods do not determine a particular mode of genetic transmission. The information obtained from genetic linkage and segregation analysis offers a more powerful method of doing this. Both approaches, however, have limited power to detect or quantify heterogeneity of underlying genetic susceptibility. For example, there may be recessive as well as dominant susceptibility genes for affective disorders without any obvious clinical markers for such subtypes.

Segregation analysis makes use of family data obtained according to various ascertainment (selection) rules. It compares the likelihood for the observed frequency of illness in a pedigree with those that can be predicted by various hypothetical models. One computer program used for complex segregation analysis is POINTER (Lalouel *et al.*, 1983). This implements the mixed model of Morton and MacLean (1974) to parameterize genetic transmission and other sources of similarity within families. The likelihood of goodness of fit for the single major locus (SML) autosomal model, the multifactorial polygenic model (MFP) and a mixed model have been tested using POINTER with data for the affective disorders. The model assumes that a phenotypic variable, such as the presence or absence of manic-depressive illness, is represented by the dichotomous expression of an underlying continuous trait which is approximately normally distributed in the population. Individuals above a certain threshold on this trait manifest the illness, and those below it will have a normal phenotype. Different factors can contribute additively to the variance of the trait, and the overall value of the variance is arbitrarily taken to be unity. The most general model tested is usually the mixed model, in which there are contributions to the variance from three sources: random environmental effects, multifactorial transmission from parent to child (comprising genetic and non-genetic factors), and a single major locus effect. The single major locus effect is usually modelled as being due to a diallelic system such that each of the three possible genotypes have a different mean liability. This effect is characterized by the gene frequency of each allele, the difference between the mean liabilities for individuals homozygous for each allele, and the position of the heterozygote mean relative to the homozygote mean (the dominance of the gene). However, Smith (1975) and Bodmer (1984) have both argued that discrimination between different modes of inheritance cannot be accomplished easily in the presence of a number of confounding factors. These include reduced or non-penetrance (the incomplete or absent manifestation of a trait in individuals who carry the genotype, phenocopies (cases who do not carry the genotype but who nevertheless manifest the disorder) and genetic heterogeneity (subtypes of the disorder caused by separate major genes). Lastly, variable age of onset of a disorder means that it is not possible to assume that a so-called unaffected person does not possess the disease gene because the gene may be penetrant at a later time. Other potential sources of error included diagnostic difficulties, ascertainment bias, sampling bias and new genetic mutations.

Another interesting issue concerns the possible effects of decade or year of birth on the susceptibility to develop affective disorder. Recent research on two generation families has suggested a birth cohort effect on the recurrence of BP and related UP affective disorder, whereby younger individuals appear to be more at risk or have an earlier age of onset (Gershon et al., 1987; Rice et al., 1987). This effect might be due to the fact that younger people have a more accurate recall of the time of onset of their depression than do older people. Alternatively, suicide or other causes of early death might have reduced the numbers of older affected individuals. Lastly, it is possible that younger people are more at risk because the Western cultures in which these cohort studies have been conducted have become more depression inducing.

There has been quite good agreement amongst the segregation analyses of families containing BP probands and their affected UP or BP relatives. The comparisons made between likelihoods have often favoured a single major locus (SML) effect, usually with multifactorial background variance as part of a 'mixed' model. (Gershon *et al.*, 1975a, 1975b; Crowe and Smouse, 1977; Lalouel *et al.*, 1983; O'Rourke *et al.*, 1983; Egeland *et al.*, 1987). For example, the study by O'Rourke *et al.* (1983) compared an SML model with a mixed model and multifactorial models to analyse 194 nuclear families selected from bipolar probands. They found that many of the models incorporating a major locus, with or without multifactorial background, were consistently associated with greater likelihoods of 'fit' than those incorporating no major locus. Rice *et al.* (1987) conducted a segregation analysis on data from 187 families selected through BP probands. They found that single major locus transmission with multifactorial background 'fitted' the patterns of transmission observed when effects of both cohort and age of onset were controlled. When a more general vertical transmission model was applied (i.e. when not constrained by the mendelian value of 50% probability that an affected heterozygote parent transmits the disease allele to one of their children), the evidence suggested that there were additional sources of within-family resemblance for affective disorders. However, some workers have favoured other modes of transmission (Slater and Tsuang, 1968; Bucher *et al.*, 1981a, 1981b). One important study combined both a linkage and segregation analysis of the Old Order Amish (Egeland *et al.*, 1987). Egeland reported that the recurrence of BP and UP illness was consistent with autosomal dominant transmission of a gene with a frequency of 0.021 and a penetrance of 0.63 at age 30 and above. These values imply that approximately 2% of the population is at risk, but amongst those who have inherited the gene 63% will have developed an affective disorder by the age of 30.

A recent segregation analysis on a sample of large Icelandic pedigrees selected for linkage analysis has been carried out (Curtis *et al.*, 1990). Five kindreds selected through probands attending an Icelandic hospital were recruited for linkage studies of manic-depression. There was a uniformly high incidence of the BP and UP forms of the disorder in all branches of the kindreds studied. The incidence of affective disorder was equal for males and females and the age of onset was predominantly in early adult life. Affection rates did not rise appreciably with age. A complex segregation analysis was performed using POINTER to obtain maximum likelihood estimates of the contributions to liability from multifactorial transmission and a single major locus. Likelihood ratios between models supported a role for a single major locus which was dominant and had moderately high penetrance with additional multifactorial transmission. Although selection bias limits the conclusions that can be drawn from this analysis, the results were broadly in line with those reported by other workers who have studied samples ascertained for segregation analysis.

9.4 The search for major genes in affective disorder using genetic linkage and association analysis

Linkage analysis is a much more powerful approach to establishing a mode of transmission than segregation analysis and much attention has recently been focused on the use of DNA polymorphisms as linkage markers to identify major gene effects. A genetic marker is a reliably measured characteristic which has a simple mode of inheritance and which is polymorphic (i.e. there are two or more alleles with measurable frequencies). Traditionally, geneticists have used polymorphic protein variants from blood (e.g. histocompatibility antigens, red blood cell types) to map potential disease loci on a chromosome. This previously limited the number of measurable markers and resulted in a low probability of assigning genes for the disorder in question to their respective chromosomal locations through linkage to a known marker. DNA technology has now enabled the detection of genetic markers at the DNA level regardless of their phenotypic expression and this has transformed genetic research. The first step in the development of recombinant DNA technology was the discovery of bacterial enzymes capable of recognizing specific DNA segments as targets for cleavage (Gurling, 1985). These restriction enzymes or endonucleases cut DNA at every point where the specific DNA sequence is present. If there are restriction enzyme sites present or absent due to base sequence variation, then the resulting differences in cutting sites will show up as variant DNA fragment sizes. These differences are inherited in a simple mendelian fashion. The inherited differences in the lengths of DNA generated by restriction enzymes are termed restriction fragment length polymorphisms (RFLPs) and represent one type of the new generation of DNA genetic markers. Another type of DNA marker is the dinucleotide repeat found to be widely dispersed throughout the human genome (Weber and May, 1989).

To detect specific RFLPs a technique known as Southern hybridization is employed (Southern, 1975). Human genomic DNA is chopped up or digested by one or more restriction enzymes. The resulting fragments can be separated according to size by electrophoresis and then transferred from the electrophoretic gel to a filter in the same relative positions. The filter is then hybridized to a radiolabelled probe (segment of DNA or gene of known sequence) and any DNA fragments with complementary base sequences to the probe will bind to it. By exposing the filter to an X-ray film, a display of the hybridized fragments will become visible as dark bands on an autoradiograph.

There are two approaches for the study of disorders using genetic markers. Studies of association can be undertaken between markers and the disorder and then compared with a general population control group. In this instance the phenomenon of allelic association or linkage disequilibrium is employed to localize a disease gene. Linkage disequilibrium refers to the evolutionary tendency for DNA segments that are close together to remain linked in successive generations despite the presence of genetic recombination between loci. In fact, DNA sequences that are less than a distance of 1% recombination (1 million base pairs) tend to stay linked over evolution. In the case of a disease there may be marker polymorphisms that tend to be co-inherited due to linkage disequilibrium. These polymorphisms are referred to as being allele specific and are indicators that the polymorphic marker is less than approximately one million base pairs from the disease mutation. Classical marker studies have focused on association studies between disease and the human leucocyte antigen (HLA) system and ABO blood groups (Flemebaum and Larson, 1976). However, these studies, reviewed by Berritini *et al.* (1984), have produced contradictory and inconsistent results. No clear association has been established. This is not surprising, for in order for a population association to be detected, the marker and aberrant gene locus must be in very close proximity to one another. Secondly, hidden population stratifications such as those due to ethnic origin may confound valid frequency estimates in both disease and control samples. In addition, there must be a significant degree of genetic homogeneity for the subtypes of the affective disorder amongst the individuals tested. Association studies are a very weak approach to the identification of a disease gene unless there is a strong a priori hypothesis that a specific gene is to blame for causing susceptibility to a disease.

Linkage studies, however, test whether there is co-segregation of markers and the disorder within a given family (Elston and Lange, 1975). Thus the establishment of linkage between a genetic marker allele and an inherited trait requires the finding of markers which are sufficiently close to the disease mutation that the two are not separated from each other by crossing over or recombination when the gametes are formed. Recombination takes place when there is an exchange of genetic material between homologous chromosomes, thereby producing the genetic variation which we observe in different individuals of the same family. The closer the marker is to the disease locus, the less likely it is that recombination will occur. The marker and disease gene will therefore be transmitted together from one generation to the next. It should be noted that the marker need not contain the gene of interest and can be up to 30–40% recombination or 30–40 million base pairs away from

319

the mutation. Whether a marker is close enough to be considered linked is estimated by the frequency of genetic recombination during meiosis. An important criterion for a genetic marker is the question as to whether it is informative for a given family. For a marker to be identified as being informative and linked to a disorder it must be possible to distinguish between maker sequences on each of the pair of homologous chromosomes that one or both of the parents possess. Such a state is termed heterozygosity. The ideal linkage marker would exist in different allelic forms on both chromosomes of one parent and also exist in two further allelic forms on the two homologous chromosomes of the other parent. The more polymorphic a genetic marker, the greater is the likelihood of heterozygosity and the more useful it will be. Once a particular allelic marker is observed to co-segregate with the disorder in different pedigrees, the results must be rationalized using some form of statistical analysis. The distance between the marker and the disease gene locus determines the probability that genetic recombination will separate them. If the two loci are far apart then independent assortment of alleles will occur, i.e. the recombination fraction will be 0.5 (50%). This situation provides the null hypothesis against which to test any data from pedigree analysis. If there is linkage between a marker allele and disease locus the likelihood of this occurring by chance can be calculated at various recombination fractions and expressed as the lod or $\log_{10}$ of the odds ratio. A lod of 3.00 has been considered significant evidence for claiming linkage between markers and a disease but the more markers that are tested and the more the disease definition is varied together with penetrance, the higher the lod must be before it is considered significant. Various mapping functions have been constructed to convert the observed recombination fraction (θ) into a physical distance (Kosambi, 1944). A lod of greater than 3.85 has been taken to demonstrate that linkage is present when penetrance is varied, and a lod of -2.00 or less that linkage is absent (Ott, 1985; Lander, 1988). The recombination fraction at which the maximum lod score is found gives a statistical measure of the proximity of the marker to the disease locus.

Another, less powerful method of evaluating linkage is to study the sharing of marker alleles in doubly affected pairs of siblings (Green and Woodrow, 1977). The markers will be more 'identical by descent' than expected if they are linked to the disease gene. Because information is obtained from individuals who must possess the disease alleles, error from obtaining information from so-called normal but potentially non-penetrant carriers of the disease alleles can be avoided. The method is therefore resistant to the problems of incomplete or non-penetrance. Also, unlike the lod score approach, the affected sib pair method does not require the mode of inheritance to be specified. Bodmer shows that the sib pair method can be quite effective in detecting linkage with disorders which are often sporadic but which nevertheless have strong genetic influences (Bodmer, 1984). However, this method is considered less efficient than the lod method for mendelian disorders. It is also not useful for estimating the recombination fraction accurately and cannot detect heterogeneity of linkage as efficiently as the lod method. Therefore, genetic subtypes of depression cannot easily be differentiated with sib pair data.

9.5 Strategies using candidate genes, markers for favoured loci and random markers

There are three types of cloned genes and gene markers that could be used in the multiply affected family (lod) score and affected sib pair approach (Gurling, 1986).

9.5.1 Cloned 'candidate genes'

These are genes which on an a priori basis may be genetically predisposing to the disorder in question. Such candidate genes can function as their own linkage markers by virtue of exhibiting polymorphism within or close to the gene itself. In this instance the problems of linkage analysis should not be too difficult to overcome. This is because the necessary linkage and association analyses only need to prove the involvement of the linkage marker itself and do not have to take into account recombination between the marker and disease alleles.

The underlying assumption in using candidate genes is either that their protein products are directly implicated in the aetiology of the disorder under study or that they are part of a multigene family that share similar functions. Thus enzymes and receptor proteins thought to be implicated in the genetics of affective disorders could be cloned and used as candidate gene markers. Some 5-HT and human dopamine D1, D2 receptor genes have been cloned (see above) as well as a D3 receptor (Sokoloff et al., 1990). The human β_1-, β_2-, α_1- and α_2-adrenoceptor genes have also been cloned and sequenced (Kobilka et al., 1986; Frielle et al., 1987; Yang-Feng et al., 1990). This means that comparisons of nucleotide sequence between receptors can be carried out to reveal how they have changed during evolution. Tyrosine hydroxylase is the rate limiting enzyme on the dopamine/noradrenaline pathway and was cloned originally in the rat (Lamouroux et al., 1982). Subsequently, the human tyrosine hydroxylase gene has been mapped to a portion of chromosome 11 very near the insulin locus on the short arm. At least three different genes that code for the opioid peptides have been cloned. One of these is the pro-opiomelanocortin gene (POMC) from which β-endorphin, adrenocorticotrophic hormone (ACTH) and melanocyte stimulating hormones are derived (Feder *et al.*, 1985). It is plausible that the products of the POMC gene have a role in the regulation of central noradrenaline metabolism (Chapter 3).

9.5.2 Cloned genes, DNA segments and protein markers mapping to a 'favoured' locus

In a 'favoured locus' approach, areas of the chromosome which have on an a priori basis been shown to have some possible involvement in affective illness can be screened by suitable markers in an attempt to detect linkage to the disorder (Ferguson-Smith and Aitken, 1982). Thus, cytogenetic studies which reveal deletions, translocations or other abnormalities may suggest the use of specific linkage markers. Secondly, weakly positive lod scores found in inconclusive linkage studies can be explored in new samples which may, with luck, be more homogeneous than the original sample. To date there have only been non-statistically non-significant reports of linkage to unipolar affective disorders with classical serum protein markers. There have been descriptions of cytogenetic abnormalities in the affective disorders on chromosomes 11, 15, and X. Two reports focused interest on the long arm of chromosome 11 as possibly containing a gene of importance in predisposing to developing psychotic illness. St Clair *et al.* (1990) have described a family in which several individuals who have developed schizophrenia and other psychiatric illnesses have a translocation from 11q25 to chromosome 1. Smith and Potkin (1989) have described a pedigree in which a translocation from 11q22.3 to 9pter co-segregates with manic depression in five individuals. In addition, disturbances of dopamine transmission have long been thought to be a possible factor in the genesis of psychotic illness and dopamine-2 receptor antagonists have anti-psychotic action. The gene for the dopamine-2 receptor is sited at the 11q22.3–q23 junction (Litt *et al.*, 1989). Holland *et al.* (1991) have also observed a family with a cytogenetic abnormality on chromosome 11q but which was thought to be at a distance from the site implicated by the cytogenetic abnormality reported by Smith and Potkin (1989).

9.5.3 Cloned genes, DNA segments and protein markers to screen the chromosome randomly

It was predicted by Botstein *et al.* (1980) that it would be feasible to map the whole human genome using random DNA markers within a few years. There is now an almost complete human genetic linkage map composed of many anonymous polymorphic DNA sequences and some human genes that display polymorphism in or near their coding regions (Donis-Keller *et al.*,

1988). Systematic screening of all the human chromosomes for linkage to any major gene disorder can now be accomplished. This approach does, however, require tenacity and also benefits from collaboration between researchers. The new technology has been successful in the task of tracking and identifying genes for disorders with mendelian patterns of inheritance, such as cystic fibrosis and Huntington's chorea. The application of linkage analysis to the spectrum of phenotypes found in the affective disorders faces specific problems related to the fact that they are very common in the general population and may be difficult to define. The problem of genetic heterogeneity, where several genes on different chromosomes are responsible for producing the same or similar phenotype in a sample of families, provides the most serious obstacle. However, statistical tests are available to refute homogeneity of lod scores within a heterogeneous family linkage sample (Ott, 1985).

Initial reports of linkage between the HLA genes on chromosome 6 and BP/UP disorders were in favour of linkage (Smeraldi et al., 1978, 1984; Smeraldi and Bellodi, 1981). Weitkamp et al. (1981) reported that a subset of 'low genetic loading' sibships, where there were two rather than three or more affected cases, showed linkage to the HLA gene family. Turner and King (1981) also found positive evidence for linkage of the HLA region to affective disorder in BP pedigrees when UP, BP and personality disorders were included as cases. However a closely linked marker only showed a statistically significant lod when linkage was calculated with stricter criteria for caseness. Targum and co-workers (1979) and Goldin et al. (Goldin and Gershon, 1983; Goldin et al., 1983) reanalysed data from a family sample using the sib pair and lod methods without finding any support for linkage with the HLA genes. Suarez and Crougham (1982) also failed to confirm the earlier suggestion of linkage with HLA. The most recent effort to confirm the original linkage with HLA (Weitkamp and Stancer, 1989) was largely negative, but certain subgroups still showed a significant linkage at the HLA loci using the sib pair method (Stancer et al., 1987, 1988, 1989). The validity of analysing subgroups, as has been carried out in these studies, has been questioned (Berretini et al., 1984). The recent linkage studies employing markers at other loci are summarized in Table 2.

The Old Order Amish religious community from south-east Pennsylvania presented a potentially ideal opportunity for genetic linkage studies of the BP and UP affective disorders. Egeland and co-workers (1987) identified several large pedigrees with a high incidence of affective disorder. Detailed geneaological records document that the community members are descendants from about 30 founder couples and have remained genetically isolated. Thus they appeared to represent a restricted gene pool with a reduced likelihood of multiple genes being responsible for affective illness. A low incidence of drug and alcohol abuse, which may complicate diagnosis, and the presence of large

Table 2 Linkage studies of affective disorders*

Source and location	No. pedigrees	Marker	Lod score†
Chromosome Xq			
Reich *et al.* (1969), USA	2	CB	> +3.00
Mendlewicz *et al.* (1972), USA	7	CB	> +2.00
Mendlewicz and Rainer (1974), USA	7	CB	> +3.00
Baron (1977), USA	1	CB	> +2.00
Gershon *et al.* (1979), USA	6	CB	< −2.00
Mendlewicz *et al.* (1979), Belgium	8	CB	> +2.00
Del Zompo *et al.* (1984), Sardinia	2	G6PD	NS
Mendlewicz *et al.* (1980), Iranian in Belgium	1	G6PD	> +3.00
Kidd *et al.* (1984), USA	5	CB	NS
Mendlewicz *et al.* (1987), Belgium	5	Factor IX	> +3.00
Baron *et al.* (1987), Israel	5	G6PD	> +3.00
Chormosome 11p			
Egeland *et al.* (1987), North America (Amish)	1	INS H-RAS-1	> +3.00
Hodgkinson *et al.* (1987b), Iceland	3	INS H-RAS-1 Tyrosine hydroxylase	< −2.00
Detera-Wadleigh *et al.* (1987), North America	3	INS	< −2.00
Kluznik *et al.* (1988),USA	1	INS	NS
Gill *et al.* (1988), Ireland	1	INS H-RAS	NS

* CB indicates Colour Blindness
INS = Insulin
NS = Not Significant
† The Lod score was calculated as the log of the probability of obscuring the given family data, assuming linkage with a recombination fraction of 0, compared with the probability of the same data assuming no linkage.

multiply affected sibships and multiple living generations were also favourable factors.

Initial linkage studies on the BP pedigree in the Amish included a number of standard polymorphic systems but could not confirm the presence of a single major locus conferring possibility to affective disorder, which had been suggested by segregation analysis (Pauls, 1985) of family data. Subsequently,

DNA techniques were used to dramatically increase the number of available polymorphic loci. This led to the publication of a reported linkage between BP illness and two markers on the tip of the short arm of chromosome 11, the H-RAS-1 oncogene locus (H-RAS) and the insulin locus (INS). Analysis incorporating data from a number of markers indicated that the affective disorder (AD) gene was most likely to be tightly linked to the INS locus on the short arm of chromosome 11. The lod scores obtained were greater than 3.00 for linkage between H-RAS-1 and the AD locus at all penetrance values greater than 0.55. This initial result was based on one large composite family with 81 individuals. Those included as affected received a diagnosis of either BP I, BP II, atypical BP, schizoaffective or major depressive disorder (MDD). RDC diagnostic criteria were used and all available relatives were interviewed. Extensive clinical data was collected to determine diagnoses.

The Amish study was later extended to include new clinical data on several individuals with recent onsets of affective disorder who had been unaffected at the time of the original study. Genotypic data was obtained on several members not previously analysed by including two extensions of the original core pedigree. Recent publication of these new data show a lowering of the lod score in the original core pedigree and rule out linkage in the complete kindred with extensions. If all new data are included, the hypothesis that a single major AD locus is linked to the marker could be excluded at 5 cM on either side of INS and 10 cM for H-RAS (Kelsoe et al., 1989). The results highlight many of the problems which could confound the localization of genes in the affective disorders. Variable age of onset of affective disorder led to two previously unaffected members of the Amish kindred becoming affected, thus reducing the lod score. This reinforces the importance of longitudinal follow-up of pedigrees and updated re-analyses of data. The most important question, though, is whether there is genetic heterogeneity of linkage present among the Amish even though they are a relatively isolated community. If affective disorder is genetically homogeneous, then throughout the whole kindred there is strong evidence against linkage with a susceptibility locus to affective disorder on the short arm of chromosome 11. However, there is the possibility that there is more than one gene responsible for affective disorder which is confounding the analysis. In fact, tracing of some of the progenitor individuals has shown that it is likely that there were a number of individuals with psychiatric disorder who were members of the original migrant group or who married into the main kindred. Therefore, there could be three or more independent disease alleles segregating in the Amish community. Many other DNA markers have now been tested in this kindred but no other linkage has yet been demonstrated. The testing of further markers covering the whole genome may reveal another linked locus. However, it may not be possible for any single affective disorder locus to generate a positive lod score over the entire pedigree if genetic heterogeneity exists. There is also the possibility that phenocopies are confounding the analysis. This would be maximal if false-positive cases were occurring in a critical part of the pedigree or if their frequency was great. Using clinical judgements rather than the RDC diagnostic scheme, the maximum lod score for the core pedigree remained positive at 2.88 at zero recombination in the re-analysis by Kelsoe *et al.* (1989). This method excluded single episode MDD and minor depression cases from the analyses and thus may have reduced the frequency of phenocopies and false recombinants.

The initial findings of the Amish study generated considerable excitement and enthusiasm, and other investigators attempted to replicate the results in different pedigrees. In a parallel study conducted in the UK, linkage of affective disorder to H-RAS, INS and a third marker, tyrosine hydroxylase, (located in the same region of chromosome 11) was excluded in three large Icelandic BP pedigrees (Hodgkinson *et al.*, 1987a, 1987b). Detera-Wadleigh *et al.* (1987) studied three kindreds of European origin from North America and also excluded linkage to H-RAS and INS. Subsequently, Gill *et al.* (1988) and Kluznick (1988) also failed to find linkage to these markers in single pedigrees from Ireland and the USA, respectively. More recently Leboyer *et al.* (1990) have reported a positive association (not linkage) between tyrosine hydroxylase polymorphisms and BP illness. This raises the question that the original lod in the Amish may still have some validity if it is indeed the tyrosine hydroxylase gene that predisposes to a subtype of bipolar disorder. However, Nothen *et al.* (1990) and Todd and O'Malley (1989) both failed to replicate the positive association.

Recent reports of a chromosomal translocation which co-segregates with manic depression and the localization of the dopamine-2 (D2) receptor gene on the long arm of chromosome 11 has suggested that a susceptibility locus for affective disorder might be located in this region of the chromosome. Smith *et al.* (1989) have described a pedigree in which a translocation from chromosome 11 to chromosome 9 ((9, 11) + (pter; q 22.3)) co-segregates with manic depression in five individuals. Because the gene for the D2 receptor is sited at 11q22.3–q23 (Bunzow *et al.*, 1988), there was speculation that the translocation might have disrupted the D2 gene. Holmes *et al.* (1991) could find no evidence for linkage in five Icelandic pedigrees between affective disorder and markers in the 11q region, thus excluding the sites of the cytogenetic abnormalities.

The first positive study to suggest X-linkage in Manic Depression was carried out two decades ago (Winokur and Tanna, 1969; Reich *et al.*, 1969). These workers reported the possibility of close linkage between colour blindness and the manic depressive phenotype. Subsequently, research using colour blindness (CB) and other X-chromosome markers also produced results suggestive of X-linkage in a proportion of families (Mendlewicz *et al.*, 1972,

1974, 1979, 1980, 1987; Baron, 1977; Baron *et al.*, 1987; Reading, 1979; Del Zompo *et al.*, 1984). Other investigators have failed to show linkage to colour blindness and the glucose-6-phosphate dehydrogenase (G6PD) gene which is localized near the colour blindness gene (Goetzl *et al.*, 1974; Gershon *et al.*, 1979; Holmes *et al.*, 1989). The absence of male-to-male transmission and an excess of affected females may sometimes be found in families showing X-linked transmission for a genetic disorder. In fact, this feature was observed in some of the early family studies of manic depression but subsequently many studies showed that male-to-male transmission was common. Some controversy has remained over whether X-linked dominant inheritance contributes to affective illness in some affective disorder pedigrees. Risch and Baron (1982) reanalysed several published data sets to test X-linked dominant inheritance and genetic heterogeneity. Their work suggested that there was genetic heterogeneity both between published studies and within them. They estimated that approximately a third of BP/UP illness was X-linked and emphasized that this was a crude estimate. RFLP data together with other markers have been used to test the X-linkage hypothesis in some very large Israeli families by Baron *et al.* (1987). They identified five large pedigrees originating from the patient population of the Jerusalem Mental Health Centre and were able to demonstrate close linkage of BP affective illness to the X-chromosome markers colour blindness and G6PD. Only those pedigrees which demonstrated a pattern of inheritance consistent with X-linkage were included. The population chosen was particularly suitable because of the relatively high prevalence of affective disorder, low rates of drug and alcohol abuse, the high frequency of G6PD deficiency among the non-Ashkenazi population and the availability of large pedigrees. All five pedigrees were Jewish, of which four were Sephardic and one Ashkenazi. The families were all derived from BP I probands. Relatives with diagnoses of BP I, BP II, MDD, SA and cyclothymia were included as affected. Diagnoses were made using RDC criteria. The pedigrees contained 161 adults, 47 of whom were affected. All the non-Ashkenazi pedigrees supported linkage, whereas the single Ashkenazi pedigree had negative lod scores. If it is assumed that there is genetic heterogeneity and that the single Ashkenazi pedigree can be excluded, the maximum lod score coincides with the CB locus. If all five pedigrees are included, the maximum lod is 7.52, which is still strongly in favour of linkage, with the affective disorder locus being placed 5 cM to the right of G6PD. The lod score results were robust with regard to assumptions about gene frequency and penetrance. It is interesting to note that reanalysis of the data using a narrower definition of the phenotype, when three individuals with cyclothymic disorder were counted as unaffected, the maximum lod scores for CB and G6PD dropped to 4.37, assuming heterogeneity, and 2.02 assuming homogeneity for all the pedigrees.

The G6PD and CB loci are assumed to be at a 2% recombination fraction apart at the distal end of the long arm of the X chromosome. The results suggest that the probable location of an affective disorder susceptibility gene is close to and possibly between these two markers. Linkage between the subterminal region of the X chromosome and affective disorder was confirmed shortly afterwards by Mendlewicz and co-workers (1987). Ten pedigrees from Belgium informative for linkage between AD and a *Taq-1* polymorphism at the factor IX locus (Xq27 region) were studied. Genetic linkage was demonstrated between this RFLP and affective disorders. The maximum lod score was 3.10 at a recombination fraction of 0.11.

X-linkage in manic depression was originally demonstrated in the USA (Winokur and Tanna, 1969) and has been found in Sardinia, Belgium, Israel, the USA and New Zealand in independent samples (Baron, 1977; Baron *et al.*, 1987; Reading, 1979; Zompo *et al.*, 1984; Mendlewicz *et al.*, 1987). Thus, at the present time, there is compelling evidence for X-linked dominant transmission and heterogeneity of linkage in manic depression. The implication is that future researchers in the field will have to obtain samples sufficiently large to test the hypothesis that there is linkage on the long arm of the X chromosome in a proportion of the families that they are studying. Although it is possible to test for heterogeneity (by refuting homogeneity) in a sample of nuclear families or affected sib pairs, large kindreds are preferred because it can reasonably be assumed that there is genetic homogeneity within a single kindred and a more accurate estimate of the recombination fraction can be made. This, however, cannot be guaranteed unless there is only a single unilateral source of the illness segregating within each kindred.

There have been two attempts to identify possible clinical features of the affective disorders that may reflect the underlying genetic subtype. A comparison of the large kindreds used in linkage studies by Gurling and others (1988) concluded that clinical variation and variable age of onset did not discriminate between X-linked, the putative 11p linked and 'non-11/non-X-linked' BP/UP affective disorders. In a collaborative effort organized by the MacArthur Foundation similar conclusions were reached (Merikangas *et al.*, 1989).

9.6 Gene–environment relationships and affective disorders

There have been very few attempts to study the joint effects of genes and environment in the AD. This is probably because systematic collection of environmental data is difficult and has therefore not been incorporated into the large twin registers that exist, or into the adoption method. Obviously it would be quite intrusive to systematically collect data about the lives of adoptees. However, one twin study and an adoption study have made a start in this area.

The fact that anxiety and depressive disorders often co-occur within the same individual is evidence that they might share some of the same genetic determinants. Twins offer good genetic control and the ability to distinguish familial environmental effects (the common environment) from non-specific (unique) environmental effects not shared by other family members. Because monozygotic twins have identical genes and because they share the same environment, then differences between twins can be attributed to unique environmental effects as well as random effects and error. Similar inferences can be drawn from dizygotic twins, except that they have additional within-twin variance attributable to genetic differences. Kendler *et al.* (1987) used multivariate statistics to study a large cohort of twins identified in Australia and found evidence that both anxiety and depression symptoms (not BP and related UP disorder) shared the same non-specific genetic cause. The authors stated that the tendency in the general population for symptoms of anxiety to co-occur with symptoms of depression is largely environmental. In other words, there were only non-specific genetic effects that made an individual liable to symptoms of 'psychiatric distress'. The environment then acted independently to produce specific symptom patterns of anxiety or depression. The authors reasoned that the environmental effects that produced these symptom patterns were unique, specific environmental variables and not parental/family effects shared at home. In a study of 48 adoptees with major depression, Cadoret and colleagues (1985) showed that both primary and secondary depression were associated with several environmental factors. An increased amount of depression was found amongst males in an adoptive home in which there was another alcoholic. Amongst females, both death of an adoptive parent prior to the age of 19 and an adoptive family having another individual with a behaviour disturbance tended to increase depression. In general, environmental factors occurring prior to the age of 18 predisposed to depression.

9.7 Conclusions

The understanding of the genetics of BP illness and related affective disorders has been advanced by linkage analysis in the past few years. The hypothesis that single major loci confer susceptibility for BP and related UP affective disorder has now been confirmed for the X chromosome. In the past, some observers have speculated that mutations predisposing to the affective disorder might serve some evolutionary purpose, such as maintaining social hierarchies (Price, 1972). It can equally be argued that such mutations are purely random and have no evolutionary advantage (Gurling *et al.*, 1989). Molecular genetic techniques can be used to move closer to susceptibility genes and should enable the cloning and sequencing of the responsible mutations. New treatments and preventive strategies will result. In contrast, our genetic understanding of non-BP disorder and the many other subtypes of depression is quite crude. Multivariate models of gene/environment effects offer a way forward to disentangle the subtle interplay between polygenic and multifactorial environmental influences. New insights into the effect of the environment on BP and related UP disorders will result when biological markers become available, enabling the joint indexation of specific genes and specific environmental factors. Such a combination will have more explanatory power than if either genes or environment are considered on their own.

References

American Psychiatric Association (1980) *Diagnostic and Statistical Manual for Mental Disorders*, 3rd edn. Washington DC, American Psychiatric Association.

Andreasen, N.C. (1977) *Arch. Gen. Psychiatry* **34**, 1229–1235.

Andreasen, N.C., Scheftner, W., Reich, T., Hirschfeld, R.M., Endicott, J. & Keller, M.B. (1986) *Arch. Gen. Psychiatry* **43**, 246–251.

Andreasen, N.C., Rice, J., Endicott, J., Coryell, W., Grove, W.M. & Reich, T. (1987) *Arch. Gen. Psychiatry* **44**, 461–469.

Angst, J. (1966) *Monogr. Neurol. Psychiatr.* **122**, 1–118.

Baron, M. (1977) *Arch. Gen. Psychiatry* **24**, 721–727.

Baron, M. (1980) *Acta Genet. Med. Gemellol.* **29**, 289–294.

Baron, M., Gruen, R., Asnis, L. & Kane, J. (1982) *Acta Psychiatr. Scand.* **65**, 253–262.

Baron, M., Risch, N., Hamburger, R. *et al.* (1987) *Nature* **326**, 289–292.

Berretini, W., Goldin, L., Nurnberger, J. & Gershon, E.S. (1984) *J. Psychiatr. Res.* **18**, 329–350.

Bertelsen, A. (1979) In *Origin, Prevention and Treatment of Affective Disorders* (eds Schou, M. & Stromgren, E.), pp 227–239. Orlando, Academic Press.

Bertelsen, A. (1987) *Br. J. Psychiatry* **130**, 330–351.

Blehar, M.C., Weissman, M.M., Gershon, E.S. & Hirschfeld, R.M. (1988) *Arch. Gen. Psychiatry* **45**, 289–292.

Bodmer, W.F. (1984) In *Banbury Report 16: Genetic Variability in Responses to Chemical Exposure*, pp 287–296. Cold Spring Harbor Laboratory.

Bohman, M. (1978) *Arch. Gen. Psychiatry* **35**, 269–276.

Botstein, D., White, R., Skolnick, M. & Davis, R.W. (1980) *Am. J. Hum. Genet.* **32**, 314–331.

Brown, G. & Harris, T. (1978) *Social Origins of Depression: A Study of Psychiatric disorder in Women*. New York, Free Press.

Bucher, K.D. & Elston, R.C. (1981a) *J. Psychiat. Res.* **15**, 53–63.

Bucher, K.D., Elston, R.C., Green, R. *et al.* (1981b) *J. Psychiat. Res.* **16**, 65–78.

Bunzow, J.R., Van Tol, H.H.M., Grandy, D.K. *et al.* (1988) *Nature* **336**, 783–785.

Cadoret, R.J. & Gath, A. (1978) *Arch. Gen. Psychiatry* **40**, 843–950.

Cadoret, R.J., O'Gorman, T.W., Heywood, E. & Troughton, E. (1985) *J. Affective Disord.* **9**, 155–164.

Cavalli-Sforza, L.L. & Feldman, M.W. (1981) *Monogr. Popul. Biol.* **16**.

Cloninger, C.R., Reich, T. & Wetzel, R. (1979) In *Alcoholism and Affective Disorders* (eds Goodwin, D.W. & Erickson, C.K.), pp 57–86. New York, Spectrum.

Coryell, W., Endicott, J., Reich, T., Andreasen, N. & Keller, M. (1984) *Br. J. Psychiatry* **145**, 49–54.

Coryell, W., Endicott, J., Andreasen, N. & Keller, M. (1985) *Am. J. Psychiatry* **142**, 817–821.

Cox, N., Reich, T., Rice, J., Elston, R., Schober, J. & Keats, B. (1989) *J. Psychiat. Res.* **23**, 109–123.

Crowe, R.R. & Smouse, P.E. (1977) *J. Psychiat. Res.* **13**, 273–285.

Curtis, D., Brynjolfsson, J., Petursson, H., Holmes, D. & Gurling, H.M.D. (1990) *Br. J. Psychiatry* (in press).

Del Zompo, M., Brochetta, A., Goldin, L.R. & Corsini, G.U. (1984) *Acta Psychiatr. Scand.* **70**, 282–287.

Detera-Wadleigh, S.D., Berretini, W.H., Goldin, L.R., Boorman, D., Anderson, G. & Gershon, E.S. (1987) *Nature* **325**, 783–787.

Donis-Keller, H. (1988) *Cell* **51**, 319–337.

Egeland, J., Gerhard, D.S., Pauls, D.L. *et al.* (1987) *Nature* **325**, 783–787.

Elston, R.C. & Lange, K. (1975) *Ann. Hum. Genet.* **38**, 341–357.

Endicott, J. (1984) *J. Affective Disord.* **8**, 17–25.

Endicott, J. & Spitzer, R.L. (1978) *Arch. Gen. Psychiatry* **35**, 837–844.

Endicott, J., Nee, J., Coryell, W., Keller, M., Andreasen, N. & Croughan, J. (1986) *Compr. Psychiatry* **27**, 1–3.

Falconer, D.S. (1985) *Ann. Hum. Genet.* **29**, 51–76.

Feder, J., Gurling, H.M.D., Darby, J. & Cavalli-Sforza, L.L. (1985) *Am. J. Hum. Genet.* **37**, 286–294.

Feldman, M.W. & Cavalli-Sforza, L.L. (1979) *Theor. Popul. Biol.* **15**, 276–307.

Ferguson-Smith, M.A. & Aitken, D.A. (1982) *Cytogenet. Cell Genet.* **32**, 24–42.

Flemebaum, A. & Larson, J.W. (1976) *Dis. Cereb. Nerv. Syst.* **37**, 581–583.

Forgin, A., Raymond, J.R., Lohse, M.J., Kobilka, B.K., Caron, M.G. & Lefkowitz, R.J. (1988) *Nature* **355**, 358–360.

Frielle, T., Collins, S., Daniel, K.W., Caron, M.G., Lefkowitz, R.L. & Kobilka, B.K. (1987) *Proc. Natl Acad. Sci. USA* **84**, 7920–7924.

Gershon, E.S., Baron, M. & Leckman, J.F. (1975a) *J. Psychiatr. Res.* **12**, 301–317.

Gershon, E., Bunney, W.E., Leckman, J.F., Van Eerdewegh, M. & DeBauche, B.A. (1975b) *Behav. Genet.* **6**, 227–261.

Gershon, E.S., Targum, S.D., Matthyse, S. & Bunney, W.E. (1979) *Arch. Gen. Psychiatry* **36**, 1423.

Gershon, E., Hamovit, S., Guroff, J.J. *et al.* (1982) *Arch. Gen. Psychiatry* **139**, 209–212.

Gershon, E.S., Hamovit, J.H., Guroff, J.J. & Nurnberger, J.I. (1987) *Arch. Gen. Psychiatry* **44**, 314–319.

Gill, M., McKeown, P. & Humphries, P. (1988) *J. Med. Genet.* **25**, 634–635.

Goetzl, V., Green, R., Whybrow, P. & Jackson, L. (1974) *Arch. Gen. Psychiatry* **31**, 665–672.

Goldin, L.R. & Gershon, E.S. (1983) *Psychiatr. Dev.* **4**, 387–418.

Goldin, L.R., Gershon, E.S., Targum, S.D., Sparkes, R.S. & McGinnis, M. (1983) *Am. J. Hum. Genet.* **35**, 274–287.

Green, J.R. & Woodrow, J.C. (1977) *Tissue Antigens* **9**, 31–35.

Gurling, H.M.D. (1985) *Psychiatr. Dev.* **3**, 257–273.

Gurling, H.M.D. (1986) *Psychiatr. Dev.* **4**, 287–309.

Gurling, H.M.D. (1989) In *Depression: An Integrated Approach* (eds Paykel, E. & Herbst, K.), pp 45–52. London, Heinemann.

Gurling, H.M.D., Oppenheim, B.E. & Murray, R.M. (1984) *Acta Genet. Med. Gemellol.* **33**, 333–339.

Gurling, H.M.D., Grant, S. & Dangl, J. (1985) *Br. J. Addict.* **80**, 269–279.

Gurling, H.M.D., Sherrington, R.P., Brynjolfsson, J. *et al.* (1988) *Mol. Neurobiol.* **2**, 1–7.

Henderson, N. (1982) *Ann. Rev. Psychol.* **33**, 403–440.

Hodgkinson, S., Gurling, H.M.D., Marchbanks, R.M., McInnis, M. & Petursson, H. (1987a) *J. Psychiat. Res.* **21**, 589–596.

Hodgkinson, S., Sherrington, R., Gurling, H.M.D. *et al.* (1987b) *Nature* **325**, 805–806.

Holland, A. (1990) *J. Psychiatr. Res.* (in press).

Holmes, D., Sherrington, R.P., Hodgkinson, S. *et al.* (1989) *Am. J. Hum. Genet.* **45**, 195A.

Holmes, D., Brett, P., Brynjolfsson, J. *et al.* (1991) *Br. J. Psychiatry* (in press).

James, N.M. & Chapman, C.J. (1975) *Br. J. Psychiatry* **126**, 449–456.

Johnson, G.F.S. & Leeman, M.M. (1977) *Arch. Gen. Psychiatry* **34**, 1074–1083.

Julius, D., MacDermott, A.B., Axel, R. & Jessel, T.M. (1988) *Science* **241**, 558–556.

Kelsoe, J.R., Ginns, E.I., Egeland, J.A. *et al.* (1989) *Nature* **342**, 238–243.

Kendler, K.S., Heath, A.C., Martin, N.G. & Eaves, L.J. (1987) *Arch. Gen. Psychiatry* **44**, 451–457.

Kidd, K.K., Egeland, J.A., Molthan, L., Pauls, D., Kruger, S.D. & Messner, K.H. (1984) *Am. J. Psychiatry* **141**, 1042–1049.

Kluznik, J.R., Orr, H., Rich, S., Koller, B. & Duvick, L. (1988) Paper presented to the *43rd Annual Meeting of the Society of Biological Psychiatry*, May 4–8, Montreal.

Kobilka, B.K., Dixon, R.A.F., Friell, T. *et al.* (1986) *Proc. Natl Acad. Sci. USA* **84**, 46–50.

Kobilka, B.K., Frielle, T., Collins, S. *et al.* (1987) *Nature* **329**, 75–79.

Kosambi, D.D. (1944) *Ann. Eugen.* **12**, 178–185.

Lalouel, J.M., Rao, D.C., Morton, N.E. & Elston, R.C. (1983) *Am. J. Hum. Genet.* **35**, 816–826.

Lamouroux, A., Biguet, N.F., Samolyk, D. *et al.* (1982) *Proc. Natl Acad. Sci. USA* **79**, 3881–3885.

Lander, E.S. (1988) *Nature* **336**, 105–106.

Leboyer, M., Malafrosse, A., Boularand, S. *et al.* (1990) *Lancet* **335**, 1219.

Leonhard, K. (1959) *Aufteiling der Endogenen Psychosen*. Berlin, Akademie Verlag.

Levitt, J.L. & Tsuang, M.T. (1988) *Am. J. Psychiatry* **145**, 926–936.

Litt, M. & Luty, J.A. (1989) *Am. J. Hum. Genet.* **44**(3), 397–401.

McGuffin, P. & Katz, R. (1989a) *Br. J. Psychiatry* **155**, (Suppl. 6), 18–26.

McGuffin, P. & Katz, R. (1989b) *Br. J. Psychiatry* **155**, 294–304.

Mendlewicz, J. & Fleiss, J.L. (1974) *Biol. Psychiatry* **9**, 261–264.

Mendlewicz, J. & Rainer, J. (1974) *Am. J. Hum. Genet.* **25**, 692–701.

Mendlewicz, J. & Rainer, J.D. (1977) *Nature* **268**, 327–329.

Mendlewicz, J., Fleiss, J.L. & Fieve, R.R. (1972) *J.A.M.A.* **222**, 1624–1627.

Mendlewicz, J., Linkowski, P., Guroff, J.J. & van Praag, H.M. (1979) *Arch. Gen. Psychiatry* **36**, 1442–1447.

Mendlewicz, J., Linkowski, P. & Wilmotte, J. (1980) *Br. J. Psychiatry* **134**, 337–342.

Mendlewicz, J., Simon, P., Sevy, S. *et al.* (1987) *Lancet* **i**, 1230–1231.

Merikangas, K.R., Leckman, J.F., Prusoff, B.A., Pauls, D.L. & Weissman, M.M. (1985) *Arch. Gen. Psychiatry* **42**, 367–372.

Merikangas, K.R., Spence, M.A. & Kupfer, D.J. (1989) *Arch. Gen. Psychiatry* **46**, 1137–1141.

Morton, N.E. & Maclean, C.J. (1974) *Am. J. Hum. Genet.* **26**, 489–503.

Nothen, M., Korner, J., Lanczik, M., Fritze, J. & Propping, P. (1990) *Lancet* **336**, 575.

O'Rourke, D.H., McGuffin, P. & Reich, T. (1983) *Am. J. Phys. Anthropol.* **62**, 51–59.

Ott, J. (1985) *Analysis of Human Genetic Linkage*. Baltimore, Johns Hopkins University Press.

Pauls, D. (1985) Paper presented at the *IVth World Congress of Biological Psychiatry*, Philadelphia.

Perris, C. (1966a) *Acta Psychiatr. Scand.* (*Suppl.*) **203**, 1544.

Perris, C. (1966b) *Acta Psychiatr. Scand.* (*Suppl.*) **42**, 194.

Pollitt, J. (1972) *Br. J. Psychiatry* **121**, 67–70.

Price, J. (1972) *Int. J. Ment. Health* **1**, 124–144.

Reading, C.M. (1979) *Orthomol. Psychiatry* **8**, 68–77.

Reich, T., Clayton, P.J. & Winokur, G. (1969) *Am. J. Psychiatry* **125**, 1358–1369.

Rice, J., Reich, T., Andreasen, N.C. *et al.* (1987) *Arch. Gen. Psychiatry* **44**, 441–447.

Risch, N. & Baron, M. (1982) *Ann. Hum. Genet.* **46**, 153–166.

St Clair, D., Blackwood, D., Muir, W. *et al.* (1990) *Lancet* **336**, 13–16.

Schuckit, M.A. (1986) *Am. J. Psychiatry* **143**, 140–147.

Shapiro, R.W. (1970) *Acta Jutlandica* **42**, 2–15.

Slater, E. & Roth, M. (1974) *Clinical Psychiatry*, pp 66–67. London, Ballière Tindall.

Slater, E. & Shields, J. (1969) In *Studies of Anxiety* (ed. Lader, M.H.), British Journal of Psychiatry Special Publications, No. 3, Ashford Kent, Headley Bros.

Slater, E. & Tsuang, M. (1968) *J. Med. Genet.* **6**, 197–199.

Smeraldi, E. & Bellodi, L. (1981) *Am. J. Psychiatry* **138**, 1232–1234.

Smeraldi, E., Negri, F., Melica, A.M. & Scorza-Smeraldi, R. (1978) *Tissue Antigens* **12**, 270–274.

Smeraldi, E., Petroccione, A., Gasperini, M., Macciardi, F. & Orsini, A. (1984) *J. Affective Disord.* **7**, 99–107.

Smith, C.A.B. (1975) *Ann. Hum. Genet.* **38**, 451–461.

Smith, M. & Potkin, S. (1989) In *Abstracts of the 1989 Annual Meeting of the American Society of Human Genetics*.

Sokoloff, P., Giros, B., Martreus, M.P., Bouthenet, M.L. & Schwarz, J.C. (1990) *Nature* **347**, 146–151.

Southern, E.M. (1975) *J. Mol. Biol.* **98**, 503–517.

Spitzer, R.L. & Endicott, J. (1977) *The Schedule for Affective Disorders and Schizophrenia, Lifetime Version*, 3rd edn. New York, New York State Psychiatric Institute.

Spitzer, R.L., Endicott, J., Robins, E. (1978) *Research Diagnostic Criteria for a Selected Group of Functional Disorders*, 3rd edn. New York, New York State Psychiatric Institute.

Stancer, H.C., Mellor, C., Weitkamp, L.R. *et al.* (1987) *Can. J. Psychiatry* **32**, 768–772.

Stancer, H.C., Weitkamp, L.R., Persad, E. *et al.* (1988) *Ann. Hum. Genet.* **52**, 279–298.

Stancer, H.C., Weitkamp, L.R., Persad, E. *et al.* (1989) *Genet. Epidemiol.* **6**, 191–194.

Suarez, B. & Croughan, J. (1982) *Psychiat. Res.* **7**, 19–27.

Sunahara, R.K., Niznik, H.B., Weiner, D.M. *et al.* (1990) *Nature* **347**, 80–83.
Targum, S.D., Gershon, E.S., Van Eerdewegh, M. & Rogentine, N. (1979) *Biol. Psychiat.* **14**, 615–636.
Todd, R.D. & O'Malley, K.L. (1989) *Biol. Psychiatry* **25**, 626–630.
Torgersen, S. (1986) *Arch. Gen. Psychiatry* **43**, 222–226.
Turner, W.J. & King, S. (1981) *Biol. Psychiat.* **16**, 417–439.
Van Knorring, A.L., Cloninger, C.R., Bohman, M. & Sigvardsson, S. (1983) *Arch. Gen. Psychiatry* **40**, 943–950.
Weber, J.L. & May, P.E. (1989) *Am. J. Hum. Genet.* **44**, 388–396.
Weissman, M.M. & Myers, J. (1978) *Arch. Gen. Psychiatry* **35**, 1304–1311.
Weissman, M.M., Wickramaratne, P., Merikangas, K.R. *et al.* (1984a) *Arch. Gen. Psychiatry* **41**, 1136–1143.
Weissman, M.M., Gershon, E.S., Kidd, K.K. *et al.* (1984b) *Arch. Gen. Psychiatry* **41**, 13–21.
Weissman, M.M., Merikangas, K.R., Wickramaratne, P. *et al.* (1986a) *Arch. Gen. Psychiatry* **43**, 430–434.
Weissman, M., Merikangas, K., John, K., Wickramaratne, P., Prusoff, B.A. & Kidd, K. (1986b) *Arch. Gen. Psychiatry* **43**, 1104–1116.
Weitkamp, L.R. & Stancer, H.C. (1989) *Genet. Epidemiol.* **6**, 305–310.
Weitkamp, L.R., Stancer, H.C., Persad, E., Flood, C. & Guttormsen, S. (1981) *N. Engl. J. Med.* **305**, 1301–1306.
Wender, P.H. & Kety, S.S. (1986) *Arch. Gen. Psychiatry* **43**, 923–929.
Wing, J.K., Cooper, J.E. & Sartorius, N. (1974) *The Measurement and Classification of Psychiatric Symptoms*. New York, Cambridge University Press.
Winokur, G. (1979) *Am. J. Psychiatry* **136**, 911–913.
Winokur, G. & Clayton, P. (1967) *Adv. Biol. Psychiatry* **9**, 5–50.
Winokur, G. & Tanna, V.L. (1969) *Dis. Nerv. Syst.* **30**, 89–93.
Winokur, G., Clayton, P. & Reich, T. (1966) *Manic-depressive Illness*. St Louis, Mossey.
Winokur, G., Tsuang, M.T. & Crowe, R.R. (1982) *Am. J. Psychiatry* **139**, 209–212.
Yang-Feng, T.L., Xue, F., Zhang, W. *et al.* (1990) *Proc. Natl Acad. Sci. USA* **87**, 1516–1520.

Index

Note

Since the main subject of this book is affective disorders, no index entry is to be found for this term, and readers are advised to seek more specific entries. Likewise limited references are to be found under "Depression". Vs. denotes differential diagnosis.

Abbreviations used in sub-entries:

ACTH = Adrenocorticotropic hormone
AMPT = α-Methyl-p-tyrosine
CRH = Corticotrophin releasing hormone
GABA = γ-Aminobutyric acid
5-HIAA = 5-Hydroxyindole acetic acid
5-HT = 5-Hydroxytryptamine (serotonin)
5-HTP = 5-Hydroxytryptophan
MDMA = 3,4-Methylenedioxymethamphetamine
MHPG = 3-Methoxy-4-hydroxyphenyl glycol
NA = Noradrenaline
PCPA = p-Chlorophenylalanine
TRH = Thyrotrophin-releasing hormone
TRP = L-Tryptophan
WHO = World Health Organization

335

Heterozygous, definition, 307
Hierarchical system of diagnosis, 5–6
Hippocampus, 5-HT$_1$ binding sites,
   in suicides, 209
Histamine, in depression, 131–132
   accumulation by platelets, 132
   H$_2$ receptors on leucocytes, 132
HLA genes, 319, 323
Homovanillic acid (HVA),
   in mania, 279
   in post-mortem studies, 200–201
Hormone, secretion, temporal
   regulation, 240
Hospital treatment, indication, 51
Hostile depression, 27
H-RAS-1 oncogene locus (H-RAS),
   325, 326
Human leucocyte antigen (HLA)
   system, 319, 323
5-Hydroxyindole acetic acid
   (5-HIAA),
   in brains,
      in depressed patients, 197–200
      of suicides, *see* Suicide victims
   cerebrospinal fluid (CSF),
      decrease in depression, 81, 98,
         149, 152, 193–194, 209
      in mania, 279–280
   marker for impulsivity, 81–82
   predictor of violent suicide, 82
5-Hydroxytryptamine (5-HT),
   abnormalities in affective disorders,
      assessment, *see* Neuroendocrine
         challenge tests
      possible sites, 149, 150
      postsynaptic, 161, 179
      predictive value absent, 179
      presynaptic, 160–161, 161,
         179
   co-requirement, in
      β-adrenoreceptor
      down-regulation, 85
   deficiency, 69, 78, 80–81
      hypothesis of affective disorders,
         77, 80–82, 97, 148
      neuroendocrine testing of
         hypothesis, 152–162
   drugs affecting, in mania, 283
   evidence for involvement in
      depression, 151–152

increase, in high carbohydrate
   intake, 251
-induced aggregation of platelets,
   130, 131
levels in post-mortem studies,
   see Suicide victims
in mania, 280, 294
-noradrenaline-glucocorticoid link
   hypothesis, 88–89, 90
-noradrenaline-linked signal
   transduction system, 86–87
raised, tricyclic action, 55
in seasonal affective depression
   (SAD), 251
supersensitivity after
   antidepressants, 85
synthesis, 152
   inhibitor, 152
transport, 127
   abnormalities in depression, 117,
      119
uptake,
   by platelets, *see* Platelets
   sites, in post-mortem studies,
      202–208
5-Hydroxytryptamine (5-HT)
   neuron, 149, 151
   cell bodies, in raphe nuclei, 151
   dysfunction, possible sites, 149,
      150
   function assessment, 149–152
   nerve terminals, 151
5-Hydroxytryptamine (5-HT)
   receptors, 86, 87
   5-HT$_1$, 153
      post-mortem studies, 208, 209
   5-HT$_{1A}$, 156
      abnormalities, 157, 161
      agonists, 156, 157
   5-HT$_2$, 87, 130, 152, 208
      in frontal cortex, 209–210
      agonists, 155–157
      down-regulation, 87
      genes, 321
      neuroendocrine abnormalities,
         161
      platelet, 130–131
      post-mortem studies, 208–210
   in signal transduction, 86
   subtypes, 151